LIPOPROTEIN METABOLISM AND ENDOCRINE REGULATION

DEVELOPMENTS IN ENDOCRINOLOGY VOLUME 4

LIPOPROTEIN METABOLISM AND ENDOCRINE REGULATION

Proceedings of a European Workshop held in Noordwijkerhout, The Netherlands, on October 2-4, 1978.
Organized by the Gaubius Institute, Health Research Organization TNO in collaboration with the University Hospital Leiden.
Sponsored by the Committee on Medical and Public Health Research of the Commission of the European Communities

L.W. Hessel *and* **H.M.J. Krans** *Editors*

1979

ELSEVIER/NORTH-HOLLAND BIOMEDICAL PRESS
AMSTERDAM · NEW YORK · OXFORD

ISBN for this volume: 0-444-80102-2
ISBN for the series: 0-444-80009-3

Published by:
Elsevier/North-Holland Biomedical Press
335 Jan van Galenstraat, PO Box 211
Amsterdam, The Netherlands

Sole distributors for the USA and Canada:
Elsevier North-Holland Inc.
52 Vanderbilt Avenue
New York, N.Y. 10017

Printed in The Netherlands

PREFACE

Research in the field of human lipid metabolism is strongly motivated by the relationship between blood lipoprotein levels and the pathogenesis of athero-sclerosis.

Although it was recognized at an early date that almost all components of the endocrine system can be intimately involved both in atherogenesis and in lipo-protein disorders, most research of the last ten years has been directed at the enzymological and cellular aspects of lipid metabolism and at unravelling the quantitative and qualitative intricacies of the circulating lipoproteins. As a result there has been a rapid development in the analytical accessibility of some major apoproteins, in the recognition of a cellular defect in familial hypercholesterolemia and a renewed interest in the role of the High Density Lipoproteins.

In endocrinology one of the most far-reaching advances is the discovery that hormone action is modulated on the target cell level by changes in receptors and that such changes can sometimes be monitored by binding studies on circulating blood cells. It seems that receptor modulation, already invoked for some time to explain insulin resistance, emerges as a general controlling mechanism. As a result the information gained from the measurement of hormone levels must in many cases be qualified by data on the receptors.

Interaction between these two rapidly growing fields of research has been weak, probably because so many promising approaches are possible within each of these areas. Yet, these same advances are of such a nature that their integration in an overall pattern is necessary for the solution of fundamental questions such as: how are lipoprotein levels in blood regulated and what consequences might be expected for the unsolved problem of atherosclerosis? Thus, when the Committee of Medical Research and Public Health of the Commission of the European Communities recognized the need of an integrated approach to these problems, the opportunity was taken to convene investigators in both fields from major European research centres to discuss lipid metabolism and its hormonal control at a workshop.

In this book the papers presented at his workshop have been collected together with short summaries of the discussions.

There are three parts:

- In section I direct hormonal control (by insulin, corticosteroids, thyroid hormones, etc.) as well as indirect influences (by GIP and other peptides, via the endocrine pancreas) and some pharmacological aspects (e.g. of oral

contraceptives) have been covered.
- Section II is devoted to the modulation of hormonal effects and receptor
  mechanisms and
- Section III deals with hormonal effects and lipid metabolism in selected
  organs, especially in the liver.

There is still a long way to go before anything like a satisfactory understanding of the interaction between the regulatory hormones, their receptors,
and lipoproteins, their synthesis, secretion, interconversions and catabolism
can be expected. Suggestions for a follow-up of this first meeting have been
received and plans in this direction might be realized in another one or two
years.

The organizers are most grateful to the Committee of Medical Research and
Public Health of the European Communities for the help that made this workshop
possible.

Leiden, November 1978
L.W. Hessel

LIST OF PARTICIPANTS

G. Assmann, Medizinische Einrichtungen der Westfälischen Wilhelms-Universität, Zentrallaboratorium, 4400 Münster (West Germany).

J.C. Birkenhäger, Department of Internal Medicine III, Division of Clinical Endocrinology and Metabolism, University Hospital "Dijkzigt", Erasmus University, Rotterdam, (The Netherlands).

D.N. Brindley, Department of Biochemistry, University of Nottingham Medical School, Queen's Medical Centre, Nottingham NG7 2UH (U.K.)

Y. Broer, Unité de Recherche de Diabétologie et d'Etudes Radio-Immunologiques des Hormones Protéiques, U.55 (Institut National de la Santé et de la Recherche Médicale), E.R.A. n° 494 (Centre National de la Recherche Scientifique), Hôpital Saint-Antoine, 184 Rue du Faubourg Saint-Antoine, Paris 12°, (France).

J.D. Brunzell, St. Thomas' Hospital, Department of Chemical Pathology and Metabolic Disorders, London SE1 7EH (U.K.) (temporary address).

K.D. Buchanan, Department of Medicine, Queen's University of Belfast, (Ireland).

R. Ebert, Medizinische Klinik und Poliklinik Göttingen, Robert-Koch-Strasse 40, 3400 Göttingen (West Germany).

D.J. Galton, Diabetes and Lipid Research Laboratory, St. Bartholomew's Hospital, London E.C.1 (U.K.)

J.A. Gevers Leuven, Gaubius Institute, Health Research Organization TNO, Herenstraat 5d, 2313 AD Leiden (The Netherlands).

J. Gliemann, Institute of Medical Physiology C, University of Copenhagen, Panum Institute, Blegdamsvej 3C, DK-200 Copenhagen N. (Denmark).

L.W. Hessel, Gaubius Institute, Health Research Organization TNO, Herenstraat
    5d, 2313 AD Leiden (The Netherlands).

W.C. Hülsmann, Department of Biochemistry I, Medical Faculty, Erasmus
    University Rotterdam, P.O. Box 1738, 3000 DR Rotterdam (The
    Netherlands).

C. Jarrouse, Unité de Recherche de Diabétologie et d'Etudes Radio-
    -Immunologiques des Hormones Protéiques, U.55 (Institut National de la
    Santé et de la Recherche Médicale), E.R.A. n° 494 (Centre National de la
    Recherche Scientifique), Hôpital Saint-Antoine, 184 Rue du Faubourg
    Saint-Antoine, Paris 12°, (France).

B. Jeanrenaud, Laboratoires de Recherches Médicales, 64 Avenue de la Roseraie,
    1205 Geneva (Switzerland).

D.G. Johnston, Endocrine Unit, Royal Victoria Infirmary, Newcastle upon Tyne
    NE1 4LP (U.K.).

H. Kather, Klinisches Institut für Herzinfarktforschung an der Medizinischen
    Universitätsklinik Heidelberg, Bergheimerstrasse 58, D-69 Heidelberg
    (West Germany).

H.J.M. Kempen, Gaubius Institute, Health Research Organization TNO, Herenstraat
    5d, 2313 AD Leiden (The Netherlands).

H.M.J. Krans, Department of Endocrinology, University Hospital Leiden (The
    Netherlands).

A.S. Luyckx, Division of Diabetes, Institute of Medicine, Hôpital de Bavière,
    Boulevard de la Constitution 66, B-4020 Liège (Belgium).

P.J. Magill, Department of Chemical Pathology and Metabolic Disorders, St.
    Thomas' Hospital Medical School, London SE1 7EH (U.K.).

M. Mancini, Semeiotica Medica, 2nd Faculty of Medicine, University of Naples,
    Naples (Italy).

G.P. Mannaerts, Laboratory of Pharmacology, School of Medicine, Katholieke
Universiteit Leuven, B-3000 Leuven (Belgium).

J. Marco, Clinica Puerta de Hierro, Universidad Autonoma de Madrid, Madrid-35
(Spain).

R.H. Michell, Department of Biochemistry, University of Birmingham, P.O. Box
363, Birmingham B15 2TT (U.K.).

S. Rössner, King Gustaf V Research Institute, Karolinska Hospital, S-104 01
Stockholm (Sweden).

V. Tomasi, Laboratory of General Physiology, University of Bologna, 40126
Bologna (Italy).

L. Vanhaelst, Metabolic Unit, Vrije Universiteit Brussel, Brussels (Belgium).

Tj. Wieringa, Department of Endocrinology, University Hospital Leiden (The
Netherlands).

CONTENTS

LIPOPROTEIN TRANSPORT AND HORMONE LEVELS

Lipoprotein Metabolism and Endocrine Regulation
L.W. Hessel and H.M.J. Krans editors
© ECSC, EEC, EAEC, Brussels-Luxembourg, 1979
Published by Elsevier/North-Holland Biomedical Press-Amsterdam

THE METABOLISM OF PLASMA LIPOPROTEINS

Gerd Assmann and Gerd Schmitz
Medizinische Einrichtungen der Westfälischen Wilhelms-Universität,
Zentrallaboratorium, 4400 Münster (West-Germany)

The plasma lipoproteins may be divided into four major classes. Their chemical and physical properties are summarized in Tables 1 and 2.

TABLE 1

CHEMICAL PROPERTIES OF HUMAN PLASMA LIPOPROTEINS

	Protein	Triglyceride (% by weight)	Cholesterol	Phospholipid
Chylomicrons	2.5	85	4	8
VLDL	10	50 - 55	15	18
LDL	20 - 25	12	30	22
HDL	50	6	15	25

TABLE 2

PHYSICAL PROPERTIES OF HUMAN PLASMA LIPOPROTEINS

	Diameter ($\mathring{A}$)	Molecular weight	Hydrated density	mobility
Chylomicrons	800	10^9	0,93	origin
VLDL	250–800	10^7	0,97	pre-ß
LDL	175–250	$2,3 \times 10^6$	1,03	ß
HDL_2	85–150	$3,6 \times 10^5$	1,09	$alpha_2$
HDL_3	70– 90	$1,7 \times 10^5$	1,15	$alpha_3$

The protein portion of the lipoproteins consists of multiple heterogeneous proteins known as apolipoproteins. Studies of the regulation of serum lipid concentration require not only consideration of the lipoproteins but also consideration of the apoprotein components of the lipoproteins (Table 3).

TABLE 3
APOLIPOPROTEINS OF HUMAN SERUM

Apolipoprotein	Density class	mol.wt. $\times 10^{-3}$	concentration (mg/dl)
A-I	HDL	28	80 – 120
A-II	HDL	17	30 – 50
A-III	HDL	21	2 – 4
B	LDL, VLDL	275	70 – 90
C-I	VLDL, HDL	7	3 – 7
C-II	VLDL, HDL	8,5	3 – 5
C-III	VLDL, HDL	8,5	8 – 12
E	VLDL, HDL	39	3 – 6
D-2	HDL	7	1 – 2

The best characterization of the apoproteins is the determination of the amino acid composition and of the terminal amino acid. Alternatively, the apolipoproteins can be characterized by their migration rate in defined polyacrylamide gel systems and/or their immunochemical properties. The major function of apolipoproteins is their ability to stabilze lipid micelles during the transport in blood and chyle. Some of the apolipoproteins have been found to have specific physiologic functions. Apoprotein C-II is an activator of lipoprotein lipase, while apoprotein A-I has been shown to be the activator of lecithin-cholesterol acyltransferase. In addition to the functions mentioned above, apolipoproteins play an important role for lipid metabolism in general. As evidenced from the disorders Tangier disease and hyperbetalipoproteinemia, both apoprotein A-I and apoprotein B are of critical importance in maintaining cellular cholesterol balance. In the absence of apoprotein A-I and HDL from plasma (Tangier disease), cholesteryl

esters accumulate in tissue macrophages, Schwann cells, and intestinal smooth muscle cells; the activity of the key enzyme in
sterol biosynthesis in man, hydroxy-methylglutaryl-coenzyme A
reductase, is regulated by a negative feedback mechanism through
apolipoprotein B.

CHYLOMICRONS

Chylomicrons are particles that in normal subjects appear
after ingestion of a fatty meal and in certain types of hyperlipoproteinemia. In serum samples they tend to separate in a
creamy layer when serum is refigerated overnight. The low density reflects their high triglyceride content. On agarose electrophoresis, they do not move from origin. The major function of
the chylomicrons is the transport of dietary or exogenous triglycerides. Chylomicrons are synthesized within the Golgi apparatus
of the intestinal mucosa and traverse the lymphatic system to
the thoracic duct where they enter the blood stream.

Valuable information concerning chylomicron formation can be
obtained from studies of the rare familial disorder, abetalipo-
proteinemia. Patients with this disorder have fat malabsorption;
apoprotein B is completely absent from the plasma and there are
no circulating chylomicrons, VLDL, or LDL. This disorder reveals
that synthesis of apoproteins and in particular the synthesis of
apoprotein B is essential for the formation and/or secretion of
triglyceride-rich particles from the liver and the gut.

Chylomicrons are removed from the circulation faster than any
of the other lipoprotein classes. The half-life of chylomicron
triglycerides in circulation is less than 1 hour in humans. Under
physiologic conditions, chylomicron catabolism proceeds in two
steps. About 80 % of the triglyceride moiety of chylomicrons is
catabolized by muscle and adipose tissue; most of the cholesteryl
ester moiety of chylomicrons is catabolized by the liver. The enzyme responsible for triglyceride hydrolysis of the chylomicrons,
extrahepatic lipoprotein lipase, is bound to the capillary endothelial cells in muscle and adipose tissue and can be released by

intravenous administration of heparin. Heparin-releasable lipolytic activity, however, contains several enzymes of hepatic and
extrahepatic origin: apoprotein C-II dependent extrahepatic lipoprotein lipase, apoprotein C-II independent hepatic triglyceride
lipase, monoglyceride hydrolase, and phospholipase A activity. To
what extent these enzymes recognize chylomicron lipids, VLDL
lipids and/or the lipids contained in the remnants of these lipoproteins is as yet unknown. The cholesterol and cholesteryl esters
contained in the remnants of the chylomicrons are taken up by the
liver and (a) converted to bile acids and secreted in the bile,
(b) secreted into the bile as neutrol sterol, or (c) incorporated
into lipoproteins and released into the plasma.

Fasting chylomicronemia is due to ineffective removal mechanisms of chylomicrons and is seen in patients with absolute
(type I hyperlipoproteinemia) or relative (type V hyperlipoproteinemia) lipoprotein lipase deficiency. A decrease in lipoprotein
lipase activity can be the result of a deficiency of either the
enzyme or the activating apoprotein. Chylomicronemia is also encountered in patients with Tangier disease (analphalipoproteinemia).
The latter condition indicates that the regular presence of HDL
in plasma is required for chylomicron clearance. The role of HDL
in chylomicron catabolism most likely relates to the ability of
these lipoproteins to provide apoprotein C-II in the initial phase
of chylomicron clearance and to act as lipid acceptor macromolecules. Chylomicronemia is also seen secondary to insulinopenic
diabetes due to decreased levels of extrahepatic lipoprotein lipase.

VLDL

The very-low-density lipoproteins (VLDL) are particles with a
diameter of 250-800 Å. These lipoproteins have prebeta mobility
on electrophoresis and are often referred to as prebetalipoproteins.
In the absence of chylomicrons, the major portion of the serum
triglyceride are transported in this fraction. The liver and, to
a lesser extent, the intestine are the source of plasma VLDL. A
major factor determining the amount of triglycerides secreted in
VLDL is the availability of free fatty acids and of carbohydrate.

Uncontrolled diabetes mellitus, adult onset (hyperinsulinemic) diabetes, carbohydrate feeding and alcoholism represent examples of increased synthesis and secretion of VLDL. Whether or not an excess of free fatty acids or increased de novo synthesis of fatty acids may simultaneously affect VLDL apoprotein synthesis is not known.

Colchicine, vincristine, and orotic acid inhibit VLDL secretion in the rat. Colchicine and vincristine are thought to block the microtubular system, and thus, the release of VLDL from the Golgi apparatus of the hepatocyte. Orotic acid is thought to interfer with the final step of VLDL secretion by inhibiting the linkage of the carbohydrate to the apoproteins.

The fate of VLDL triglycerides in plasma is thought to be similar to those from chylomicrons. It is generally assumed that VLDL triglycerides are hydrolyzed at extrahepatic tissue sites by the lipoprotein lipase system. During the catabolism of VLDL, more than 90 % of apoprotein C is transferred to HDL, whereas essentially all of apoprotein B remains with the original lipoprotein particle. In man, the transformation of VLDL to LDL occurs through the formation of lipoproteins of intermediate density (d 1.006 – 1.019; IDL). It has been calculated that as much as 60-80 % of the phospholipids and unesterified cholesterol molecules and 90 % of the C apoproteins originally present in VLDL particles are removed from the lipoprotein during the formation of LDL. The precise mechanisms of removal of lipids and apoproteins from the triglyceride rich macromolecules are yet obscure; in particular, whether phospholipid hydrolysis or phospholipid transfer to HDL predominates in VLDL catabolism in vivo is unknown. Part of the phospholipid, cholesterol and apoprotein moieties may be directly taken up by tissue cells during the interconversion process.

Hypertriglyceridemia in the absence of chylomicronemia may be due to increased rates of synthesis or decreased rates of catabolism of VLDL. In most patients with hypertriglyceridemia, the lipid abnormality is due to altered metabolic pathways of VLDL rather than to an abnormal composition or structure of the lipoprotein.

Occasionaly, synthesis and secretion of VLDL particles with excess triglycerides may be observed. It is generally accepted that in-effective delipidation and removal pathways of the triglyceride-rich lipoproteins are the most prevalent mechanisms responsible for the different disorders manifested by elevated VLDL levels. The molecular basis for the slow delipidation is not understood in most patients with endogenous or exogenous hyperlipidemia. In these patients, heparin-released lipolytic enzymes are within the range observed among normotriglyceridemic subjects. Therefore, factors other than absolute levels of lipolytic enzymes are of importance in the removal of VLDL. The precise molecular mecha-nisms, by which insulin and glucagon affect VLDL concentrations, are as yet unknown. Both insulin deficiency (impaired VLDL cata-bolism) and hyperinsulinemia (VLDL overproduction) may lead to hypertriglyceridemia in diabetes.

LDL

Low-density lipoproteins (LDL) constitute 40-50 % of the plasma lipoprotein mass in man. They transport about two thirds of the serum cholesterol, and in diseases when serum cholesterol is in-creased, LDL are usually elevated. Apoprotein B comprises appoxi-mately 25 % by weight of LDL. The molecular weight of apoprotein B is unknown, and published estimates range between 10.000 and 250.000. Technical problems in solubilizing and dissociating apo-protein B have made progress in the characterization slow as compared with the other apoproteins.

Formation of LDL occurs primarily from the catabolism of VLDL. To what extent additional pathways of LDL synthesis, such as di-rect hepatic secretion or catabolism of chylomicrons, contribute to circulating LDL mass needs to be determined. The body tissues in which plasma LDL is catabolized in man are unknown. It seems likely, that both the liver and nonhepatic tissues degrade LDL. Since the liver provides the major secretary pathway of choleste-rol from the body and constitutes the site of disposal of excess cholesterol, it should assume a major role in LDL catabolism. The hypothesis that LDL can be degraded in tissues other than the liver has been supported by the finding that a variety of nonhe-patic human cells in culture, such as fibroblasts, arterial smooth

muscle cells, lymphoid cells, and endothelial cells are able to
degrade LDL. These cells possess specific receptors on the cell
surface that bind plasma LDL. As a consequence of this binding,
cholesteryl ester and cholesterol are transferred to the cellular
compartment where it is found largely associated with cell membranes. The accumulation of unesterified cholesterol within the cell
regulates the activities of two microsomal enzymes: (a) it suppresses hydroxy-methylglutaryl coenzyme A reductase, causing a reduction of cellular cholesterol synthesis, and (b) it activates an
acyl-CoA: cholesteryl acyltransferase, facilitating cellular
cholesterol esterification. The binding of LDL to its receptor
probably involves an ionic interaction between the protein component of LDL and the surface receptor. Recent evidence indicates
that the receptor binding of apoprotein B is not limited to this
apoprotein and that at least one other apoprotein, the "arginine-
rich" apoprotein (=apoprotein E), harbors regions that are homologous with apoprotein B. Therefore, apoprotein B-and apoprotein E
containing lipoproteins may be functionally similar in their ability to deliver cholesterol to cells through an interaction with
the same cellular receptors.

Of particular importance, patients with familial hyperbetalipoproteinemia are either deficient in specific LDL receptors or else
the receptors are defective. The impairment of specific receptor
interaction leads to decreased rates of disappearance of LDL particles from the circulation. Besides the defective removal of LDL
from the circulation in certain patients with familial hyperbetalipoproteinemia, ineffective removal of IDL may be operative to a
significant degree in patients with elevated LDL levels. Clearly,
the possible role of the conversion of IDL to LDL in the pathogenesis of hypercholesterolemia and the regulation of plasma LDL
merits further study.

HDL

High-density lipoprotein (HDL) particles isolated in the density range 1.063 to 1.21 g/ml are 75 to 150 Å in diameter, and in the human can be divided into two subclasses: HDL_2 (d = 1.063 to 1.112 g/ml) and HDL_3 (d = 1.112 to 1.21 g/ml). Approximately 50 % of the HDL mass is protein; the other major constituents are cholesterol and cholesteryl esters (about 20 %) and phospholipids (about 30 %). Apoprotein A-I and apoprotein A-II are the major proteins in HDL. Apoprotein C and apoprotein D are also present.

No information is avaiable on the nature of newly synthesized HDL particles in humans and the quantitative contribution of different organs (intestine, liver) to apoprotein A synthesis is not completely understood. Preliminary studies with isolated mucosal cells from the small intestine of humans by direct and indirect immunofluorescence have revealed a strong drop-shaped fluorescence pattern of both A apoproteins. In isolated human hepatocytes, however, specific apoprotein A fluorescence is weak and exhibits a fine granular pattern. Apoprotein A can not be detected in fibroblasts, lymphocytes or plasma cells. The observation of a strong apoprotein A immunofluorescence in tissue slices and isolated mucosal cells of the small intestine is in agreement with the present hypothesis of the intestine as the origin of a major portion of the A apoproteins. The role of apoprotein synthesis in the integrity of HDL is illustrated by patients with Tangier disease. In the homozygous form of the disease, apoprotein A-I levels are reduced to about 1 % of normal and HDL is virtually absent from plasma. The patients demonstrate mild hypertriglyceridemia and accumulation of cholesteryl oleate in tissue macrophages. The cumulative evidence of recent biochemical findings links the defect in Tangier disease to a structural mutation of apoprotein A-I. The observations in patients with Tangier disease raise the interesting suggestion that HDL may play an important role in the transport of cholesterol from certain tissues to the liver. Biochemical, clinical and epidemiological data on a specific role of HDL in atherogenesis seem to further support this view.

In several respects HDL seem to be involved in the enzymatic
reaction catalyzed by LCAT which accounts for most of the cholesteryl esters in plasma. It is generally assumed that HDL is the major
substrate for the LCAT reaction and that virtually all of the plasma cholesteryl esters are formed in the plasma HDL. The general
view held is that esterified cholesterol in other plasma lipoprotein
fractions is transferred from HDL. Such transfer of esterified
cholesterol from HDL to both VLDL and LDL has been demonstrated by
in vitro experiments; however, the mechanism of cholesteryl ester
transfer from HDL to other lipoproteins is not yet understood.
Both C apoproteins and the arginine-rich protein may participate
in such transfer reactions. More recent evidence suggests that
there is heterogeneity of esterified cholesterol in HDL. It has
been proposed that the newly secreted HDL from the liver (rat liver perfusion experiments) are the true substrates for the LCAT
reaction, and that the cholesteryl esters formed on the surface
of the HDL bilayer discs may move into the core thereby converting
the discs into spherical mature HDL. In addition to the substrate
and operator roles of HDL in cholesteryl ester formation, the activity of LCAT in vitro is highly dependent upon the presence of apo
A-I as activator apoprotein.

The major site of HDL degradation is the liver; specific removal
mechanisms, however, have not yet been identified. In humans, the
biological half-life of the two A apoproteins is similar or identical,   suggesting that HDL is catabolized as a unit.

HDL levels may vary considerably among individuals with normal
plasma lipid levels and patients with hyperlipidemia. HDL and apoprotein A-I levels are higher in menstruating females than in males of the same age. In pregnancy, HDL concentrations may approach
twice the normal concentration. In subjects with primary chylomicronemia or excessive hypertriglyceridemia HDL levels are usually
low. Most of these observations are as yet unexplained. The further elucidation of factors involved in the regulation of HDL
synthesis and degradation is required to better understand the
metabolism of these and the other plasma lipoproteins.

Lipoprotein Metabolism and Endocrine Regulation
L.W. Hessel and H.M.J. Krans editors
© ECSC, EEC, EAEC, Brussels-Luxembourg, 1979
Published by Elsevier/North-Holland Biomedical Press-Amsterdam

HIGH-DENSITY LIPOPROTEINS IN RELATION TO ENDOCRINE FACTORS

ESKO A. NIKKILÄ
Third Department of Medicine, University of Helsinki, 00290 Helsinki 29
(Finland)

ABSTRACT

Little is known so far on the biochemical control of plasma high-density
lipoprotein levels. Endocrine factors may have an important role in this
respect and at least sex steroids and insulin have been found to exert an
influence on HDL levels.

INTRODUCTION

Upon recognition of the important role of plasma high-density lipoproteins
(HDL) in the pathogenesis of coronary heart disease and other atherosclerotic
disease[1,2] attention was drawn to a significant sex difference in the concentration of HDL cholesterol. It was suggested that relative protection of
women from coronary atherosclerosis could at least partly be accounted for
by their higher HDL levels. This view has been strongly supported by more
recent prospective data indicating that there is little sex difference in the
incidence of CHD when men and women are compared at similar HDL levels[3].
It is thus obvious that endocrine and metabolic factors influence the plasma
HDL levels and these may have important implications in the pathogenesis of
atherosclerotic vascular disease.

PRINCIPLES OF REGULATION OF PLASMA HDL

Circulating HDL (and its subfractions HDL_2 and HDL_3) has a relatively constant chemical composition and structure but it is not turned over as a single
compound. Its component lipids and apoproteins are derived from different
sources and they also leave the particle at different sites and by different
rates (Fig. I). These features make the HDL appropriate for transport of
lipids as e.g. for transfer of cholesterol from tissues and from triglyceride-
rich lipoproteins into liver[4-6]. However, these complex turnover kinetics
have made it difficult to define the biochemical mechanisms which are responsible for individual plasma HDL levels and for their variations.

It is currently believed that the primary HDL particle is secreted by the
liver[7]. This "nascent" HDL contains arginine-rich apoprotein, unesterified
cholesterol and phospholipids. Within plasma it is transformed to the major

14

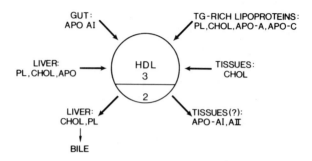

Fig. 1. Sites of origin and removal of the components of HDL.

circulating forms of HDL by incorporation of apoprotein A-I in exchange for
the arginine-rich protein and by esterification of cholesterol with LCAT.
In circulation HDL takes up cholesterol, phospholipids and apoproteins from
triglyceride-rich lipoproteins during their degradation by endothelial lipoprotein lipase (LPL). Additional cholesterol is also derived from peripheral
tissues and the excess cholesterol and phospholipids is evidently released
from HDL in the liver and secreted into bile[6].

   Little is known as yet on the mechanisms by which the plasma HDL concentration is regulated. It has been suggested[5] that major factors responsible for
HDL levels would be (1) the splanchnic production rate of nascent HDL and of
apoprotein A-I (coming mainly from intestine), (2) the rate of catabolism of
triglyceride-rich lipoproteins, and (3) the rate of degradation of HDL apoproteins, notably that of apo A-I. Major variations of HDL occur in the
lipid-rich subfraction HDL_2[8,9] while the concentration of HDL_3 is relatively
much more stable.

   There is a definite positive correlation between plasma HDL (cholesterol
and apoprotein A-I) levels and the activity of adipose tissue LPL activity[10].
It is not yet known as to whether HDL in some way promotes the synthesis of
endothelial LPL or whether the HDL level is regulated by the LPL activity.
We have been inclined to favour the latter alternative on the basis of
numerous clinical studies where changes of HDL have been clearly secondary
to alterations of LPL activity[11].

INFLUENCE OF SEX AND OF GONADAL STEROIDS

Early studies established that women have consistently higher concentrations of HDL cholesterol and phospholipids than men[2,12,13]. This difference
applies mainly to HDL_2 while concentrations of HDL_3 are rather similar in the
two sexes[8,14,15]. HDL_2 contains more cholesterol in relation to apoprotein
A-I (or total protein) than HDL_3 and this accounts for the higher HDL cholesterol levels of women in comparison with men[16]. On the other hand, there is
no significant sex difference in the composition of either HDL_2 or HDL_3[16].
It seems likely that the higher HDL_2 levels in women are related to a better
transport of cholesterol from tissues and from triglyceride-rich lipoproteins
into the liver. The underlying mechanisms of this sex difference are far
from clear, however. Recent studies suggest that women do not have higher
synthetic rates or lower catabolic rates of apoprotein A-I than men[17] and,
if confirmed, this finding would indicate that the sex difference is not
based on differences in apoprotein metabolism. Another possibility is that
the increased HDL levels of women could result from higher LPL activity of
adipose tissue[10]. This view is consistent with the hypothesis that cholesterol in HDL (particularly HDL_2) is partly derived from catabolism of triglyceride-rich lipoproteins. Women would thus have higher HDL and lower VLDL
levels than men because they have higher endothelial LPL activity and, accordingly, more rapid turnover of chylomicrons and VLDL. However, the difference
in HDL levels persists also when men and women are compared at similar LPL
activity or at similar VLDL levels[18] indicating that the above concept cannot
be the sole explanation for the sex difference in HDL.

Administration of gonadal hormones induces changes of HDL which are largely
consistent with the observed sex difference in the concentration of this lipoprotein. Thus, conjugated and synthetic estrogens increase the HDL cholesterol, phospholipid and protein concentrations in men[19,20] while androgenic
steroids cause an opposite change[19,20]. Natural estrogens have also been
shown to increase the HDL cholesterol levels as illustrated by Table 1[21].
On the other hand, progestins evidently cause a decrease of HDL cholesterol[22].
Oral contraceptive agents may either decrease or increase the HDL depending
on their estrogen and progestin content[22].

The mode of action of gonadal steroids on HDL metabolism is still obscure.
Estrogenic hormones specifically increase the synthesis of VLDL (apoproteins)
in the liver but they have not been shown to induce production of apoprotein A-I. Estrogens are also without significant effect on LPL activity in
man[23]. It is somewhat perplexing that estrogen-containing oral contraceptive

TABLE 1

EFFECT OF TREATMENT WITH ESTRADIOL VALERIANATE ON HDL CHOLESTEROL
AND TRIGLYCERIDE CONCENTRATIONS (MEAN $\pm$ S.D.) IN POSTMENOPAUSAL
HYPERCHOLESTEROLEMIC WOMEN (mmol/l)

	Before treatment	After 3 months of treatment	After 6 months of treatment
Cholesterol	1.42 $\pm$ 0.31	1.59 $\pm$ 0.32	1.84 $\pm$ 0.42[x]
Triglyceride	0.13 $\pm$ 0.16	0.25 $\pm$ 0.08	0.25 $\pm$ 0.05[x]

Values significantly different from pre-treatment concentration (paired
t test): [x] $p < 0.05$.

drugs have been reported to cause mainly an increase of HDL_3 and little change
in HDL_2[24], a result opposite to that expected from the male/female difference.
Undoubtedly more detailed studies on the effects of individual steroids are
needed.

RELATION OF HDL TO INSULIN

In patients with clinical diabetes Barr et al.[1] found HDL cholesterol
levels ranging from low to normal but the average value was decreased compared
to non-diabetics. No systematic studies on serum lipoprotein patterns in
different types of diabetes have been carried out. Recently, low HDL cholesterol levels have been observed in noninsulin-requiring diabetes[25-27] and in
untreated juvenile diabetes with ketosis[28]. Upon initiation of insulin treatment the HDL values are slowly increased[28] and in diabetics receiving long-
term insulin treatment the HDL cholesterol levels may be even higher than
those of non-diabetics[29]. Table 2 presents data obtained in our laboratory
on serum lipoproteins in different forms of clinical diabetes.

Obesity is associated with a decrease of HDL cholesterol levels[30] and with
insulin resistance. On the other hand, highly physically active people
represent an opposite extreme having increased HDL levels[31,32] and insulin-
sensitivity[33]. These findings suggest that HDL levels could be controlled
not only by amount of insulin secretion but also by insulin sensitivity of
peripheral tissues or liver. The mechanism of this association between insulin
and HDL is not clear but it could be mediated by lipoprotein lipase activity
of adipose tissue which is known to be highly sensitive to variations in
insulin responsiveness. This possibility is supported by the observation
that both HDL levels and adipose tissue LPL activity are elevated in runners

TABLE 2

SERUM HDL CHOLESTEROL AND VLDL TRIGLYCERIDE IN DIABETES (MALES)

Group	HDL cholesterol	VLDL triglyceride
	mmol/l	
Juvenile ketotic (untreated)	1.10^x	2.16^x
" (treated)	1.14	1.12
Long-term insulin treated	1.52^x	0.75^x
Adult onset, non-obese	1.20	0.81
" obese	1.00^x	1.98^x
Non-diabetic males	1.24	0.92

x) Significantly different from control values at $p < 0.05$

with endurance type physical training but are normal in sprinters with mainly athletic activity[34].

Since it appeared that insulin could be one important factor in the control of plasma HDL levels we determined plasma insulin levels during a conventional oral glucose tolerance test in 32 obese non-diabetic subjects, who underwent lipoprotein studies. There was no significant correlation between the individual values of basal or one-hour postglucose plasma insulin levels and HDL cholesterol but by grouping the subjects according to the magnitude of plasma insulin responses one was able to find an increasing trend of HDL cholesterol with decreasing plasma insulin responses (Table 3). Of another 15 healthy subjects having HDL cholesterol in the upper quintile of a basic population 12 had one-hour plasma insulin levels less than 50 µU/ml and none

TABLE 3

RELATION OF HDL CHOLESTEROL TO PLASMA INSULIN RESPONSE DURING ORAL GLUCOSE TOLERANCE TEST

One-hour plasma insulin	Mean HDL cholesterol
µU/ml	mmol/l
< 50	1.16
50 to 100	1.05
> 100	0.81

had a response in excess of 100 µU/ml. It thus seems that insulin sensitivity (low plasma insulin values combined with low blood glucose during oral glucose tolerance test) is associated with increased HDL levels at least in comparison with people having insulin resistance and hyperinsulinemia.

ACKNOWLEDGEMENTS

The studies summarized in this review have been supported by grants from Finnish State Medical Research Council (Academy of Finland), from Sigrid Jusélius Foundation, Helsinki, Finland and from Nordisk Insulinfond, Copenhagen, Denmark. The collaboratorion of Drs. Marja-Riitta Taskinen, Pirkko Hormila, Kari Harno and Matti Tikkanen is appreciated.

REFERENCES

1. Barr, D.P., Russ, E.M. and Eder, H.A. (1951) Amer. J. Med., 11, 480-493.
2. Nikkilä, E.A. (1953) Scand. J. Clin. Lab. Invest. 5, Suppl. 8, 1-101.
3. Castelli, W.P., Doyle, J.T., Gordon, T., Hames, C.G., Hjortland, M.C., Hulley, S.B., Kagan, A. and Zukel, W.J. (1977) Circulation, 55, 767-772.
4. Glomset, J.A. (1970) Amer. J. Clin. Nutr., 23, 1129-1136.
5. Nikkilä, E.A. (1978) Eur. J. Clin. Invest., 8, 111-113.
6. Schwartz, C.C., Halloran, L.G., Vlahcevic, Z.R., Gregory, D.H. and Swell, L. (1978) Science, 200, 62-64.
7. Hamilton, R.L., Williams, M.C., Fielding, C.J. and Havel, R.J. (1976) J. Clin. Inv. 58, 667-680.
8. Nichols, A.V. (1967) in Advances in Biological and Medical Physics, Lawrence, J.H. and Gofman, J.W., eds., Academic Press, New York and London, pp. 109-158.
9. Anderson, D.W., Nichols, A.V., Pan, S.S. and Lindgren, F.T. (1978) Atherosclerosis, 29, 161-179.
10. Nikkilä, E.A., Taskinen, M.-R. and Kekki, M. (1978) Atherosclerosis, 29, 497-501.
11. Nikkilä, E.A. (1978) in High Density Lipoproteins and Atherosclerosis, Gotto, A.M.,Jr., Miller, N.E. and Oliver, M.F., eds., Elsevier, Amsterdam, pp. 177-192.
12. Russ, E.M., Eder, H.A. and Barr, D.P. (1951) Amer. J. Med., 11, 468-479.
13. Barr, D.P. (1955) J. Chron. Dis., 1, 63-85.
14. deLalla, O.F., Elliott, H.A. and Gofman, J.W. (1954) Amer. J. Physiol., 179, 333-337.
15. Barclay, M., Barclay, R.K. and Skipski, V.P. (1963) Nature, 200, 362-363.
16. Cheung, M.C. and Albers, J.J. (1977) J. Clin. Invest., 60, 43-50.
17. Shepherd, J., Packard, C.J., Patsch, J.R., Gotto, A.M.,Jr. and Taunton, O.D. (1978) Eur. J. Clin. Invest., 8, 115-120.

18. Nikkilä et al., unpublished data.

19. Russ, E.M., Eder, H.A. and Barr, D.P. (1955) Amer. J. Med., 19, 4-24.

20. Furman, R.H., Alaupovic, P. and Howard, R.P. (1967) in Progress in Biochemical Pharmacology, Kritchevsky, D., Paoletti, R. and Steinberg, D. eds., Karger, Basel and New York, Vol. 2, pp. 215-249.

21. Tikkanen, M.J., Nikkilä, E.A. and Vartiainen, E. (1978) Lancet, ii, 490-491.

22. Bradley, D.B., Wingerd, J., Petitti, D.B., Krauss, R.M. and Ramcharan, S. (1978) New Engl. J. Med. 299, 17-20.

23. Applebaum, D.M., Goldberg, A.P., Pykälistö, O.J., Brunzell, J.D. and Hazzard, W.R. (1977) J. Clin.Invest. 59, 601-608.

24. Krauss, R.M., Lindgren, F.T., Silvers, A., Jutagir, R. and Bradley, D.D. (1977) Clin. Chim. Acta, 80, 465-470.

25. Gordon, T., Castelli, W.P., Hjortland, M.C., Kannel, W.B. and Dawber, T.R. (1977) Amer. J. Med., 62, 707-714.

26. Lopes-Virella, M.F.L., Stone, P.G. and Colwell, J.A. (1977) Diabetologia, 13, 285-291.

27. Howard, B.V., Savage, P.J., Bennion, L.J. and Bennett, P.H. (1978) Atherosclerosis, 30, 153-162.

28. Taskinen, M.-R. and Nikkilä, E.A. (1979) Diabetologia (submitted for publication).

29. Nikkilä, E.A. and Hormila, P. (1978) Diabetes, 27 (in press).

30. Miller, G.J. and Miller, N.E. (1975) Lancet, i, 16-19.

31. Hoffman, A.A., Nelson, W.R. and Goss, F.A. (1967) Amer. J. Cardiol., 20, 516-524.

32. Lopez-S, A., Vial, R., Balart, L. and Arroyave, G. (1974) Atherosclerosis, 20, 1-9.

33. Björntorp, P., Fahlén, M., Grimby, G., Gustafson, A., Holm, J., Renström, P. and Scherstén, T. (1972) Metabolism, 21, 1037-1044.

34. Nikkilä, E.A., Taskinen, M.-R., Rehunen, S. and Härkönen, M. (1978) Metabolism, 27 (in press).

Lipoprotein Metabolism and Endocrine Regulation
L.W. Hessel and H.M.J. Krans editors
© ECSC, EEC, EAEC, Brussels-Luxembourg, 1979
Published by Elsevier/North-Holland Biomedical Press-Amsterdam

THE EFFECTS OF HORMONES ON LIPOPROTEIN KINETICS

P.J. MAGILL AND B. LEWIS
Department of Chemical Pathology and Metabolic Disorders,
St. Thomas's Hospital Medical School, London SE1 7EH, England.

INTRODUCTION

The scheme of lipoprotein interconversions shown in fig. 1 is
an attempt to summarise the present concepts gained from a large
number of studies in man and laboratory animals. Liver and
small intestine are the main sources of lipoproteins, the former
secreting very low density lipoproteins (VLDL) and the latter

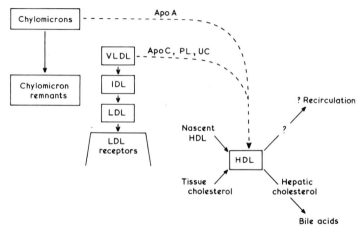

Fig. 1. Lipoprotein interconversions.

chylomicrons. Perfusion of the rat liver and ileum has shown
also the secretion of "discoidal high density lipoprotein" (HDL),
containing phospholipid (PL), unesterified cholesterol (UC),
apoprotein E and apoprotein A[1]. Apoprotein A, in HDL is further
derived from chylomicrons during the peripheral lipolysis which
results in the smaller chylomicron remnant[2].

In normal circumstances at least 90 percent of VLDL apoprotein B is converted to LDL in man, and all LDL apoprotein B is
derived from VLDL. However in some subjects with hypertriglyceridaemia the turnover of VLDL exceeds that of LDL[3,4], while
in familial hypercholesterolaemia the turnover of LDL exceeds
that of VLDL[5,6]. It therefore seems that in some circumstances

a separate pathway for catabolism of triglyceride-rich lipoproteins becomes active, and direct secretion of cholesterol-rich
lipoproteins can take place. Insight into the mechanisms of
catabolism of VLDL has been provided by the evidence that VLDL
from hypertriglyceridaemic patients suppresses hydroxy-methylglutaryl CoA reductase activity in cultured fibroblasts[7].

Hydrolysis of VLDL triglyceride by lipoprotein lipase in vitro
releases discoidal structures containing phospholipid, unesterified cholesterol and apoprotein C which accumulate in the
1.04 - 1.21g/ml density range[8]. One concept is that these discoidal structures may fuse or bind to preexisting high density
lipoprotein[9]. But "nascent HDL" itself is difficult to isolate
in normal metabolism, and concepts of its structure derive
greatly from study of particles found in the HDL density range
in abnormal situations - obstructive jaundice, LCAT deficiency,
or in rat liver perfusion systems incorporating an LCAT inhibitor.
It seems likely that HDL components arise from more than one
source, and that HDL particles, themselves heterogeneous and
labile in composition may represent a pool into which, and from
which, many components transfer, at rates influenced by the
metabolism of triglyceride-rich lipoproteins.

Removal of LDL from plasma is largely mediated by specific
receptors in peripheral cells, permitting regulated internalization and degradation; the ultimate fate of HDL is not known.
Bile acids[11] and biliary cholesterol[12] are derived, at least
in part, from HDL cholesterol and there is also evidence for a
specific receptor for HDL, located, not unexpectedly, in the
liver[13].

TURNOVER STUDY METHODS

Relatively few studies have explored the relationship between
lipoprotein metabolism and hormones using kinetic techniques.
Either the lipid or protein components can be labelled. Radioactive iodine has been used to label apoprotein B or apoprotein A
by the method of McFarlane[14], while tritiated glycerol[15] and 14C
palmitate have been used for the in vivo labelling of triglyceride.
After injection, decay of specific activity is measured in serial
blood samples. Plotted against time apoprotein labelled material
may show one exponential curve for triglyceride rich lipoproteins

and two for LDL or HDL. Lipid labelled VLDL has been reported to decay as a single major exponential, but in some hands its disappearance curve is complex and requires multicompartmental analysis. The fractional catabolic rate (FCR) derived from these curves when multiplied by the pool size of lipid or protein gives the turnover rate.

The FCR is a measure of the efficiency of clearance of protein or lipid, but it must be interpreted cautiously if the removal mechanism is saturable. The drawback of protein labelling is that the kinetics do not necessarily reflect lipid turnover, while the half life of tritiated triglyceride may be prolonged if incorporation of labelled glycerol is not very rapid in comparison with its rate of removal.

THYROID HORMONES

The half life and FCR of ^{131}I labelled LDL has been studied by Walton et al[16] in hypo- and hyperthyroid patients. In five hypothyroid patients the half life was prolonged and in 2 of these it was shown to be corrected after replacement therapy. Conversely the half life was reduced in 3 hyperthyroid patients, and corrected in the 2 patients restudied after treatment. Calculations were not extended to include synthetic rates of LDL, but clearly the prolonged half life of LDL would account for the hypercholesterolaemia commonly found in hypothyroidism if no increase in synthetic rate is assumed. Nikkila et al[17] found a significantly decreased FCR of plasma triglyceride in hypothyroid patients. Triglyceride synthetic rate was not significantly changed, and the hypertriglyceridaemia present was therefore attributed to a low rate of removal. Post heparin lipolytic activity was also reduced, in keeping with diminished triglyceride clearance, while later work has demonstrated diminished LDL receptor binding in hypothyroidism[18], in keeping with prolonged apoprotein B half life. In hyperthyroidism Nikkila et al also reported mild hypertriglyceridaemia resulting from increased production rates with normal FCR. However the increase in production rate did not correct after successful treatment of the hyperthyroidism.

OESTROGENS AND ORAL CONTRACEPTIVES

The hypertriglyceridaemia found during oestrogen therapy with or without progestogen is usually mild; the occasional patients who develop massive hypertriglyceridaemia probably suffer a primary hyperlipidaemia aggravated by oestrogen. Kekki et al[19], studying triglyceride kinetics in premenopausal women on oral contraceptive therapy found an increase in triglyceride synthetic rate which was compensated to some extent by an increase in the efficiency of removal. The increase in removal efficiency was tentatively attributed to the progestogen component of the contraceptives, but very similar findings were reported by Glueck et al[20] using oestrogens alone in postmenopausal women. Further evidence for an effect of oestrogens on the removal of triglyceride rich lipoproteins, comes from studies of patients with broad beta disease, in whom defective removal of VLDL remnants is corrected by oestrogen therapy[21].

INSULIN AND DIABETES

Mild hypertriglyceridaemia is not uncommon in untreated diabetes, levels falling during treatment. A more severe hypertriglyceridaemia is found in a few patients in whom triglyceride levels fall but do not usually enter the normal range following treatment. Studies of the families of these patients frequently reveal a familial form of hypertriglyceridaemia, which has been aggravated by untreated diabetes[22].

Studies of turnover rates have demonstrated increased synthesis of triglyceride in diabetes. Nikkila et al[23] found increased turnover rates in 8 out of 9 patients with diabetic ketoacidosis, the turnover rates falling in the four patients restudied after treatment, in whom the hypertriglyceridaemia was totally corrected. Sigurdsson et al[24] found very high turnover rates of apoprotein B in three newly diagnosed diabetic patients with marked hypertriglyceridaemia. Kissebah[25], studying newly diagnosed maturity onset diabetics found increased production rates only in a group of obese patients, lean patients having normal production rates.

In all three series fractional catabolic rates were reduced in hypertriglyceridaemic diabetics, but the interpretation of FCR as a measure of efficiency of removal mechanisms is difficult because of the saturable nature of the mechanisms combined with an increased pool size[28]. Support for a removal defect mediated

through reduced lipoprotein lipase activity comes from the studies
of Bagdade[26] and Brunzell[27] but the importance of increased production rates as a mechanism of hypertriglyceridaemia in diabetics
is less clear.

HIGH DENSITY LIPOPROTEINS

Recently published studies of the kinetics of apoprotein A
metabolism in HDL have not, with one exception, studied their
interrelation with hormones. Shepherd et al[29] found an increased
$HDL_2:HDL_3$ ratio in females versus males, but found no significant
differences between sexes for apoprotein A_1 half life or absolute
catabolic rate.

A further relationship between HDL cholesterol levels and insulin replacement in diabetics has been described[30], and it seems
hopeful that kinetic studies will help to illuminate the mechanisms of such relationships.

REFERENCES

1. Hamilton, R.L., Williams, M.C., Fielding, C.J. and Havel, R.J.
    (1976) J. Clin. Invest. 58, 667-680.

2. Havel, R.J. (1978) High Density Lipoproteins and Atherosclero-
    sis, Elsevier North-Holland, pp. 21-36.

3. Sigurdsson, G., Nicoll, A. and Lewis, B. (1976) Europ. J.
    Clin. Invest. 6, 167-177.

4. Reardon, M.F., Fidge, N.H. and Nestel, P.J. (1978) J. Clin.
    Invest. 61, 850-860.

5. Janus, E.D. In preparation.

6. Soutar, A.K., Myant, N.B. and Thompson, G.R. (1977) Athero-
    sclerosis 28, 247-256.

7. Gianturco, S.H., Gotto, A.M., Jackson, R.L., Patsch, J.R.,
    Sybers, H.D., Taunton, O.D., Yeshuran, D.L. and Smith, L.C.
    (1978) J. Clin. Invest. 61, 320-328.

8. Chajek, T. and Eisenberg, S. (1978) J. Clin. Invest. 61, 1654-65

9. Eisenberg, S. (1978) High Density Lipoproteins and Athero-
    sclerosis, Elsevier North-Holland, pp. 67-75.

10. Goldstein, J.L. and Brown, M.S. (1977) Ann. Rev. Biochem.
    46, 897-930.

11. Halloran, L.G., Schwartz, C.C., Vlahcevic, Z.R., Nisman, R.M.
    and Swell, L. (1978) Surgery 84, 1-7.

12. Schwartz, C.C., Halloran, L.G., Vlahcevic, Z.R., Gregory, D.H.
    and Swell, L. (1978) Science 200, 62-64.

13. Nakai, T., Otto, P.S., Kennedy, D.L. and Whayne, T.F. (1976)
    J. Biol. Chem. 251, 4914-4921.

14. McFarlane, A.S. (1958) Nature (Lond.) 182, 53.

15. Reaven, G.M., Hill, D.B., Gross, R.C. and Farquhar, J.W. (1965) J. Clin. Invest. 44, 1826.

16. Walton, K.W., Scott, P.J., Dykes, P.W.,and Davies, J.W.L. (1965) Clin. Sci. 29, 217-238.

17. Nikkila, E.A. and Kekki, M. (1972) J. Clin. Invest. 51, 2103-2114.

18. Chait, A., Albers, J.J. and Bierman, E.L. (1978) Clin. Res. 26, 303.

19. Kekki, M. and Nikkila, E.A. (1971) Metabolism 20, 878-889.

20. Glueck, C.J., Fallat, R.W. and Scheel, D. (1975) Metabolism 24, 537-545.

21. Chait, A., Hazzard, W.R., Albers, J.J., Kushwaha, R.P. and Brunzell, J.D. (1978) Metabolism 27, 1055-1066.

22. Brunzell, J.D., Hazzard, W.R., Motulsky, A.G. and Bierman,E.L. (1975) Metabolism 24, 1115-1122.

23. Nikkila, E.A. and Kekki, M. (1973) Metabolism 22, 1-22.

24. Sigurdsson, G., Nicoll, A. and Lewis, B. (1976) Europ. J. Clin. Invest. 6, 167-177.

25. Kissebah, A.H., Adams, P.W. and Wynn, V. (1974) Diabeto-logia 10, 119-131.

26. Bagdade, J.D., Porte, D. and Bierman, E.L. (1967) New Eng. J. Med. 276, 427.

27. Brunzell, J.D., Porte, D. and Bierman, E.L. (1975) Meta-bolism 24, 1123-1138.

28. Brunzell, J.D., Hazzard, W.R., Porte, D. and Bierman, E.L. (1973) J. Clin. Invest. 52, 1578.

29. Shepherd, J., Packard, C.J., Patsch, J.R., Gotto, A.M. and Taunton, O.D. (1978) Europ. J. Clin. Invest. 8, 115-120.

30. Paisey, R., Elkeles, R.S., Hambley, J. and Magill, P. (1978) Diabetologia 15, 81-85.

Lipoprotein Metabolism and Endocrine Regulation
L.W. Hessel and H.M.J. Krans editors
© ECSC, EEC, EAEC, Brussels-Luxembourg, 1979
Published by Elsevier/North-Holland Biomedical Press-Amsterdam

ENDOCRINE DISORDERS AND ADIPOSE TISSUE LIPOPROTEIN LIPASE

John D. Brunzell
St. Thomas' Hospital, Department of Chemical Pathology and
Metabolic Disorders, London SE1 7EH, England.

ABSTRACT

Lipoprotein lipase activity in human subcutaneous adipose tissue
is under the control of various hormones. It is increased in
obesity, and further increases in individuals who have lost weight
and have maintained this weight loss. It is decreased in insulin
deficient and thyroxin deficient states and returns to normal with
hormone replacement. No abnormality in lipoprotein lipase is
seen with estrogen therapy.

INTRODUCTION

Lipoprotein lipase is an enzyme that hydrolyses triglyceride
contained in the triglyceride-rich lipoproteins, chylomicrons and
very-low density lipoproteins[1] .   It is synthesized in tissues
such as muscle or adipose tissue that utilize triglyceride fatty
acids for energy or storage.   In the adipocyte the enzyme is
synthesized and stored in the cytosol. Subsequently, it is
secreted from the cell by an energy requiring process and is
transferred to nearby capillary endothelial cells where it interacts with the triglyceride-rich lipoproteins.   The uptake by the
fat cell of very low density lipoprotein triglyceride fatty acids
and free fatty acids has been shown to be highly correlated with
adipose tissue lipoprotein lipase levels[2]. Since very little
fatty acid synthesis occurs in human adipose tissue, the uptake of
fatty acids probably accounts for the majority of adipose tissue
triglyceride fatty acids. It is interesting to note that the
uptake of fatty acids has been reported to be twice as great for
triglyceride fatty acids as for free fatty acids[2] .

Studies with rat adipose tissue lipoprotein lipase suggest that
it is under multifactorial endocrine control[1] .   However, marked
species differences have been noted in the effects of hormones on
lipoprotein lipase in rats and humans[3] .   This review will be

directed towards studies of abnormalities in adipose tissue lipoprotein lipase in human endocrine disorders only.

Many studies have been performed on human adipose tissue
obtained by needle suction biopsy from subcutaneous tissue. Lipoprotein lipase in adipose tissue can be measured in several
different ways. One, an estimate of the total activity of the
enzyme can be made by measuring the activity present in extracts
of adipose tissue powders that have been defatted with acetone
and ether. The second is estimated by the incubation of adipose
tissue with heparin in vitro which elutes the enzyme activity
from the cell into the incubation medium where it can then be
measured. This activity may represent the functional form of
the enzyme. The measurement of heparin elutable adipose tissue
lipoprotein lipase activity (HE-LPL) has been performed in two
different ways. One is to incubate the adipose tissue, heparin,
and the substrate in the same tube and measure the rate of
appearance of the fatty acids in the one stage incubation
system[4,5]. The other is a two stage system in which the adipose
tissue and heparin are first incubated together, followed by
incubation of the elution medium containing only the enzyme with
the substrate[2,4,6-8]. Whether or not the difference in these
techniques is important is not known[4]. The HE-LPL correlates
with the activity measured in the extracts of the acetone-ether
powders obtained from the same piece of tissue[6,7,9]. This is not
surprising, since the HE-LPL is probably a major component of the
enzyme activities measured in the total tissue extract. From
studies in certain endocrine disorders[9,10] and in hypertriglyceridemic subjects on chronic maintenance hemodialysis[11] it
appears that the major abnormality in these disorders in humans is
in HE-LPL. The intracellular form of the enzyme appears to be
normal. In contrast both the HE-LPL and the activity in the
acetone-ether powders are essentially zero in patients with
familial lipoprotein lipase deficiency[3]. The HE-LPL has been
reported as activity per gram of adipose tissue[4,7,12] and as
activity per cell in adipose tissue[2,5,7,8,13]. Since with
varying degrees of obesity and adipocyte cell size the number of
cells per gram of adipose tissue is quite different the method
of reporting of activity can have an effect on the interpretation

of results (see below under obesity).

OBESITY

HE-LPL per cell is increased in obesity in adults[7-9,13-15]. It is linearly correlated with fat cell size (μg TG/cell) over the range of cell size seen in man in which most of the difference in adipose tissue mass is dependent on cell size without a change in cell number[16]. In this range of from 80 to 180 per cent of ideal body weight the decision to report LPL activity per gram of adipose tissue is important. Some groups have reported a decrease[4,7,17] and some groups have reported no change[5,8,14,15] in HE-LPL per gram of adipose tissue in obesity. If the enzyme is distributed uniformly throughout the cell, including the triglyceride droplet, this would be an appropriate way of reporting the data. However, it seems unlikely that the enzyme is present in the triglyceride droplet. Rather, one would expect the enzyme to be located either in the cytosol or on the surface of the cell, which for practical purposes, are the same. Thus, the decrease in the number of cells per gram of adipose tissue in obese individuals, as opposed to thin ones, would explain the decrease in LPL per gram in obesity in some studies and an increase in LPL per cell in others. The importance of LPL in determining or regulating cell size can be surmised from the studies of subjects who were formerly obese and are now thin and weight stable[18]. It is now important to differentiate between the state of on going weight loss and the state after weight loss, in which enough calories are consumed to maintain this reduced weight. During active weight loss adipose tissue LPL (per cell or per gram) is decreased from that found prior to beginning weight loss[8,19]. A different situation is found in an individual who has undergone weight loss and now is consuming enough calories to maintain weight. This individual has to be constantly aware of an increase in appetite to prevent the return to his former level of obesity and this is almost always unsuccessful. If the increase in LPL per cell in obesity were secondary to the increase in the fat cell size then one would expect the LPL per cell in weight reduced individuals to fall to levels seen in normally thin individuals of the same weight. In fact this is not the case. The LPL per cell in these weight reduced individuals has been found to be

increased three fold above expected[18]. A higher center, the
hypothalamic "weight stat", itself controlled by some unknown
factor(s), may regulate LPL levels by some humoral or neural means.
The LPL in adipose tissue may then be the subsequent regulator of
fat cell size. This increase in adipose tissue LPL after weight
loss might explain the marked difficulty and lack of success of
obese individuals in maintaining weight loss.

A direct relationship between obesity and fasting insulin levels
and between fasting and stimulated insulin levels has been noted[20].
In the type of obesity usually seen in adult humans the increase
in fat cell size is probably a major determinant of the fasting
and, perhaps, the stimulated insulin levels. This conclusion is
based on the parallel decrease in insulin levels and fat cell size
seen in individuals after weight loss[21]. It has previously been
proposed by us that a combination of fasting and stimulated insulin
levels are the major determinants of fasting adipose tissue LPL in
man[22] in a way similar to that reported for rats[1]. However, as
stated above, the LPL per cell may be somehow regulated by the
hypothalmus which subsequently determines fat cell size. Fat
cell size would then determine insulin resistance, which would
then be a regulator of insulin secretion.

The relationship between fat cell LPL and plasma insulin appears
to be more complex than this, however. In the insulin deficient
state seen with fasting hyperglycemia in diabetes, LPL in adipose
tissue is reduced (see below). Also it has been demonstrated
that LPL per cell in thin individuals increases in the fed state
as a function of the amount of insulin secreted which itself was
determined by the amount of carbohydrate fed[9]. To further complicate matters, the change in adipose tissue LPL with feeding is a
negative one in obese, hyperinsulinemic subjects[11,23,24]. And
finally, while rat adipose tissue LPL increases in vitro when
incubated with insulin, no such effect on human adipose LPL was
demonstrable[25]. The final analysis of the relationships between
LPL and insulin still remains to be made

UNTREATED DIABETES MELLITUS

Patients with untreated diabetes who have fasting plasma glucose
levels persistantly above 10mM/L have decreased levels of

adipose tissue LPL per cell[8,9] or per gram of adipose tissue[12,26]. Although the LPL found in extracts of acetone-ether powders is also decreased, this decrease is probably due to a lowering of the HE component only[9]. The decrease in HE-LPL seen in the fasting state in untreated diabetes returns to normal with insulin or oral sulfonylurea therapy and is associated with a decrease in plasma triglyceride levels to that seen in their non-diabetic relatives . These diabetics also can be demonstrated to have a decrease in HE-LPL in the fed state that is related to the degree of insulin deficiency[9]. An unusual and as yet unexplained finding relates to the delay for 4-10 weeks after initiating antidiabetic therapy in the return of LPL and triglyceride levels completely to normal. With chronic insulin or oral sulfonylurea therapy, without an intervening episode of ketoacidosis, no abnormality in LPL has been demonstrated.

HYPOTHYROIDISM

Both hypercholesteremia and hypertriglyceridemia have been reported in hypothyroidism, and often an increase in VLDL and LDL occur simultaneously. A decrease in post-heparin plasma hepatic lipase has been reported, while post-heparin plasma LPL was found to be normal[27]. Interestingly, adipose tissue HE-LPL is low in hypothyroidism[10]. Furthermore, the decreased LPL returns to normal over 1-3 months of therapy with thyroxin and the increase in LPL correlates with the simultaneous decrease in plasma trigly- ceride levels. Whether the abnormality in adipose tissue LPL is a function of the decrease in circulating thyroxine levels or due to an increase in TSH levels is unknown.

ESTROGEN THERAPY

Even though estrogen decreases adipose tissue LPL in rats and may account for part or all of the hypertriglyceridemia in this species, neither adipose tissue nor post heparin plasma LPL in humans are effected by estrogen therapy[26,28]. The hypertrigly- ceridemia seen in estrogen treated humans is probably due to increased triglyceride production,or,less likely,to the associated decrease in post-heparin plasma hepatic triglyceride lipase[26,28].

SUMMARY

Although a number of hormones have been demonstrated to regulate LPL in rats[1,25] the effects of insulin and estrogen and the hypothyroid state seem to be different in man[2,25]. We have yet to learn of the effects on human adipose tissue LPL of such hormones as glucocorticoids, glucagon, testosterone, or prolactin.

ACKNOWLEDGEMENTS

This work was supported by NIH Grants HL 18687 and AM 02456. The excellent technical assistance of Ms. Martha Kimura was an important contribution to this work. I would also like to thank Dr. R. James St.Hilaire for his assistance in preparing this manuscript.

REFERENCES

1. Robinson, D.S. (1970) The function of the plasma triglycerides in fatty acid transport. In Comprehensive Biochemistry. Vol.18. Lipid Metabolism. Florkin, M. and Stotz, E.H. eds. Elsevier, Amsterdam, p.51.

2. Taskinen, M.-R.and Nikkila, E.A. (1977) Lipoprotein lipase activity in adipose tissue and in postheparin plasma in human obesity. Acta Med. Scand. 202:399.

3. Brunzell, J.D. and Goldberg, A.P. (1977) Hormonal regulation of human adipose tissue lipoprotein lipase. In Atheroscler- osis IV. Schettler,G., Goto, Y., Hata, Y., and Klose, G. eds. Springer-Verlag, New York, p.336.

4. Persson, B., Schroder, G., and Hood, B. (1972) Lipoprotein lipase in human adipose tissue: Assay methods. Atherosclerosis 16:37

5. Lithell,H. and Boberg, J. (1977) A method of determining lipoprotein-lipase activity in human adipose tissue. Scand. J. Clin. Lab. Invest. 37:551.

6. Nilsson-Ehle, P. (1974) Human lipoprotein lipase activity: comparison of assay methods. Clin. Chem. Acta 54:283.

7. Pykalisto, O.J., Smith, P.H., and Brunzell, J.D. (1975) Human adipose tissue lipoprotein lipase: Comparison of assay methods and expressions of activity. Proc. Soc. Exp. Biol. Med. 148:297.

8. Guy-Grand, B. and Bigorie, B. (1975). Effect of fat cell size, restrictive diet and diabetes on lipoprotein lipase release by human adipose tissue. Horm. Metab. Res. 7:471.

9. Pykalisto, O.J., Smith, P.H., and Brunzell, J.D. (1975)
    Determinants of human adipose tissue lipoprotein lipase:
    Effects of diabetes and obesity on basal and diet induced
    activity. J. Clin. Invest. 56:1108.

10. Pykalisto, O.J., Golberg, A.P., and Brunzell, J.D.,(1976)
    Reversal of decreased human adipose tissue lipoprotein
    lipase and hypertriglyceridemia after treatment of hypo-
    thyroidisin. J. Clin. Endo. Metab. 43:549.

11. Goldberg, A.P., Sherrard, D.J., and Brunzell, J.D. (1978)
    Adipose tissue lipoprotein lipase in chronic hemodialysis:
    Role in plasma triglyceride metabolism. J.Clin. Endo.
    Metab. (December 1978)

12. Jaillard, J., Sezille, G., Fruchart, J.C. Dewailly, P.,
    and Romon, M. (1976). Etude de l'activite de la lipoproteine-
    lipase et de la cellularite au niveau du tissu adipeux humain.
    Diabete Metabolisme (Paris) 2:5.

13. Bjorntorp, P., Enzi, G., Persson, B., Sponbergs, P. and
    Smith, U. (1975). Lipoprotein lipase activity and uptake of
    exogenous triglycerides in fat cells of different size.
    Horm. Metab. Res. 7:230.

14. Lithell,H., Boberg, J., Hellsing, K. and Waern, U. (1978).
    Lipoprotein-lipase activity in subcutaneous, adipose tissue
    in healthy subjects. Variation of activity in a population of
    60 year-old men. Ups. J. Med. Sci. 83:45.

15. Lithell, H., and Boberg, J. (1978). The lipoprotein-lipase
    activity of adipose tissue from different sites in obese
    women. Relationship to cell size.
    Intern. J. Obesity 2:47.

16. Sjostrom,L., and Bjorntorp,P.(1974) Body composition and
    adipose tissue cellularity in human obesity.
    Acta Med. Scand. 195:201.

17. Persson, B. (1973). Lipoprotein lipase activity of human
    adipose tissue in health and in some diseases with hyper-
    lipidemia as a common feature.
    Acta Med. Scand. 193:457.

18. Schwartz,R.S., and Brunzell, J.D. (1978) Increased adipose
    tissue lipoprotein lipase in moderately obese men after
    weight reduction. Lancet 1:1230.

19. Persson,B., Hood, B., and Angervall, G. (1970). Effects of
    prolonged fast on lipoprotein lipase activity eluted from
    adipose tissue. Acta Med. Scand. 188:225

20. Bagdade, J.D., Bierman, E.L., and Porte, D., Jr. (1967) The significance of basal insulin levels in the evaluation of the insulin responses to glucose in diabetic and non-diabetic subjects. J. Clin. Invest. 46:1549.

21. Bagdade, J.D., Porte, D., Jr., Brunzell, J.D., and Bierman,E.L. (1974).Basal and stimulated hyperinsulinism: reversible metabolic sequelae of obesity. J. Lab. Clin. Med. 83:563.

22. Goldberg, A.P. Chait,A., and Brunzell, J.D. (Submitted for publication). Adipose tissue lipoprotein lipase and insulin in the regulation of triglyceride metabolism in normal and hypertriglyceridemic man.

23. Dahms, W.T., Nilsson-Ehle,P., Atkinson, R.L.,Garfinkel, A., Schotz, M., and Bray, G. (1976) Lipoprotein lipase is unresponsive to glucose in obesity. Proc. Endo. Society Abstract 494.

24. Goldberg,A.P., Sherrard, D.J., and Brunzell, J.D.,(1976) Abnormal regulation of adipose tissue lipoprotein lipase in uremic hypertriglyceridemia. Clin. Res. 24:155 (Abstract).

25. Elkeles, R.S. (1974) Lipoprotein lipase in human adipose tissue. Clin. Sci. Mol. Med. 46:753.

26. Nikkila, E.A. (1978) Metabolic and endocrine control of plasma high density lipoprotein concentration. In High Density Lipoproteins and Atherosclerosis, Gotto, A.M. Jr., Miller,N.E., and Oliver, M.F. eds. Elsevier/North Holland Biomedical Press, Amsterdam, p 177.

27. Krauss, R.M., Levy, R.I., and Fredrickson, D.S. (1974) Selective measurement of two lipase activities in post heparin plasma from normal subjects and patients with hyperlipoprotein-emia. J. Clin. Invest. 54:1107.

28. Applebaum, D.M., Goldberg, A.P., Pykalisto, O.J., Brunzell,J.D. and Hazzard, W.R. (1977). Effect of estrogen on post-heparin lipolytic activity; selective decline in hepatic triglyceride lipase. J. Clin. Invest. 59:601.

Lipoprotein Metabolism and Endocrine Regulation
L.W. Hessel and H.M.J. Krans editors
© ECSC, EEC, EAEC, Brussels-Luxembourg, 1979
Published by Elsevier/North-Holland Biomedical Press-Amsterdam

EFFECT OF PROLONGED FASTING ON PLASMA LIPOPROTEIN COMPOSITION IN OBESE
PATIENTS.

M. Mancini, P. Strazzullo, F. Contaldo, A. Postiglione, G. Riccardi, N. Per-
rotti, C. Iovine.
Semeiotica Medica, 2nd Faculty of Medicine, University of Naples, Naples,
Italy.

ABSTRACT

Changes in plasma lipoprotein (Lpt) composition during prolonged fast,
in the treatment of massive obesity, were evaluated in 5 obese females in a
metabolic ward. Plasma lipoprotein cholesterol (CHOL) and triglyceride (TG)
concentration of the three major Lpt classes, isolated by preparative ultracentrifugation, was determined weekly for six weeks. Plasma immunoreactive
insulin (IRI) and glucagon (IRG) levels were also estimated.

Mean weight loss during treatment was 15 kg. Very low density lipoprotein
(VLDL) concentration decreased stepwise with no change in TG/CHOL ratio.
Low density lipoprotein (LDL)-CHOL, after a transient elevation during the
first week, decreased until the end of the fourth week, showing a trend to
higher values thereafter. LDL-TG slightly increased with inverse relation
to VLDL-TG and a net increase in LDL TG/CHOL ratio. A slight decrease in
CHOL content of high density lipoprotein (HDL) was also observed.

For a more detailed evaluation of lipid changes in the early phase of
fasting, quantitative analysis of plasma lipoprotein was also carried out
on a daily basis in four obese males fasting for 2 weeks.

Plasma IRI decreased during treatment in all patients while plasma IRG
showed a peak at the first week and thereafter remained slightly above
baseline values.

INTRODUCTION

Some studies have indicated effects of caloric restriction or prolonged
fasting on blood lipid concentration in obese patients[1-3]. In particular
it was observed that a fall in total serum CHOL and TG concentration took

place until the end of the fourth week of fasting while a progressive rise towards pretreatment values could be seen thereafter[4].

This work aims to study this phenomenon in more details by evaluating changes in plasma Lpt composition in fasting obese patients, because very little information is now available in this regard. Changes in plasma IRI and IRG during this type of treatment were also investigated as these hormones play a fundamental role in lipid metabolism[5].

PATIENTS AND METHODS

Five obese females with body weight (B.W.) between 117 and 124 kg and body mass index (B.M.I., w/h^2) between 48.7 and 55.9 were studied while fasting for 6 weeks. In addition a short term evaluation was carried out in four obese males with B.W. between 80 and 124 kg and B.M.I. between 31.3 and 38.5. Normal range for B.M.I. is 18-23 for females and 20-24 for males. All patients were normolipidemics, except G.R., who had hyperlipoproteinemia type IIB (W.H.O., 1970). Patient C.O. was overtly diabetic (Table 1).

TABLE 1

PATIENTS DATA

NAME	SEX	AGE (yrs)	B.W. (kg)	B.M.I. (w/h^2)	CHOL (mg/dl)	TG
D.M.	M	46	80	31.3	180	133
D.R.	M	26	124	37.8	211	130
V.A.	M	33	104	38.5	207	182
D.I.	M	24	99	33.5	222	123
C.O.	F	40	118	55.9	156	75
G.R.	F	36	117	48.7	250	302
M.O.	F	31	124	55.1	208	116
D.C.	F	38	117	51.4	152	141
B.O.	F	29	117	50.5	145	126

Patients were hospitalized in a metabolic ward for weight reduction by prolonged fasting (0-80 Kcal=0-17g Protein). A liberal fluid intake, poly-vitamin tablet and 30-60 mEq oral potassium were given every day.

Quantitative analysis of plasma lipoproteins was carried out weekly in the 5 females, while in the 4 males, who fasted for two weeks, it was carried out daily. Plasma lipoproteins (VLDL,d<1.006; LDL, 1.006<d<1.063; HDL, 1063<d<1.210) were isolated by preparative ultracentrifugation[6] and extracted by isopropanol for estimation of CHOL[7] and TG[8] concentration. Also Lpt protein moiety was estimated by the method of Lowry et al.[9]. Haematocrit was assayed by the micro-fuge method (Clay Adams). Plasma IRI was determined by the method of Hales and Randle[10] and plasma IRG by the method of Aguillar Parada et al.[11].

RESULTS

Fasting was well tolerated by all patients with improvement of their general conditions. Blood glucose was normalized within few days in patient C.O..

No significant change in haematocrit was observed in any case during the fasting treatment.

Average weight loss in females fasting six weeks was 15 kg (Table 2).

TABLE 2

WEIGHT LOSS IN OBESE PATIENTS DURING FASTING

NAME	WKS OF FASTING	WEIGHT LOSS (kg)
D.M.	2	6
D.R.	2	12
N.A.	2	10
D.I.	2	8
C.O.	6	17
G.R.	6	17
M.O.	6	14
D.C.	6	14
B.O.	6	16

Changes in total plasma CHOL and TG concentration were similar to those

38

previously described[4]. Changes in CHOL content of the three isolated lipoprotein fractions are shown in figure 1.

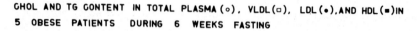

CHOL AND TG CONTENT IN TOTAL PLASMA (o), VLDL(□), LDL(•),AND HDL(■)IN 5 OBESE PATIENTS DURING 6 WEEKS FASTING

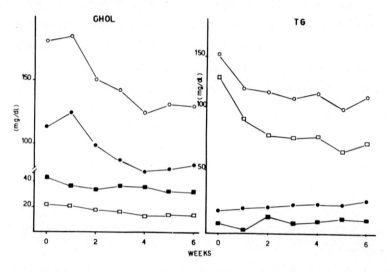

LDL-CHOL, after a transient increase above the baseline value at day 7, dropped regularly until the end of the fourth week (p<0.01) with an upward trend to higher values thereafter. VLDL-and HDL-CHOL content were also progressively reduced altough to a lesser degree (p<0.05).

A marked stepwise fall in VLDL-TG was observed, which accounted for the decrease in TG concentration of total blood. A slight increase of LDL-TG was found with a progressive rise of LDL TG/CHOL ratio (figure 2).

Plasma IRI decreased during the fasting regimen (fig. 3) and remained below baseline values during all the period of study. Viceversa plasma IRG showed a peak level at the first week and thereafter remained above pretreatment values (fig. 3).

A more detailed evaluation of lipoprotein changes in the early phase of fasting could be observed in the 4 male patients who lost on the average 9 kg in 2 weeks (Table 2). VLDL-CHOL and VLDL-TG decreased stepwise since the beginning with a mean reduction of 10 mg/dl and 65 mg/dl respectively

TG/CHOL RATIO IN
PLASMA LIPOPROTEINS

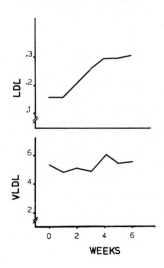

CHANGES IN PLASMA IRI
(o) AND IRG (•) DURING
PROLONGED FASTING

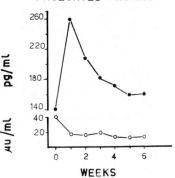

GHOL AND TG GONTENT IN TOTAL PLASMA(o), VLDL(□), LDL(•) AND HDL(■)IN
4 OBESE PATIENTS DURING 2 WEEKS FASTING

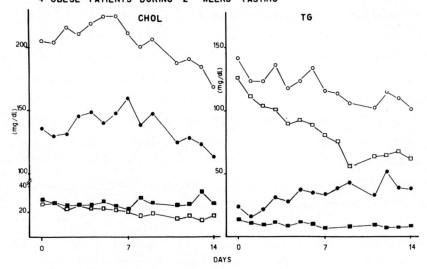

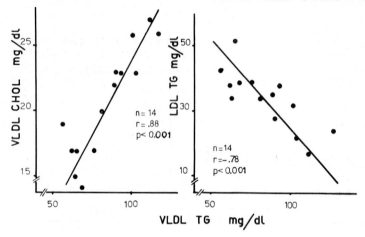

CORRELATIONS BETWEEN DAILY CHANGES IN LIPID CONSTITUENTS OF PLASMA LIPOPROTEINS IN 4 OBESE MALES DURING 2 WEEKS FASTING

($p < 0.01$), while LDL-TG concomitantly increased of about 14 mg/dl ($p < 0.01$) (fig. 4).

LDL-CHOL rose up to day 7, to fall below baseline values during the second week. No significant decrease occurred in HDL-CHOL and HDL-TG.

Daily changes of different components of the three lipoprotein fractions were correlated each other. As follow-up period was 2 weeks, 14 pairs of observations have been plotted, each point representing the daily mean of the data from 4 patients.

Strong positive correlation between VLDL-CHOL and VLDL-TG ($r=.88$, $p < 0.001$) and inverse relationship between VLDL-TG and LDL-TG ($r=-.78$, $p < 0.001$) were found (fig. 5).

Changes in VLDL-TG and in LDL-CHOL were parallel to changes in protein content of these lipoprotein molecules (fig. 6).

DISCUSSION

The reduction of total plasma CHOL and TG concentrations already observed by some authors and by one of us in fasting obese patients[1-4] has been confirmed

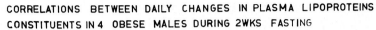

CORRELATIONS BETWEEN DAILY CHANGES IN PLASMA LIPOPROTEINS
CONSTITUENTS IN 4 OBESE MALES DURING 2WKS FASTING

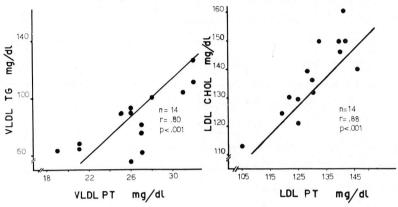

in the present study. According to the findings of this study the fall in
total CHOL concentration during prolonged fasting is essentially due to a
drop of LDL-CHOL; this is accompanied by minor changes in the other two major
Lpt fractions. The temporary increase in total plasma CHOL observed during
the first week is due to a transient elevation in LDL-CHOL concentration.

On the other hand the stepwise decrease in plasma TG concentration is
largely to be attributed to decrease in VLDL-TG and to a much smaller extent
in HDL-TG. Viceversa it has been seen that LDL-TG content tends to increase
in our patients during fasting: this phenomenon was more marked when studied
in obese males. The parallel decrease of CHOL and TG moieties in VLDL with
unchanged TG/CHOL ratio indicates an overall reduction of plasma concentration
of this Lpt molecule . This view is also supported by the observation of a
concomitant decrease of VLDL protein. Reduced concentration of VLDL-TG is
in keeping with studies which have shown decreased endogenous synthesis of
TG despite increased flux of free fatty acids (FFA) to the liver[12]. This may
be at least partly explained by the reduced ratio IRI/IRG in the plasma
observed in our patients[12-13]. Moreover, as it has been recently shown,

42

hepatic ketogenesis, certainly enhanced during prolonged fasting, is inversely
related to TG production rate[14].

Plasma concentration of LDL is also reduced as judged by the concomitant
reduction of its CHOL and protein moieties. Increased TG/CHOL ratio in this
fraction indicates a TG rich low density lipoprotein, possibly explained by
the observed reduction of lipoprotein lipase activity in adipose tissue and
skeletal muscle during prolonged fasting[15-16].

This brings about an impaired catabolism of VLDL and increased concentrations of   the intermediate lipoprotein fraction[17]. This view
is further supported by the strong inverse correlation found between VLDL-TG
and LDL-TG in our male patients during fasting.

A slight fall in HDL-CHOL concentration is predictable since lipoprotein
lipase activity is reduced and VLDL catabolism impaired[18]. The absence of
lipoprotein secretion in the gut during the fasting regimen may also contribute
to reduced plasma lipoprotein levels under these circumstances.

In conclusion the results of this study essentially indicate reduced plasma
lipoprotein biosynthesis during prolonged fasting well in accordance with
the reduced plasma insulin level and reduced insulin glucagon ratio[12-19].
In addition they provide some evidence in favour of an associated impairment
in VLDL catabolism as suggested by the accumulation of an intermediate lipoprotein TG rich.

REFERENCES

1. Martin, B.L., Man, E.B., Winkler, A.W. and Peters, J.B. (1944) J. Clin.
   Invest., 23:824-835.

2. Rubin, L. and Aladjem, F. (1954) Am.J.Physiol., 178:263-266.

3. Mancini, M., Oriente, P., Moro, C.O., Cerqua, R., de Divitiis, O. and
   Cioffi, L.A. (1968) Boll.Soc.Ita.Biol.Sper., 44:2234-2238.

4. Mancini, M., Postiglione, A., Di Marino, L. (1977) Nutr.and Metab.,
   21:13-25.

5. Lewis, B. (1976) In the Hyperlipidaemias, Blackwell Scient.Publ.Oxford,
   London, Edinburgh, Melbourne, pp 155-160.

6. Carlson, K. (1973) J.Clin.Path., Suppplement 26,5, 32-37.

7. Abell, L.L., Levy, G.B., Brodie, B.B., and Kendall, F.E. (1952) J.Biol. Chem., 195, 357-366.

8. Pantulu, G.A., Anderson, J.T. and Keys, A. (1964) Fed.Proc., 24:438-441.

9. Lowry, O.H., Rosenbrough, N.J., Farr, A.L. and Randall, R.J. (1951) J. Biol.Chem., 193:265-275.

10. Hales, C. and Randle, P. (1963) Biochem. J., 88: 137-146.

11. Aguilar Parada, E., Eisentrant, A.M. and Unger, R.H. (1969) Am.J.Med.Sci., 257:415-419.

12. Streja, D.A. and Steiner, G. (1977) Metabolism, 26:505-516.

13. Heimberg, M., Weinstein, I., Kohout, M. (1969) J.Biol.Chem., 244: 5131-5139.

14. Mc Garry, J.D., Meier, J.M. and Foster, D.W. (1973). J.Biol.Chem., 248: 270-278.

15. Huttunen, J.K., Enholm, C., Nikkila, E.A. and Onta, M. (1975) Europ. J.Clin.Invest., 5: 435-446.

16. Taskinen, M.R. and Nikkila, E.A. (1978), 5èmes Journées Internationales d'Endocrinologie de Marseille (Abstract).

17. Sailer, S. and Patsch, J. (1974) in Atherosclerosis III, Schettler, G. and Weizel, A., eds. Springer-Verlag, Berlin, Heidelberg, New York pp. 691-693.

18. Nikkila, E.A., Taskinen, M.R. and Kekili, M. (1978) Atherosclerosis, 29: 497-501.

19. Eaton, R.P. (1976) Metabolism, 25: 1415-1417.

Lipoprotein Metabolism and Endocrine Regulation
L.W. Hessel and H.M.J. Krans editors
© ECSC, EEC, EAEC, Brussels-Luxembourg, 1979
Published by Elsevier/North-Holland Biomedical Press-Amsterdam

GLUCAGON : CONTROL OF SECRETION AND POSSIBLE ROLE IN LIPOPROTEIN METABOLISM

PIERRE J. LEFEBVRE and ALFRED S. LUYCKX

Division of Diabetes, Institute of Medicine, Hôpital de Bavière, Blv. de la Constitution 66, B-4020 Liège (Belgium)

ABSTRACT

A concise review is presented on the nature of glucagon, the methods for studying its secretion, the factors affecting its release, the mechanisms involved, and the possible role of glucagon in lipoprotein metabolism.

INTRODUCTION

For the chemist, glucagon is a 29 amino acid polypeptide with a molecular weight of 3485. The amino-acid sequences of porcine, bovine and human glucagons are identical and recent data on rabbit, camel and rat glucagons suggest their identity with porcine glucagon. There are known differences between the amino-acid sequences of guinea-pig and certain types of bird or fish glucagons (review in Sundby[1]). Recent X-ray analyses of Blundell et al.[2] have shown that the structure of glucagon in the crystals is largely helical with molecules associated in a complex arrangement of trimers, and have also provided evidence in favor of the existence of such helical trimers in α-granules of the islets of Langerhans and the formation of a helical conformer at the level of the glucagon receptor.

In contrast with these precise chemical or physicochemical data, glucagon for the physiologist (or the clinician) is still a poorly characterized concept as recently emphasized by Unger[3]. It is accepted that glucagon is a circulating polypeptide hormone originating mainly but not exclusively from the A-cells of the islets of Langerhans ; it is detected in plasma and tissues by radioimmunoassay : thus, the term "immunoreactive glucagon" or IRG should be used.

The radioimmunoassay of glucagon has always been a hazardous enterprise[4], not only due to the difficulties in obtaining appropriate antisera and the lability of the iodinated glucagon tracer, but mainly because of the presence in the digestive tract of a family of polypeptides which possess different physicochemical, immunological and biological properties than glucagon but which cross-react with many of the antisera raised against this hormone. These polypeptides are usually refered to as "glucagon-like immunoreactive material" (GLI) or, erroneously, as "enteroglucagon" ; they have obscured for many years the whole field of glucagon research. It is now accepted that an antiserum which is to be used in a glucagon radioimmunoassay should not (or at most very poorly) cross-react with gut-GLI : 30K antibody raised by Dr Unger in Dallas is a world-wide accepted example of an antiserum "specific" for glucagon.

The extensive studies of Heding et al.[5] have shown that the antigenic site in glucagon is located within the 24-29 section of the molecule but have also shown that biologically inactivated glucagon may retain immunoreactivity in spite of the loss of receptor-binding activity.

When a plasma or tissue extract is run on an appropriate chromatography column and then assayed using a so-called "specific" antiserum, 3 to 4 fractions of apparently different molecular weight are found : beside IRG ^{3500} which is probably related to what the chemist calls glucagon, a fraction of about 2000 daltons probably represents a degradation product, a fraction of about 9000 daltons might be a glucagon precursor and a fraction of about 200.000 daltons probably represents what Weir et al.[6] have called the "interference factor" or what Valverde et al.[7] have called "big plasma glucagon" or BPG. The physiological significance of this last compound is completely unknown.

Glucagon originates essentially in the A cells of the islets of Langerhans of the pancreas. It has recently been shown that identical cells are present in the gastro-intestinal tract, and indeed, a material which, according to all criteria, is identical to pancreatic glucagon has been extracted from the digestive tract of

some animal species[8]. This "glucagon" is particularly abundant in
the dog gastric fundus, and in the pig is present not only in the
gastric cardia but also in the duodenum, small intestine and
colon[9]. The **existence** of such **extra**-pancreatic "true glucagon"
in man is still a matter of controversy. Finally, a glucagon
related peptide has also been found in the salivary glands of some
species, mainly the rodents[10].

METHODS FOR STUDYING GLUCAGON SECRETION

Glucagon secretion has been investigated using isolated tissues,
isolated perfused organs, in situ organs or entire organisms.

Isolated tissues include pancreas slices as such (an inadequate
procedure because of the damage caused to glucagon by the proteolytic enzymes simultaneously released) or slices from a duct-liga-
ted pancreas (to obviate the preceeding artefact), and isolated
islets of Langerhans prepared either by microdissection or by
collagenase digestion of pancreatic pieces (using this last procedure caution must be taken to avoid damage to the A cells which
in species such as the rat are located at the periphery of the
islets).

Isolated organs systems use isolated rat or dog pancreas or
stomach, preparations which are perfused by artificial media or
blood.

Appropriate catheterizations permit simultaneous measurements
of blood flow and net pancreatic or gastric glucagon production
in large animals such as the dog or the pig. Finally, at the
level of the whole organism, samples can be taken at the portal
vein or peripherally ; in this last instance, one should remember
that liver glucagon uptake may represent 30 to 85 % of liver glucagon inflow[11].

STIMULANTS AND INHIBITORS OF GLUCAGON SECRETION

Table 1 lists those factors demonstrated to stimulate glucagon
secretion.

TABLE 1

STIMULANTS OF GLUCAGON SECRETION

1. Substrates : Hypoglycemia or cytoglycopenia (2 deoxy-glucose)
   Low circulating levels of free fatty acids (FFA)
   Most amino acids
   Fumarate and glutamate

2. Neural factors : Stimulation of adrenergic and cholinergic
   nervous systems ; stimulation of the ventro-medial
   hypothalamic structures

3. Local transmitters or factors : adrenalin, noradrenalin, acetylcholine, dopamine, vasoactive intestinal peptide (VIP), neurotensin, substance P, prostaglandins, bombesin, (cyclic nucleotides ?)

4. Hormones : gastrin, cholecystokinin-pancreozymin, gastric
   inhibitory peptide (GIP), growth hormone

5. Ions : total absence of calcium ; lack of phosphate

6. Situations : starvation, exercise, stress, balanced meal

The increase in glucagon plasma levels observed during or after muscular exercise results from adrenergic stimulation in mild-to-moderate exercise[12] but in more severe exercise is also due to glucose lack since it is markedly inhibited and delayed when glucose is simultaneously given[13]. The rise in glucagon circulating levels after a balanced meal is probably due to amino-acid induced glucagon release.

The factors and conditions inhibiting glucagon release are listed in Table 2.

MECHANISMS INVOLVED IN THE CONTROL OF GLUCAGON SECRETION

The intimate mechanisms which control the release of glucagon are still poorly understood.

Some studies seem to indicate that the mechanisms controlling glucagon release are, in one way or an other, linked to substrate availability at the level of the A cell : when energy substrates are lacking (hypoglycemia, starvation..) glucagon is released, when they are abundant (glucose administration, FFA infusion...)

glucagon secretion is inhibited.

TABLE 2

INHIBITORS OF GLUCAGON SECRETION

1. Substrates : Hyperglycemia (also fructose and xylitol)

                    High circulating levels of FFA (and ketone bodies ?)

2. Local transmitters or factors : serotonin, somatostatin

3. Hormones : secretin, estrogens (insulin)

4. Pharmacological agents : atropine, β-receptor blocking agents,

                    procaïne, diazepam, phenformin, diazoxide (?),

                    sulfonylureas (?)

5. Situations : carbohydrate meal, pregnancy

Numerous investigations have suggested that glucose-induced glucagon inhibition may be an insulin requiring process. There is evidence that glucose entry into the A cell may require insulin and, indeed, Östenson and Hellerström[14] using "A-cell rich guinea-pig islets" (prepared by streptozotocin destruction of most of the B-cells) have demonstrated that insulin simultaneously increases glucose utilization by the A cells, augments their ATP formation and permits glucose to inhibit glucagon secretion.

This concept that the amount of energy substrates within the A cell plays a crucial role in the control of glucagon secretion is further supported by older observations made by Edwards and Taylor[15] who demonstrated that various metabolic inhibitors stimulate glucagon secretion.

A role for cyclic nucleotides in the control of glucagon secretion has been suggested but not proved as yet[16, 17]. Some reports indicate that calcium ions and the microfilamentous microtubular system of the A-cells might be involved[18]. The role of calcium in glucagon secretion appears complex : small amounts of calcium are normally required for glucagon secretion but glucagon suppression by glucose is a calcium-requiring process. In the total absence of calcium, a paradoxical stimulation of glucagon release by glucose has been reported[19]. There is a tremendous

need for careful histological investigations of the A-cells
under various stimulatory or inhibitory conditions. The recent
investigations of Carpentier et al.[20] have started to fulfil this
gap. In their study, arginine-stimulated glucagon release was
associated with a significant increase in morphological events
linked to exocytosis. In contrast, the paradoxical release of
glucagon observed in the presence of glucose and the absence of
calcium, although accompanied by a significant decrease in granule
stores, was not associated with an increase in morphologically
detectable exocytosis. Thus, the release of similar quantities
of glucagon in different conditions is not accompanied by similar
morphological events, suggesting that different mechanisms are
involved, and that our search for a unicist concept explaining
the control of glucagon release might be in vain.

A ROLE FOR GLUCAGON IN LIPOPROTEIN METABOLISM

A plasma hypolipemic action of glucagon was first described
by Amatuzio et al.[21]. As recently emphasized by Eaton[22], the
physiologic significance of this effect in normal man and the
implications for lipoprotein regulation during pathologically
altered glucagon secretion are still not clear. A role for glucagon in the physiologic regulation of plasma lipids in the rat
is suggested on the basis of the observations of Gey et al.[23].
It has been suggested that a basic function of glucagon may
consist in augmenting FFA availability to the liver while simultaneously "shifting" hepatic fatty acid metabolism into oxidative
pathways of ketogenesis and away from synthetic pathways of
lipoprotein production[22]. This suggestion is supported by the
recent observation that during perfusion of rat liver with oleate,
pharmacologic doses of glucagon induce a significant decrease in
triglyceride and an increase in β-hydroxybutyrate output[24].
Another explanation for the hypotriglyceridemic effect of glucagon could be a decrease in the synthesis of the VLDL protein
carriers[25].

Increased plasma glucagon concentrations are usually found in
hypertriglyceridemias (review in Eaton[22] and Tiengo et al.[24]).

Similarly, the glucagon response to arginine infusion is usually enhanced in hyperlipoproteinemia[26, 27]. Clofibrate-induced reduction in plasma triglyceride levels is associated with a reduction in basal plasma glucagon concentrations ; in contrast the glucagon response to arginine is enhanced after successful treatment of the hypertriglyceridemia by clofibrate[24]. The interpretation of the hyperglucagonemia of hyperlipoproteinemia is still a matter of discussion : it is viewed by EATON and SCHADE[28] as manifestation of "glucagon resistance" while TIENGO et al.[24] see it as the expression of a primitive hyperactivity of the A-cell.

ACKNOWLEDGMENTS

A.L. is Maître de Recherches du F.N.R.S. (Belgium). This work was supported by research grants of the F.N.R.S. and F.R.S.M. (Belgium). We are indebted to E. Vaessen-Petit for secretarial help.

REFERENCES

1. Sundby, F. (1976) Metabolism, 25 (suppl. 1), 1319-1321.

2. Blundell, T.L., Dockerill, S., Sasaki, K., Tickle, I.J. and Wood, S.P. (1976) Metabolism, 25 (suppl. 1), 1331-1336.

3. Unger, R.H. (1976) Metabolism, 25 (suppl. 1), IX.

4. Luyckx, A.S. and Lefèbvre, P.J. (1976) in Hormones in Human Blood, Antoniades, H.N. ed., Harvard Univ. Press, Cambridge Mass, pp 293-324.

5. Heding, L.G., Frandsen, E.K. and Jacobsen, H. (1976) Metabolism, 25 (suppl. 1), 1327-1329.

6. Weir, G.C., Knowlton, S.D. and Martin D.B. (1975) J. Clin. Endocrinol. Metab., 40, 296-302.

7. Valverde, I., Villanueva, M.L., Lozano, I. and Marco, J. (1974) J. Clin. Endocrinol. Metab., 39, 1090-1098.

8. Sasaki, H., Rubalcalva, B., Baetens, D., Blazquez, E., Srikant, C.B., Orci, L. and Unger, R.H. (1975) J. Clin. Invest., 56, 135-145.

9. Holst, J.J. (1977) Diabetologia, 13, 159-169.

10.Lawrence, A.M., Tan, S., Hojvat, S. and Kirsteins, L. (1977) Science, 195, 70-72.

11.Fischer, U., Luyckx, A.S., Jutzi, E., Hommel, H. and Lefèbvre, P.J. (1978) in Diabetes, Obesity and Hyperlipidemias, Alberti, K.G.M.M., Crepaldi, G. and Lefèbvre, P. eds., Academic Press,

London, New-York, in press.

12. Luyckx, A.S., Dresse, A., Cession-Fossion, A. and Lefèbvre, P.J. (1975) Am. J. Physiol, 229, 376-383.

13. Luyckx, A.S., Pirnay, F. and Lefèbvre, P.J. (1978) Europ. J. Appl. Physiol., 39, 53-61.

14. Östenson, C.G. and Hellerström, C. (1976) Diabetologia, 12, 413.

15. Edwards, J.C., Howell, S.L. and Taylor, K.W. (1970) Biochim. Biophys. Acta, 215, 297-309.

16. Weir, G., Knowlton, S.D. and Martin, D.B. (1975) Endocrinology, 97, 932-936.

17. Wollheim, C.B., Blondel, B., Renold, A.E. and Sharp, G.W.G. (1976) Diabetologia, 12, 269-277.

18. Leclercq-Meyer, V., Marchand, J. and Malaisse, W.J. (1974) Diabetologia, 10, 215-224

19. Leclercq-Meyer, V., Rebolledo, O., Marchand, J. and Malaisse, W.J. (1975) Science, 189, 897-899.

20. Carpentier, J.L., Malaisse-Lagae, F., Muller, W. and Orci, L. (1977) J. Clin. Invest., 60, 1174-1182.

21. Amatuzio, D.S., Grande, F. and Wada, S. (1962) Metabolism, 11, 1240-1249.

22. Eaton, R.P. (1977) in Glucagon : Its Role in Physiology and Clinical Medicine, Foà, P.P., Bajaj, J.S. and Foà, N.L. eds, Springer-Verlag, New-York, Heidelberg, Berlin, pp. 533-550.

23. Gey, F., Georgi, H. and Buhler, E. (1977) in Glucagon : Its Role in Physiology and Clinical Medicine, Foà, P.P., Bajaj, J.S. and Foà, N.L. eds, Springer-Verlag, New-York, Heidelberg, Berlin, pp. 517-532.

24. Tiengo, A., Nosadini, R., Garotti, M.C., Fedele, D., Muggeo, M. and Crepaldi, G. (1977) in Glucagon : Its Role in Physiology and Clinical Medicine, Foà, P.P., Bajaj, J.S. and Foà, N.L. eds., Springer-Verlag, New-York, Heidelberg, 735-757.

25. Eaton, R.P. (1973) J. Lipid Res., 14, 312-318.

26. Eaton, R.P. (1973) Metabolism, 22, 763-767.

27. Tiengo, A., Muggeo, M., Assan, R., Fedele, D. and Crepaldi, G. (1975) Metabolism, 24, 901-914.

28. Eaton, R.P. and Schade, D.S. (1973) Lancet, i, 973-974.

Lipoprotein Metabolism and Endocrine Regulation
L.W. Hessel and H.M.J. Krans editors
© ECSC, EEC, EAEC, Brussels-Luxembourg, 1979
Published by Elsevier/North-Holland Biomedical Press-Amsterdam

OCCURRENCE OF HYPERGLUCAGONISM IN THE ELDERLY

JOSE MARCO, JOSE A. HEDO, and MARIA L. VILLANUEVA

Clínica Puerta de Hierro, Universidad Autónoma de Madrid, Madrid-35 (Spain)

ABSTRACT

Glucagon and insulin responses to oral glucose and to intravenous arginine were compared in young (<25 years of age, n=19) and elderly (>64 years of age, n=21) healthy male subjects.

The mean basal glucagon levels were 191±20 (SEM) pg/ml in the elderly group and 143±11 pg/ml in young controls. After oral glucose, the depression of glucagon values found in the controls (-36 pg/ml) was absent in the aged group. Intravenous arginine elicited a greater elevation of circulating glucagon in old than in young individuals (maximal difference: 217 pg/ml). In the elderly group the insulin response to glucose was delayed and arginine-induced insulin secretion was decreased. Finally, elderly subjects also showed higher fasting blood sugar levels than young controls along with a more pronounced rise of glycemia after glucose ingestion.

The hyperglucagonism of the elderly may represent A-cell hyperfunction and/or diminished metabolic clearance of glucagon. In any case, glucagon excess could be considered as a causative factor in the reduction of glucose tolerance of aged man.

INTRODUCTION

Fasting blood sugar increases and glucose tolerance declines with advancing age[1]. In the evaluation of this phenomenon several factors have been considered, including reduced insulin secretion[2], decreased conversion of proinsulin to insulin by the aging pancreas[3] and, as reviewed recently by Palmer and Ensinck[4], peripheral insulin resistance due to physical inactivity and augmented adiposity. According to Seltzer[5], the low carbohydrate intake of the elderly is a major determinant in the development of glucose intolerance since this could be reversed by appropriate dietary preparation.

Given that glucagon is a potentially diabetogenic hormone whose secretion is increased in diabetes mellitus and other states characterized by abnormal glucose tolerance[6], we have investigated the possible contribution of A-cell dysfunction in the altered carbohydrate handling of aged man. For this reason, we have compared the glucagon responses to oral glucose and to intravenous arginine in elderly and young subjects.

54

MATERIALS AND METHODS

Subjects and procedures. All participants who volunteered in this study
were male, without a known history of diabetes in their families, weighing
±10% of the ideal body weight according to the Metropolitan Life Insurance
Company tables. They appeared to be in good health as assessed by routine
clinical examination and a normal laboratory profile including erythrocyte
sedimentation rate, red and white cell count, hemoglobin, hematocrit, calcium,
inorganic phosphorus, blood urea nitrogen, uric acid, cholesterol, total
protein, albumin, total bilirubin, alkaline phosphatase, lactic dehydrogenase
and serum aspartate aminotransferase.

The elderly group consisted of 21 subjects whose ages ranged from 65 to 90
years (mean 72.3±1.6) and the young group of 19 subjects from 19 to 24 years of
age (mean: 20.9±0.4). It should be mentioned that the former group, in general,
was of lower socioeconomic status. Informed consent was obtained.

The oral glucose tolerance test (OGTT) was performed by administering 1.75 g
glucose per kilogram of body weight (25% solution) in five minutes. Arginine
monohydrochloride (Arginina Hermes, 10% solution) was infused intravenously at
a dose of 468 mg per kilogram of body weight over a 10-minute period. There was
an interval of three to five days between the two tests in each subject.

Volunteers reported to the laboratory between 9 and 10 a.m. after an overnight fast. The collection and processing of blood samples has been previously
reported[7].

Analytical methods. All samples were tested in duplicate. Plasma glucose
was determined by means of a commercial glucose-oxidase preparation (Biochemica
Test Combination, Boehringer Mannheim GmbH). Insulin was measured by radioimmunoassay with use of the charcoal separation method of Herbert et al.[8].
Glucagon and intestinal glucagon-like immunoreactivity (GLI) in plasma were
assayed radioimmunologically[9] by means of a highly specific antiserum for true
glucagon (30K) - kindly donated by Dr. R.H. Unger - and antiserum R-8, which
exhibits great affinity for acid-alcohol extracts of intestinal mucosa[10].

Results are expressed as means±SEM. Differences between values were tested
for significance by Student's t test.

RESULTS

Glucagon and insulin plasma levels during an oral glucose tolerance test in
young and elderly subjects (Fig. 1)

In a group of 21 elderly subjects fasting glucagon levels ranged from
191±20 to 207±21 pg/ml, and in 19 young controls from 143±11 to 157±11 pg/ml.

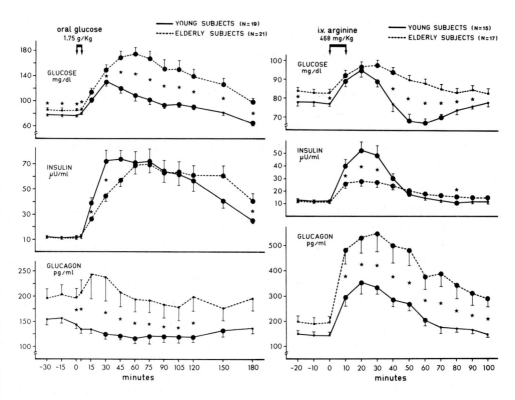

Fig. 1. Glucagon and insulin plasma
levels during an oral glucose tolerance test in young and elderly subjects (means±SEM)*.

Fig. 2. Glucagon and insulin responses to intravenous arginine in
young and elderly subjects (means±
SEM)*.

The differences were statistically significant at the zero point (p=0.03). In
the young volunteers, oral glucose was followed by a decline of circulating
glucagon which was statistically significant from 30 to 150 minutes (maximal
decrease from basal: 36 pg/ml at 60 minutes, p=0.001). However, in the elderly
glucose ingestion did not significantly depress glucagon values. Actually, a
paradoxical increase in plasma glucagon (at 15 and 30 minutes) was found,
although it did not attain the five per cent level of statistical significance.

The mean basal GLI concentration in the elderly individuals (700±50 pg/ml)
did not differ significantly from that of the young controls (600±60 pg/ml),
and its elevation after the glucose load was also very similar (100-200 pg/ml).

---

*The large dots represent statistically significant differences from the base-
line value (mean of three determinations) and the asterisks statistically significant differences between both groups at a given time.

The insulin response to oral glucose was delayed and more prolonged in aged subjects than in controls, with statistically significant differences at 15 minutes (-12 μU/ml, p=0.007), at 30 minutes (-28 μU/ml, p=0.005), and at 120 minutes (+16 μU/ml, p=0.017).

Old subjects also showed higher fasting blood sugar levels than young controls (85±3 vs. 77±2 mg/dl, p=0.04) and displayed a more pronounced rise of glycemia during the OGTT, which was statistically significant from 30 minutes until the end of the test (175±10 vs. 109±8 mg/dl at 60 minutes, p=0.0001; 140±11 vs. 91±4 mg/dl at 120 minutes, p=0.0004).

Glucagon and insulin responses to intravenous arginine in young and elderly subjects (Fig. 2)

The subjects studied in this experiment had participated in the preceding series. Basal glucagon levels of both groups were very similar to those previously detected (189±22 to 198±23 pg/ml in the elderly, and 141±15 to 149±14 pg/ml in the young group). The elevation in plasma glucagon evoked by arginine was more marked in aged individuals than in young controls, with differences varying from 143 to 217 pg/ml (p<0.05 at 10, 20 and 30 minutes; p<0.01 at the other points).

Arginine-induced insulin secretion was considerably reduced in old subjects as compared to controls (-14 μU/ml at 20 minutes; -24 μU/ml at 30 minutes, p=0.02). In the aged group, insulin levels returned to basal values more slowly than in the controls. At 80 minutes, a significant difference was observed (+5 μU/ml, p=0.01).

After arginine, the rise in plasma glucose was more sustained in elderly than in young subjects. In the former group, the late relative hypoglycemic phase was absent.

DISCUSSION

With respect to young controls, the group of elderly subjects under study showed a small elevation of fasting plasma glucose concentration as well as decreased oral glucose tolerance confirming previous reports[1]. In the aged men, basal glucagon levels were higher than in controls and these values were not depressed by the hyperglycemia subsequent to glucose ingestion which might suggest a defect in glucose recognition by the A-cell.

It is known that oral glucose stimulates the release of an intestinal factor which possesses glucagon-like immunoreactivity (GLI), and great amounts of GLI in plasma may interfere with the glucagon immunoassay yielding spuriously high concentrations of this hormone[10]. This possibility, however, seems unwarranted for the elderly individuals whose GLI response during the OGTT was similar to that of the young volunteers.

Further evidence for hyperglucagonism in aged subjects is provided by their hyperresponsiveness to i.v. arginine. In the evaluation of this phenomenon it should be considered not only an increased reactivity of the A-cell versus the aminogenic stimulus but also diminished metabolic clearance of the circulating hormone, as has been reported for other hyperglucagonemic states, such as uremia and starvation[11,12].

Recently, Dudl and Ensinck[13] have reported that arginine-induced glucagon secretion is not perceptibly altered during aging. However, in the subjects examined by these authors there was no age gradient in plasma glucose level and, therefore, their elderly group does not seem to be comparable with ours. On the other hand, the protocol used by Dudl and Ensinck included a dietary preparation ensuring a daily carbohydrate intake of 300 g for three days prior to the tests while in our study all participants were on a free diet which, as assessed by a questionnaire, was lower in carbohydrate content for the elderly than for the young subjects as was their total caloric ingestion. Since carbo-hydrate restriction is followed by an increase of basal plasma glucagon and by a slightly augmented glucagon response to exogenous amino acids[14], the hyper-glucagonism of the elderly individuals we have studied might be in part due to their alimentary habits; in any case, this would be representative of daily life dietary status.

As summarized by Andres and Tobin[2], the reports dealing with the evaluation of insulin secretion in the aged are conflicting. In our study no difference was detected between fasting insulin levels of the young and elderly subjects. However, the latter group exhibited a delayed and prolonged response to oral glucose as well as a frank reduction of arginine-induced insulin release, findings which would indicate diminished insulin reserve and/or decreased sen-sitivity of the B-cell to hyperglycemia and hyperaminoacidemia.

In conclusion, the coexistence of impaired insulin secretion and hyperglu-cagonism in the elderly offers a hormonal picture identical to that character-istic of maturity-onset diabetes[15], which could be contributory to the decrea-sed tolerance to glucose in these subjects. Nevertheless, extrapancreatic fac-tors can also be implicated.

ACKNOWLEDGEMENTS

We are indebted to Drs. N.R. Tobares, J.L. García, F. Guillén and M. Alvarez for their help in the selection of the aged group. The technical assistance of Ms. P. García, Ms. M.I. Sánchez de Molina, Ms. A. Ramírez and Ms. B. Samper is gratefully appreciated. The study was supported by a grant (12-240-76) from the Instituto Nacional de Previsión, Spain, by a research-contract (1551/RB/R2) from the International Atomic Energy Agency, Austria, and by a gift from the Alexander von Humboldt Stiftung, Federal Republic of Germany.

REFERENCES

1. O'Sullivan, J.B. (1974) Diabetes, 23, 713-715.

2. Andres, R. and Tobin, J.D. (1974) in Advances in Experimental Medicine and Biology, Cristofalo, V., Roberts, T. and Adelman, R. eds., Plenum, New York, pp. 239-249.

3. Duckworth, W.C. and Kitabchi, A. (1976) J. Lab. Clin. Med., 88, 359-367.

4. Palmer, J.P. and Ensinck, J.W. (1975) J. Clin. Endocrinol. Metab., 41, 498-503.

5. Seltzer, H.S. (1970) in Diabetes Mellitus: Theory and Practice, Ellenberg, M. and Rifkin, H. eds., McGraw-Hill, pp. 436-507.

6. Unger, R.H. (1974) Metabolism, 23, 581-593.

7. Marco, J., Diego, J., Villanueva, M.L., Díaz-Fierros, M., Valverde, I. and Segovia, J.M. (1973) N. Engl. J. Med., 289, 1107-1111.

8. Herbert, V., Lau, K-S., Gottlieb, C.W. and Bleicher, S.J. (1965) J. Clin. Endocrinol. Metab., 25, 1375-1384.

9. Faloona, G.R. and Unger, R.H. (1974) in Methods of Hormone Radioimmunoassay, Jaffe, B.M. and Behrman, H.R. eds., Academic Press, New York, pp. 317-330.

10. Marco, J., Hedo, J.A. and Villanueva, M.L. (1977) J. Clin. Endocrinol. Metab., 44, 695-698.

11. Sherwin, R.S., Bastl, C., Finkelstein, F.O., Fisher, M., Black, H., Hendler, R. and Felig, P. (1976) J. Clin. Invest., 57, 722-731.

12. Fisher, M., Sherwin, R.S., Hendler, R. and Felig, P. (1976) Proc. Natl. Acad. Sci. (USA), 73, 1735-1739.

13. Dudl, R.J. and Ensinck, J.W. (1977) Metabolism, 26, 33-41.

14. Muller, W.A., Faloona, G.R. and Unger, R.H. (1971) N. Engl. J. Med., 285, 1450-1454.

15. Muller, W.A., Faloona, G.R., Aguilar-Parada, E. and Unger, R.H. (1970) N. Engl. J. Med., 283, 109-115.

Lipoprotein Metabolism and Endocrine Regulation
L.W. Hessel and H.M.J. Krans editors
© ECSC, EEC, EAEC, Brussels-Luxembourg, 1979
Published by Elsevier/North-Holland Biomedical Press-Amsterdam

GLUCOSE TOLERANCE AND HORMONE SECRETION IN TWO AGED, SEX MATCHED GROUPS FROM EDINBURGH AND STOCKHOLM.

KEITH D. BUCHANAN
Department of Medicine, Queen's University of Belfast on behalf of the Edinburgh-Stockholm Study.
R. L. LOGAN, R.A. RIEMERSMA, M. THOMSON, M.F. OLIVER,
Department of Cardiology, Dietetics and Medicine, Royal Infirmary, Edinburgh.
A. G. OLSSON, G. WALLDIUS, S. RÖSSNER, L. KAIJSER, E. CALLMER, L. A. CARLSON
King Gustav V Research Institute, Department of Nutrition, Karolinska Institute and Departments of Medicine and Clinical Physiology, Karolinska Hospital, Stockholm.
L. Lockerbie, W. Lutz
Medical Computing and Statistics Unit, University of Edinburgh.

There is a greater incidence of ischaemic heart disease in Edinburgh compared to Stockholm and this has been shown by contrasting the findings of two recent community surveys.[1,2] Figures strongly suggested that deaths from ischaemic heart disease in younger men on a relative basis are between 2.5 and 3 times more common in Edinburgh than Stockholm. A pilot study was therefore designed to compare the prevalance of major risk factors, hyperlipidaemia, hypertension and cigarette smoking on young healthy men in the two cities[3]. This pilot survey was followed by a more detailed survey some of the results of which were recently published[4]. In the pilot study a number of risk factors for ischaemic heart disease were increased in Edinburgh compared with Stockholm. Among possible risk factors noted was an elevation in fasting serum insulin levels in Edinburgh compared with Stockholm and also a greater decrease from the fasting level in the blood glucose two hours after a standard glucose load in Edinburgh compared with Stockholm. In the second study therefore a more detailed analysis of glucose tolerance, insulin and other hormone secretion was undertaken. In addition multiple other measurements and tests were made which will not be referred to in detail in this paper unless relevant to the hormone data.

Men aged 40 years were approached by a random method to participate in the study. In Edinburgh the names were obtained at random from the general registry office. In Stockholm the names were obtained from the central files of the Stockholm Office of Statistics. 147 persons were asked to participate in the study in Edinburgh and 107 (73%) completed the study. In Stockholm 106 men were approached and of that 82 (77%) completed the study.

This present report will examine only the possible implications of hormones in the analysis.

Oral glucose tolerance test was carried out with a 30% solution of glucose (30 g/m^2 squared area). Blood was taken at 0, 15' and then at ½ hourly intervals for assay of glucose, insulin, glucagon, secretin, free fatty acids (FFA) and free glycerol.

The measurements of insulin and glucagon and secretin were performed by radioimmunoassay. The insulin assay was performed using an antibody GP25 which does not discriminate between pro-insulin and insulin and has a sensitivity of 0.5 mU/l. The glucagon assay uses a plasma extraction method and two antibodies YY89 and YY57 with different regional specificities for the glucagon molecule. YY89 has C-terminal regional specificity for the molecule and YY57 N-terminal specificity. The glucagon-like immunoreactivity (GLI) measured in the blood by these two antibodies is therefore referred to as N-terminal glucagon-like immunoreactivity (N-GLI) and C-terminal glucagon-like immunoreactivity (C-GLI) Sensitivity of the glucagon assay is 10 ng/l. Secretin radioimmunoassay also used an extraction method and antibody BB101 which appears to be highly specific for secretin. The secretin assay has a sensitivity of 5 ng/l.

The relevance of insulin, glucagon and secretin to fat metabolism has been reviewed by the author (K.D.B.) elsewhere in this issue. The relationship of abnormal circulating insulin levels to atherosclerosis has been extensively reviewed recently by Stout[5]. The review would suggest that there is evidence that subjects who have atherosclerosis or who are at risk of developing atherosclerosis have elevated circulating insulin levels. The high insulin levels may be associated with other metabolic abnormalities such as obesity and hypertriglyceridaemia or maybe of exogenous origin as in an insulin treated diabetic. There is increasing evidence that the arterial wall is an insulin sensitive tissue and exposure of the arterial tissue to insulin may result in changes which could lead to the development of lipid filled lesions similar to those of early atherosclerosis. Glucagon and gut hormones such as secretin also have effects in lipid metabolism and may also alter insulin secretion through the entero-insular axis.

RESULTS

The glucose tolerance test

There were no significant differences between the two cities in the peak concentration of plasma glucose and the total plasma glucose (area under the curve above baseline).

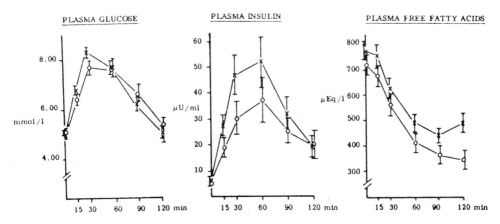

Fig. 6—Plasma glucose, insulin, and free fatty-acid responses to a standardised glucose tolerance test (30 g/m² surface area).

Edinburgh x————x   Stockholm o————o

Figure 1 reproduced by kind permission of the Lancet.
Edinburgh men had a higher peak plasma insulin concentration (p<0.001) and greater total release of insulin (area under the curve above baseline) (p<.025). The release of insulin during the first 60' was also significantly greater in Edinburgh men (p<0.001). Plasma FFA and free glycerol responses (areas under the curves below baseline) to the glucose load were also different for the two populations with Edinburgh men showing significantly less inhibition of lipolysis as reflected by higher FFA (p<0.001) and free glycerol (p<0.025).

In addition to the glucose tolerance and hormone secretion a great number of other measurements were made including fasting lipid measurements and other risk factors including cigarette smoking, alcohol, height-weight index etc. This allowed a great number of correlations to be made between insulin and some of these factors. This is shown in Table 1. In summary in Edinburgh the insulin area correlated significantly with cigarette smoking (p<.05) height-weight index (p<0.025) and adipose tissue linoleic acid percentage (p<0.001). In Stockholm there was a correlation between log VLDL triglyceride (p<0.025) HDL cholesterol (p<0.0025) fat cell size (p<0.001) and height-weight index (p<0.001).

62

TABLE 1

CORRELATION BETWEEN AREA UNDER INSULIN CURVE WITH OTHER MEASUREMENTS

Insulin area	Edinburgh (r)	Stockholm (r)
Log V.L.D.L. T.G.	0.04 (N.S.)	0.32 (p<0.025)
HDL-Cholesterol	-0.06 (N.S.)	-0.24 (p<0.025)
Cigarette smoking	-0.20 (p<0.05)	-0.05 (N.S.)
Fat cell size	0.05 (N.S.)	0.36 (p<0.001)
Wt-Ht index	0.23 (p<0.025)	0.37 (p<0.001)
Adipose tissue linoleic acid	0.33 (p<0.001)	0.16 (N.S.)
Alcohol	-0.08 (N.S.)	-0.06 (N.S.)

Tests for significance of differences in the correlations (r-values) between the two cities were performed only if at least in one of the two cities a significant correlation was found. No significant differences between the two cities was found, except for the correlation between insulin area vs fat-cell size (p<0.05).

The glucagon data has not yet been completely analysed. However, a preliminary analysis would suggest that the fasting levels of N-terminal glucagon between Edinburgh and Stockholm are identical but that there is a tendency for elevation of fasting C-terminal glucagon in Edinburgh as compared with Stockholm. The Edinburgh men show a rise in N-terminal glucagon which would appear to be greater than Stockholm. Slight suppression of C-terminal glucagon is noted in the Edinburgh subjects whereas this is not found in the Stockholm subjects.

A great deal of correlations were performed with the glucagon areas and only the most significant correlations will be reported. Correlations between C-terminal glucagon and the following in Edinburgh men were noted:- the percentage of linoleic acid in adipose tissue and in Stockholm men, plasma HDL cholesterol and plasma uric acid. Correlations for N-terminal glucagon in Edinburgh were noted with fat cell size, percentage linoleic acid in adipose tissue, plasma FFA and plasma glycerol and in Stockholm, N-terminal glucagon correlated with percentage linoleic acid in plasma triglycerides.

With respect to the glucagon results comparison between the city correlations was done by Fisher's test. Significant differences were noted between the glucose area and N-terminal glucagon area at 15 and 60' after the glucose.

Analysis of the secretin data is only very preliminary but would suggest that there are not differences between the two populations.

The data therefore clearly show that despite normal glucose tolerance Edinburgh subjects have higher insulin secretion following an oral glucose load than Stockholm subjects. This would tend to support the concept that Edinburgh men require more insulin to retain normal glucose tolerance than Stockholm men. The reason for the insulin resistance is not apparent from the study but several hypotheses are suggested. The plasma FFA responses to the glucose tolerance test showed in Edinburgh men a delayed and poor response to the glucose load whereas there was a sharper and deeper decline in Stockholm subjects. Therefore one could then say that despite higher insulin levels in Edinburgh, improved glucose tolerance and improved inhibition of lipolysis was not noted. It is conceivable that circulating metabolites such as fatty acids could have inhibited the action of insulin at the peripheral level. Another possibility is that hormones antagonist to insulin may be increased in Edinburgh subjects as compared with Stockholm subjects. However, glucagon which is known to have several antagonist actions to insulin did not appear to be significantly different in the basal state between the two cities.

The reason for the greater insulin response in Edinburgh compared to Stockholm is also not apparent from these subjects. Insulin resistance as discussed above could be a factor in stimulating further insulin secretion. Not only may insulin secretion be altered but also insulin degradation may be different in the two populations. It is possible that the entero-insular axis system could be different in the two cities, Edinburgh having a greater stimulation of insulin secretion via the entero-insular axis as compared with Stockholm. If such were the case then the key hormone to study in this case would be gastric inhibitory polypeptide possibly the major stimulus of the entero-insular axis and which has been discussed elsewhere in this conference.

Elevated glucagon levels have been noted in hypertriglyceridaemia[6] and the slightly elevated C-terminal glucagon levels in Edinburgh as compared with Stockholm could be in keeping with this. In addition there appeared to be a greater N-terminal glucagon response to oral glucose in Edinburgh men as compared with Stockholm. GLI molecules responsible for this N-terminal glucagon response are multiple and complex[7] and it is unlikely that this response is related to the entero-insular axis or insulin secretion. Because of the lack of knowledge of the biological activities of all the different gut GLI molecules released by oral glucose it is very difficult to conceive what the significance is of the greater gut GLI response in Edinburgh subjects as compared with Stockholm. However, this greater hormonal response in the Edinburgh subjects may be the same factor as is determining the greater insulin response in the Edinburgh subjects as compared with Stockholm subjects.

IN CONCLUSION

1.   In 2 matched populations of men aged 40 years in Edinburgh and Stockholm the Edinburgh men have demonstrated increased insulin secretion and increased N-terminal glucagon responses to oral glucose compared with the Stockholm men.

2.   A degree of insulin resistance is evident in the Edinburgh subjects in that the glucose tolerance is the same as Stockholm men despite higher insulin levels and because of a slow decline in FFA and glycerol levels after glucose they appear to have a poor inhibition of lipolysis following the oral glucose.

3.   It is possible that the increased insulin secretion in Edinburgh may predispose this population to ischaemic heart disease. Several hypotheses are constructed to explain the increased insulin secretion including insulin resistance related to elevations of circulating metabolites and/or hormone antagonist to insulin and also a more active entero-insular axis in the Edinburgh subjects as compared with Stockholm.

REFERENCES

1.   Armstrong, A., Duncan,B., Oliver, M.F., Julian, D.G., Donald, K.W., Fulton, M., Lutz, W., Morrison, S.L. (1972).
       Brit. Heart J. 34 page 67.

2.   Wikland, B. (1969)
       Acta Med. Scand. Suppl. page 524.

3.   Oliver, M.F., Nimmo, I.A., Cooke, M., Carlson, L.A., Olsson, A.G. (1975)
       Europ. J. Clin. Invest. 5, pp 507-514.

4.   Logan, R.L., Riemersma, R.A., Thomson, M., Oliver, M.F., Olsson, A.G., Walldius, G., Rossner, S., Kaijser, L., Callmer, E., Carlson, L.A. (1978)
       Lancet 1, pp 949-956.

5.   Stout, R.W. (1977)
       Atherosclerosis 27, pp 1-13.

6.   Tiengo, A., Nosadini, R., Garotti, M.C., Fedele, D., Muggeo, M., Crepaldi, G. (1978)
       In Glucagon: Its Role in Physiology and Clinical Medicine, Edited by Foa, P.P., Bajaj, J.S. and Foa, N.L., Springer-Verlag, pp 735-757.

7.   Buchanan, K.D. (1976)
       J. Endocrinol. 70, p 6-7.

Lipoprotein Metabolism and Endocrine Regulation ·
L.W. Hessel and H.M.J. Krans editors
© ECSC, EEC, EAEC, Brussels-Luxembourg, 1979
Published by Elsevier/North-Holland Biomedical Press-Amsterdam

GIP IN OBESITY, DIABETES AND HYPERLIPOPROTEINEMIA

W. CREUTZFELDT and R. EBERT
Division of Metabolism, Department of Medicine, University of
Göttingen, Robert-Koch-Straße 4o, D-34oo Göttingen (FRG)

The gut hormone gastric inhibitory polypeptide (GIP) has
insulin-releasing activity in vivo and in vitro[1,2]. GIP is
released after ingestion of glucose and augments glucose
induced secretion of insulin, thereby acting as 'incretin'[1].
At present, GIP is the most likely candidate for the entero-
insular axis.

Besides oral glucose, secretion of GIP is observed after
ingestion of fat[1] and amino acids[3]. The rise of GIP after oral
fat may be the reason for the increased release of insulin after
an intravenous glucose load during fat ingestion as compared to
insulin levels achieved by intravenous glucose alone[1]. On the
other hand, during the i.v. glucose load the fat induced rise of
GIP is markedly inhibited, probably due to the release of
endogenous insulin[1,4]. From this observation a negative feedback
between insulin and GIP has been proposed[1].

Little is known about the mechanisms involved in the releasing
process of GIP from the GIP cells of the gut. Perfusion studies
with a fixed glucose concentration revealed that the amount of
GIP released was greater in the duodenum than in the jejunum,
and smallest in the ileum[5]. An important factor for the release
of GIP by nutrients is the process of absorption: Under conditions
of diminished absorption (e.g. coeliac disease, pancreatic
steatorrhea) a decreased secretion of GIP is seen as compared to
the respective hormone levels of normal subjects[6]. In animal
experiments absorption of glucose form the gut was blocked by
phlorizin or prenylamine. Concomitantly, the rise of IR-GIP and
insulin was drastically inhibited[7].

While the insulinotropic effect of GIP has been demonstrated
in several laboratories, the effect of GIP on glucagon release is
still a matter of discussion: A direct glucagonotropic effect of
GIP has been found in rats. In normal man infusion of GIP does

TABLE 1

FASTING SERUM LEVELS OF IMMUNOREACTIVE GIP (IR-GIP) IN DIFFERENT DISEASES

	n	IR-GIP (pg/ml) mean ± SEM	p
Normal controls	92	287 ± 59	
Obese subjects, normal oral glucose tolerance	52	418 ± 89	n.s.
Obese subjects, pathological glucose tolerance	47	664 ± 76	< 0.05
Obese subjects, starving for 6 days	23	1762 ± 189	< 0.005
Maturity-onset diabetics	108	469 ± 23	< 0.02
Untreated ketotic juvenile diabetics	14	1612 ± 202	0.005
Juvenile diabetics after insulin treatment	6	209 ± 43	n.s.
Hyperlipoproteinemia type IV	11	609 ± 42	< 0.05
Hypercholesterinemia type IIa	6	401 ± 50	n.s.

p indicates significant difference from normal controls

not release substantial amounts of glucagon, however, indirect
evidence has been presented that GIP released glucagon in man
after ingestion of nutrients that lack direct effects on the A-
cells of the pancreas[8].

GIP SECRETION IN OBESITY

Hyperinsulinemia is a frequent finding in obesity, both in the
fasting state and following stimulation of insulin release. An
overactive rise of GIP may be responsible for this[9].

Obese subjects exhibited elevated fasting levels of IR-GIP
(Table 1). Following ingestion of loo g glucose obese subjects
with normal glucose tolerance showed no significant difference
of IR-GIP secretion as compared to normals, whereas in obese
subjects with pathological glucose tolerance IR-GIP and insulin
responses were significantly greater than in normals. Fat
induced release was augmented in obese subjects with normal and
pathological glucose tolerance. Similarly, after ingestion of a
mixed high caloric test meal which produces maximal stimulation
of IR-GIP a graded augmentation of IR-GIP release was observed
in the obese subjects with highest levels in obese subjects with
pathological glucose tolerance. In this group peak IR-GIP levels
reached nearly 5 ng/ml, in normal subjects IR-GIP levels peaked
at 1.2 ng/ml[9].

In order to elucidate the interplay between serum levels of
insulin and IR-GIP in normal and obese subjects a small dose of
glucose (3o g) and a large fat load (loo g triglyceride) were
given alone or in combination. The results are shown in Figure 1.
The increase of IR-GIP levels after 3o g glucose was small and of
the same magnitude in controls and obese subjects. The IR-GIP
increase after loo g fat was much larger and significantly
greater in obese subjects than in controls. If glucose and fat
were given together, the IR-GIP increase of normals was markedly
lower than after fat alone, but not influenced in obese subjects.
Serum levels of insulin did not change after fat ingestion, but
increased after 3o g glucose. If glucose was given together with
fat, more insulin was released in both controls and obese subjects. The results suggest that the exaggerated rise of insulin
in obesity might be due to the augmented secretion of IR-GIP. In

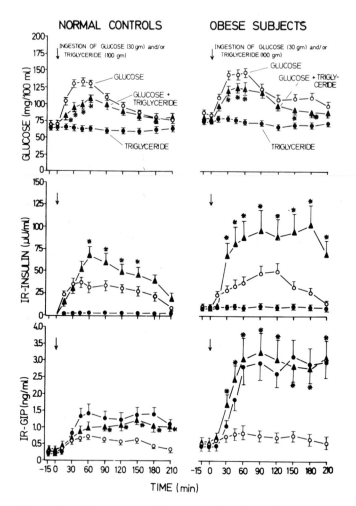

Fig. 1. Increase of serum levels of IR-GIP, IRI and glucose to the ingestion of 3o g glucose (o——o), loo g triglyceride (•——•) and 3o g glucose plus loo g triglyceride (▲——▲) in the same normal weight controls (n = 16) and obese (42 % overweight) subjects with normal glucose tolerance (n = 16). Significant differences between glucose and glucose plus triglyceride are indicated (* = p < o.o2 or less). (Creutzfeldt et al.[9])

addition, they support the contention that the proposed feedback between insulin and GIP is defective in obesity, since glucose induced insulin secretion inhibits fat induced IR-GIP secretion in normals, but not in obese subjects.

Subsequent investigations revealed that both the exaggerated rise of insulin and IR-GIP were reversed by starvation or reduced caloric intake (800 cal) for 21 days[10]. During fasting basal levels of IR-GIP increased from 527 pg/ml to a peak of 1762 $\pm$ 189 pg/ml (after 6 days of fasting). Concomitantly, the insulin levels decreased. The exaggerated response of IR-GIP and insulin in obese subjects following ingestion of the test meal became much smaller after starvation for 21 days. Similar observations were made using oral glucose (100 g) as stimulator[10].

In order to separate the effect of weight loss and food restriction a group of obese subjects with pathological glucose tolerance reduced their caloric intake for five days (800 cal) followed by complete starvation for 21 days. After 5 days of food restriction the integrated IR-GIP response to the test meal was already significantly smaller and decreased further after the starvation period. The integrated insulin levels did not significantly change after the short period of food restriction, but did so after subsequent starvation. When in obese subjects oral (100 g glucose) and i.v. glucose loads (1.1 g/kg over 90 min) were compared before and after food restriction for 14 days, it was apparent that the exaggerated release of insulin and IR-GIP after the oral glucose load were reversed, whereas the insulin levels after the intravenous glucose were only marginally influenced (Figure 2). This result indicates that the augmented release following oral glucose may be mediated by the exaggerated secretion of IR-GIP, whereas the augmented insulin secretion following the i.v. glucose load is unrelated to intestinal factors and possibly due to islet hyperplasia.

Intravenous insulin inhibits fat induced IR-GIP secretion in normal subjects[1], but not in obese subjects with pathological glucose tolerance[4]. This confirms the contention that the feedback between insulin and GIP is defective in obesity and would explain at least in part the exaggerated release of IR-GIP following ingestion of the test meal.

These findings in obese persons suggest that an overactive entero-insular axis contributes to the hyperinsulinemia of obesity.

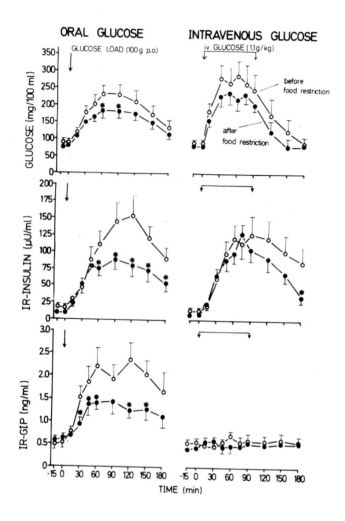

Fig. 2. Increase of serum levels of IR-GIP, IRI and glucose in 9 obese subjects with glucose intolerance following ingestion of loo g glucose or intravenous infusion of 1.1 g/kg body weight of glucose over 9o min. The tests were repeated after reduced caloric intake for 14 days and one week unrestricted diet. All values are means ± SEM. Significant differences between the serum levels before and after weight reduction of 5.2 ± o.7 kg (* = p < o.o2 and less) are indicated. o—o = before, ●—● = after weight reduction (Willms et al.[10])

GIP SECRETION IN DIABETES MELLITUS

Decreased activity of the entero-insular axis could be one
factor in the pathogenesis of diabetes, especially of the
maturity-onset type. Therefore, the role of GIP in diabetes
mellitus was studied. In maturity-onset diabetics an exaggerated
response of IR-GIP after ingestion of the test meal as well as
after ingestion of the glucose load was observed (Table 2).
However, in contrast to the IR-GIP levels in obese subjects with
pathological glucose tolerance, where peak levels of IR-GIP in
the range of 5 ng/ml were observed the mean peak levels in
maturity-onset diabetics never exceeded 2.3 ng/ml. After oral fat
(loo g) the serum concentrations of IR-GIP were only marginally
above those of controls. This is in contrast to the data obtained
in obese subjects with pathological glucose tolerance. The
insulin secretion was delayed in all diabetics after ingestion of
the test meal, showing no differences in the absolute insulin

TABLE 2
INTEGRATED IR-GIP RESPONSE IN MATURITY-ONSET DIABETICS (MOD)
AFTER A MIXED LIQUID TEST MEAL, ORAL GLUCOSE (loo g) OR ORAL
FAT (loo g)

	n	IR-GIP (ng/ml·18o min) mean ± SEM	p
Test meal			
Normal controls	32	1o9.4 ± 11.1	
MOD	68	297.8 ± 16.5	< o.o2
Glucose load			
Normal controls	19	82.9 ± 8.9	
MOD	2o	19o.4 ± 14.3	< o.o1
Fat load			
Normal controls	21	175.9 ± 18.6	
MOD	2o	2o9.3 ± 13.1	n.s.

P indicates significant difference from the corresponding controls

levels late in the course of the test between normals and
diabetics. Following starvation the insulin response to the test
meal was increased in diabetics, while the release of IR-GIP
decreased.

Untreated juvenile-onset diabetics with ketonuria exhibited
enormously elevated basal levels of IR-GIP (Table 1). Following
ingestion of the test meal the IR-GIP levels did not significantly rise above the fasting concentrations. After treatment with
insulin for 5 days, the elevated fasting IR-GIP levels were normalized (Table 1) and the response of IR-GIP to the test meal was
nearly normal. This observation shows that the release of IR-GIP
is under the control of insulin (in a direct or undirect manner).

In order to investigate further the role of insulin on IR-GIP
release juvenile-onset diabetics received an oral glucose (loo g)
or an oral fat (loo g) load in the absence or presence of
insulin. Exogenous insulin significantly inhibits the fat induced
release of IR-GIP, but not the glucose induced rise of this
hormone. The data do not support the contention that GIP
deficiency is responsible for maturity-onset diabetes.

GIP SECRETION IN HYPERLIPOPROTEINEMIA

In subjects with hyperlipoproteinemia type IV the basal levels
of IR-GIP were elevated (Table 1). Also the response to ingestion
of loo g glucose was exaggerated. Simultaneously, an augmented
release of insulin occurred late in the course of the test.
However, after oral fat (loo g) the subjects with hypertriglyceridemia showed a markedly smaller and delayed release of IR-GIP
as compared to normal subjects.

In contrast to the data obtained in subjects with hypertriglyceridemia, patients with hypercholesterinemia (type IIa) had a
normal glucose tolerance when tested after a loo g glucose load.
The insulin levels were slightly elevated during the test when
compared with normals; the IR-GIP secretion following the oral
glucose load was only marginally enhanced late in the course of
the test.

These results indicate that in hypertriglyceridemia a disturbed
secretion pattern of IR-GIP (exaggerated response after oral
glucose, diminished response after oral fat) exists. At present

it cannot be answered whether this altered IR-GIP secretion is causally related to the defects of lipoprotein metabolism or whether the observed hormonal changes are rather a consequence of the abnormal lipoprotein pattern.

REFERENCES

1. Brown, J.C., Dryburgh, J.R., Ross, S.A., Dupré, J. (1975) Rec.Progr.Horm.Res. 31, 487-531.

2. Schauder, P., Brown, J.C., Frerichs, H., Creutzfeldt, W. (1975) Diabetologia 11, 483-484.

3. Thomas, F.B., Sinar, D., Mazzaferri, E.L., Cataland, S., Mekhjian, H.S., Caldwell, J.H., Fromkes, J.J. (1978) Gastroenterology 74, 1261-1265.

4. Ebert, R., Frerichs, H., Creutzfeldt, W. (in press) Europ.J.clin.Invest.

5. Thomas, F.B., Shook, D.F., O'Dorisio, T.M., Cataland, S., Mekhjian, H.S., Caldwell, J.H., Mazzaferri, E.L. (1977) Gastroenterology 72, 49-54.

6. Creutzfeldt, W., Ebert, R., Arnold, R, Frerichs, H., Brown, J.C. (1976) Diabetologia 12, 279-286.

7. Creutzfeldt, W., Ebert, R. (1977) in Proceedings of the IX Congress of the International Diabetes Federation New Delhi 1976, J.S. Bajaj, ed., Excerpta Medica, Amsterdam, p.p. 63-75.

8. Ross, S.A., Dupré, J. (1978) Diabetes 27, 327-333.

9. Creutzfeldt, W., Ebert, R., Frerichs, H., Brown, J.C. (1978) Diabetologia 14, 15-24

10. Willms, B., Ebert, R., Creutzfeldt, W. (1978) Diabetologia 14, 379-387.

Lipoprotein Metabolism and Endocrine Regulation
L.W. Hessel and H.M.J. Krans editors
© ECSC, EEC, EAEC, Brussels-Luxembourg, 1979
Published by Elsevier/North-Holland Biomedical Press-Amsterdam

PROBLEMS IN EVALUATION OF THE EFFECT OF GUT HORMONES ON THE ENDO-
CRINE PANCREAS ("INCRETIN").

JENS F. REHFELD

Institute of Medical Biochemistry, University of Aarhus,

DK-8000 Aarhus C, Denmark.

ABSTRACT

In the last years gut hormones have proved very complex. The
complexity impedes evaluation of their activity, including their
incretin-effect. Thus, gut hormones are highly heterogenous;
they are often produced outside the gut - in islet-cells and
nerves; their different molecular forms interact greatly with
other hormones, neurotransmitters and nutrients. In the following the problems of assessing the incretin effect is illustrated
by an example, the gastrins.

INTRODUCTION

It is an old thought that gut factors may regulate the endocrine pancreas. Thus, in 1906, Moore et al.tried to treat diabetes mellitus with extracts of porcine duodenum[1]. Unfortunately, their attempt failed; but Zunz and La Barre in 1927 resur-
rected the idea[2], and coined the word "incretin" on gut hormone(s)
that might stimulate the endocrine pancreas. Renewed interest
in incretins emerged 15 years ago[3,4,5], when measurement of insulin in serum became feasible by introduction of the radioimmunoassay technique[6]. In the flood of incretin studies reported
since then, only few deserves attention by delineating the clinical impact and physiological nature of incretin.

Perley and Kipnis suggested in 1967[7] that abnormal incretin
function contributed significantly to the inappropriate insulin
secretion in maturity-onset diabetes and obesity. Motivated by
this important report, several groups have during the last decade tried to study the mechanism of incretin under circumstances
of physiological relevance. However, the complexity of gut hormones recognized in the same decade have delayed the progress
seriously; and there is still much work to be done until we have

a valid picture of the nature and significance of incretin in health and diseases.

   The following review outlines the difficulties in determining the incretin effects of hormonal peptides from the gut. Since the number of gut hormones is steadily increasing, it is at present nearly impossible to review the incretin effect of all known gut hormones. Instead, I have as model chosen one group of peptides, the gastrins, to illustrate the problems. The choice is justified for at least two reasons: 1) The chemical and physiological nature of the gastrins is known better than for any other gut hormone. 2) The other important incretin, GIP, is thoroughly discussed in the previous paper.

MOLECULAR HETEROGENEITY

   Per definition gastrin is any peptide released from the antrum, that stimulates gastric acid secretion. The biological active site of the previously isolated gastrins is accurately confined to the COOH-terminal tetrapeptide amide sequence (Trp-Met-Asp-Phe·NH_2). Thus, peptides released from antrum contatinig this sequence, are true gastrins. At present five main forms of gastrin have been found in blood and antral tissue:

   Component I   contain as mid- and COOH-terminal region gastrin$_{34}$, whereas the NH_2-terminus presumably is a sequence of further 10-15 still unknown amino acid residues[8].

   Component II correspond to gastrin$_{34}$[9] (Pyr-Leu-Gly-Pro-Gln-Gly-His-Pro-Ser-Leu-Val-Ala-Asp-Pro-Ser-Lys-Lys-gastrin$_{17}$).

   Component III correspond to gastrin$_{17}$[10] (Pyr-Gly-Pro-Trp-Leu-Glu-Glu-Glu-Glu-Glu-Ala-Tyr-Gly-Trp-Met-Asp-Phe·NH_2).

   Component IV correspons to gastrin$_{14}$[11,12], the COOH-terminal tetradecapeptide of gastrin$_{17}$.

   Component V is gastrin$_4$, the COOH-terminal tetrapeptide amide, which we recently discovered as a free peptide[13].

In addition to the five main components, pronounced micro-heterogeneity of each component is also present[14]. Thus Single amino acid residues are modified, for instance by sulphation and amidation. We have firm reasons to believe that the molecular heterogeneity of secreted gastrins reflects posttranslational cleavage and amino acid derivatization of the polypeptide chain synthetized on the ribosomes[15]. Since all structural modifications may affect biological activity, each molecular form has to be studied, separately and in combination. Moreover, it is also necessary to study the target in focus specifically. That means that it is not possible to extrapolate the ratio of biological activities of different molecular forms from one system (i.e. gastric acid secretion) to another (i.e. insulin secretion). Thus, $gastrin_{17}$ stimulates acid secretion more potent than $gastrin_4$; whereas $gastrin_4$ stimulates insulin secretion more powerful than $gastrin_{17}$[16].

LOCAL ENDOCRINE RELEASE IN ISLETS

Fetal and neonatal islets contain substantial amounts of gastrin and G-cells[17]. The number of G-cells decrease after birth[17]. That a few gastrin cells persist in the islets in adults is possible. Such cells might well be the origin of the relatively frequent pancreatic G-cell tumours that causes the Zollinger-Ellison syndrome. It also appears that the pancreatic D-cells in addition to somatostatin produce gastrin[18]. Irrespective of the cellular source of pancreatic gastrin, its presence in the islets makes interpretation of incretin-studies using exogenous gastrin difficult. The role of islet-gastrin is unknown. However, the large production of gastrin in fetal and neonatal islets[17] suggests that gastrin is an important regulator of islet growth. Accordingly, we have found excessive islet-hyperplasia and nesidioblastosis in diseases with hypergastrinaemia (achlorhydria and the Zollinger-Ellison syndrome)[19]. A trophic effect on the endocrine pancreas correspond well with the extensively studied gastrinergic regulation of mucosal growth in the gut[20].

LOCAL NEUROCRINE RELEASE IN ISLETS

We have shown that the gastrins like other hormonal peptides also is located in central[21] as well as peripheral peptidergic nerves[22]. It is likely that gastrinergic, vagal fibers[22] also innervate the pancreas (unpublished). The significance of gastrin-nerves in the pancreas is at present unknown. But again, as for islet cell-gastrin, a local neurocrine release of gastrin would interact significantly with stimulation from non-pancreatic

gastrin, either exogenous or of antral origin. Thus future studies of the incretin effect of gastrin require due attention paid
to local release of gastrin in the islets. Since other gut peptides like VIP and cholecystokinin (CCK) also are located in pancreatic nerves[23], it is of general importance to evaluate the incretin concept with respect to peptidergic nerves. Thus, it is
an unsettled but crucial question whether nerves to the pancreas
containing gut peptides exert a constant tone on the islets, or
increase the release during eating.

INTERACTIONS

   A key concept in studies of the activity of all gut hormones
is interaction. The interaction can be competitive (if the
hormone is structurally related to other peptides at the receptor-
bound sequence) or non-competitive (when the substances act on
different receptors). For gastrin of gastrointestinal origin the
following kind of interactions have to be considered:
   1. Competitive interaction with gastrins released locally by
       neuro- or endocrine secretion within the pancreatic islets.
   2. Competitive interaction between different molecular forms
       of circulating gastrin.
   3. Competitive interaction with structurally homologous hor-
       mones, the cholecystokinins.
   4. Non-competitive interaction with structurally different
       hormonal incretins like GIP, bombesin and substance P.
   5. Non-competitive interaction with structurally different
       neurotransmitters (acetylcholine, amines).
   6. Potentiation of the effect of absorbed nutrients, glucose,
       amino acids and fatty acids.
Apparently glucose concentrations have to be raised above basal
levels in order to obtain any effect on insulin secretion by the
gastrins and other gut hormones; whereas the gastrins apparently
are without effects on the amino acid induced insulin- and glucagon secretion[24]. The other kinds of interaction remain to be
studied.

CRITERIAS FOR ASSESSMENT OF THE PHYSIOLOGICAL EFFECT OF GUT HOR-
MONES ON THE ENDOCRINE PANCREAS.

The slow progress in incretin research is partly due to the
above mentioned complex character of gut hormones (molecular
heterogeneity, dual endocrine production, neurocrine release,
interactions), partly to transgression of obvious conditions for
physiological meaningful studies of incretin. As previously
pointed out[25], some often overlooked prerequisites are:

1. Use of pure hormone preparations as exogenous stimulants.
2. Elimination of species-differences by using hormone preparation from the same species, as the object to be studied. Since many gut hormones are purified only from pig
   intestines, porcine islet-function has to be studied so far
   using these hormones.
3. Use of relevant molecular forms. Some molecular forms isolated from intestinal tissue are not released, but function
   merely as intracellular biosynthetic precursors. Thus, the
   form cholecystokinin originally isolated, CCK_{33}[26], is neither released in the basal state nor after stimulation, it
   is only the small COOH-terminal octa- and tetrapeptides
   that are secreted from porcine intestines[27]. Similarly
   $gastrin_{34}$ is not released into circulation in the cat[15].
4. Administration of the pure, molecular forms from the correct species in doses that enhance the hormone levels within concentration limits of the actual endogenous molecular
   form measured under physiological circumstances. Specific
   radioimmunoassays are necessary to monitor such studies.
5. Selection of suitable pancreas preparations. An example of
   an unsuited preparation is the collagenase treated isolated
   islets that have lost the receptors for gut hormones during
   preparation.
6. In order to elucidate the kinetics of interaction of a gut
   hormone with other stimulants (competitive and non-competitive interactions), dose-response studies are generally
   necessary.

PRESENT STATE OF THE ART - EXAMPLIFIED WITH GASTRIN.

Physiological studies in man. So far reliable studies have been performed only using non-sulphated human component III, (gastrin 17). The results indicate that gastrin$_{17}$ in physiological concentrations may potentiate the glucose-induced insulin secretion[28] and possibly also the release of glucagon[24] during mixed meals. A single early study showed that component V, (gastrin$_4$) stimulated insulin secretion with greater potency than gastrin$_{17}$[16]. Recent unpublished studies have confirmed this observation.

Physiological studies in the hog. Extensive dose-response studies on the isolated, perfused porcine pancreas with all five gastrin components support the above studies in man[29]. Component III and IV displayed minor potentiating effects on insulin and glucagon release in physiological concentrations. The large molecular forms components I and II required slightly supraphysiological doses in order to act significantly. So far only interactions with glucose have been studied[29].

Pathophysiological studies. We have shown that patients with endogenous hypergastrinaemia (pernicious anaemia[30] and the Zollinger-Ellison syndrome[31]), display abnormalities in glucose tolerance and insulin secretion in accordance with the results obtained during the dose-response studies. The hypergastrinaemic patients also display the previously mentioned islet-cell hyperplasia. Since many diabetics have hypo- and achlorhydria with ensuing hypergastrinaemia, it appears likely that the hypergastrinaemia may contribute to the poor glucose tolerance in some diabetics. However, extensive clinical studies are now required to decide whether the incretin effect of gastrin or any other gut hormone is of pathogenetic significance.

REFERENCES

1. Moore, B., Edie, E.S. and Abram, J.H. (1906) Biochem. J., 1, 28-38.

2. Zunz, E. and La Barre, J. (1927) Compt. Rend. Soc. Biol., 96, 421-423.

3. McIntyre, N., Holdsworth, C.D. and Turner, D.S. (1964) Lancet, II, 20-21.

4. Elrick, H., Stimmler, L., Hlad, C.J. and Arai, Y. (1964)
   J. Clin. Endocr. Metab. 24, 1076-1084.

5. Dupré, J. (1964) Lancet II, 672-673.

6. Berson, S.A. and Yalow, R.S. (1960) J. Clin. Invest., 39,
   1157-1175.

7. Perley, M.J. and Kipnis, D.M. (1967) J. Clin. Invest., 46,
   1954-1962.

8. Rehfeld, J.F. (1972) Biochim. Biophys. Acta, 285, 364-372.

9. Gregory, R.A. and Tracy, H.J. (1975) in Gastrointestinal
   Hormones, Thompson, J.C. ed., University of Texas Press,
   Austin, pp. 13-24.

10. Gregory, R.A. and Tracy, H.J. (1964) Gut 5, 103-117.

11. Rehfeld, J.F. and Stadil, F. (1973) Gut, 14, 369-373.

12. Gregory, R.A. and Tracy, H.J. (1974) Gut, 15, 683-685.

13. Rehfeld, J.F. and Larsson, L.-I. (1978) Acta Physiol. Scand.
    in press.

14. Rehfeld, J.F., Stadil, F., Malmström, J. and Miyata, M. (1975)
    in Gastrointestinal Hormones, Thompson, J.C. ed., University
    of Texas Press, Austin, pp. 43-58.

15. Rehfeld, J.F. and Uvnäs-Wallensten, K. (1978) J. Physiol.
    in press.

16. Rehfeld, J.F. (1971) Acta Endocrinol. 66, 169-176.

17. Larsson, L.-I., Rehfeld, J.F., Håkanson, R. and Sundler, F.
    (1976) Nature 262, 609-610.

18. Greider, M.H. and McGuigan, J.E. (1971) Diabetes 20, 389-396.

19. Larsson, L.-I., Ljungberg, O., Sundler, F., Håkanson, R.,
    Svensson, S.O., Rehfeld, J.F., Stadil, F. and Holst, J. (1973)
    Virchows Arch. Abt. A. 360, 305-314.

20. Johnsson, L.R. (1976) Gastroenterology 70, 278-288.

21. Rehfeld, J.F. (1978) Nature, 271, 771-773.

22. Uvnäs-Wallensten, K., Rehfeld, J.F., Larsson, L.-I. and
    Uvnäs, B. (1977) Proc. Natl. Acad. Sci. USA 74, 5707-5710.

23. Larsson, L.-I., Rehfeld, J.F., Childers, S. and Snyder, S.H.
    (1979) Digestion, in press.

24. Rehfeld, J.F., Holst, J.J. and Kühl, C. (1978) Eur. J. Clin.
    Invest. 8, 5-9.

25. Rehfeld, J.F. (1972) Scand. J. Gastroenterol. 7, 289-292.

26. Mutt, V. and Jorpes, J.E. (1968) Biochem. Biophys. Res. Comm.
    26, 392-397.

27. Rehfeld, J.F., Holst, J.J. and Jensen, S.L. (1979) Submitted.

28. Rehfeld, J.F. and Stadil, F. (1973) J. Clin. Invest. 52,
    1415-1426.

82

29. Jensen, S.L., Rehfeld, J.F., Fahrenkrug, J., Holst, J.J., Nielsen, O.V., Schaffalitzky de Muckadell, O.B. (1979) Amer. J. Physiol., in press.

30. Rehfeld, J.F. (1976) J. Clin. Invest. 58, 41-49.

31. Rehfeld, J.F., Lauritsen, K.B. and Stadil, F. (1976) Scand. J. Gastroenterol. 11, suppl. 37, 53-56.

Lipoprotein Metabolism and Endocrine Regulation
L.W. Hessel and H.M.J. Krans editors
© ECSC, EEC, EAEC, Brussels-Luxembourg, 1979
Published by Elsevier/North-Holland Biomedical Press-Amsterdam

RELATIONSHIP BETWEEN GUT AND LIPID METABOLISM IN OBESITY AND CROHN'S DISEASE.
EFFECTS OF BYPASS AND RESECTION

STEPHAN RÖSSNER, DAG HALLBERG AND CATJA JOHANSSON
King Gustaf V Research Institute, Karolinska Hospital, S-104 01 Stockholm
(Sweden)

ABSTRACT

   Serum lipoproteins were analysed in grossly obese patients (n=29) before and
after jejuno-ileal bypass surgery and in patients with Crohn's disease (n=37),
in whom ileal resection had been performed. The patients were all studied in a
quiscent phase after surgery. Elevated VLDL-TG concentrations in the obese
patients were normalised, LDL-cholesterol concentrations were dramatically reduced by about 40%, whereas HDL-cholesterol did not increase, in spite of mean
weight losses of about 35 kg. In patients with Crohn's disease the TG concentrations in the major lipoprotein classes were normal, whereas LDL cholesterol
was markedly reduced. Significant negative relationships were found between
LDL- as well as HDL-cholesterol concentrations and the length of the resected
intestine. These data suggest indirectly that also in man, HDL secretion from
the intestinal tract may contribute to the concentration of circulating HDL
particles.

   The small intestine participates directly in the lipoprotein metabolism both
by the absorption of dietary fat and cholesterol from the intestinal lumen and
by the secretion into plasma of very low density lipoproteins[1] and, at least
in the experimental animal, also high density lipoproteins[1,2,3]. Indirectly the
small intestine takes part in the regulation of the cholesterol pool size
through the ileal reabsorption of bile acids[4]. Interference with the intestinal
regulation with resulting changes of the plasma lipid composition can be induced by intestinal surgery[5] and has found clinical application in the by-pass
operation for treatment of familial hypercholesterolaemia[6,7] and extreme obesity[9,8]. The present report summarizes some of the studies performed at our
Lipid Unit in order to further elucidate some of the mechanisms, by which lipoprotein metabolism and gastrointestinal functions are interrelated.

METHODS FOR LIPOPROTEIN SEPARATION

Serum lipoproteins were determined quantitatively by preparative ultracentrifugation from blood, drawn after an overnight fast[10]. After centrifugation for 16 h at d=1.006, VLDL was harvested in the top fraction by tube slicing.
After precipitation of LDL with heparin $MnCl_2$ HDL was recovered in the supernatant. TG and cholesterol concentrations were determined in whole serum, in
the VLDL, the LDL+HDL and the HDL fractions by the Technicon Auto-analyzer[11,12].
The LDL concentrations were then calculated by subtraction. Recovery of both
TG and cholesterol ranged from 90 to 110%.

CONTROLS

A sample of randomly selected males and females served as controls[13]. These
subjects (61 males and 56 females) had previously been repeatedly examined and
found to be without signs of disease. All had a Broca index below 1.1 (body
weight in kg/length in cm-100). The mean index ($\pm$SD) was 0.96 ± 0.09 for males
and 0.92 ± 0.10 for females. The lipoprotein data were age adjusted.

LIPOPROTEINS BEFORE AND AFTER JEJUNO-ILEAL SHUNT OPERATION IN OBESITY

An increased concentration of serum triglycerides (TG) is a common finding
in obese individuals. Even in moderately overweight subjects the incidence of
hypertriglyceridaemia is high. The serum cholesterol concentration may be
slightly elevated in obese subjects, but this is not a consistent finding[14].

At the Department of Surgery, Karolinska Hospital, subjects with massive
obesity have been screened for possible jejuno-ileal shunt operation. As part
of the preoperative metabolic analysis, serum lipid and lipoprotein concentrations were determined.

After jejuno-ileal shunt operation, total serum cholesterol is markedly
lowered[15]. In a previous study, we observed a reduction of 36% when the
patients had become weight-stable[16]. However, no significant change was found
in the total serum TG concentration, but in this subsample of 12 grossly obese
patients hypertriglyceridaemia was not found before surgery. This suggests
that the malabsorption, induced by surgery, influenced the composition of
several lipoproteins.

We studied the serum lipoprotein patterns in detail before and after surgery
in 10 men and 19 women[17]. These patients were all more than 50% above normal
weight, and after careful investigations, a shunt-operation was considered as
a suitable method to treat their massive obesity. The patients were restudied
after a mean time interval of about one year. The mean weight loss was from

145 ± 17 (S.D.) to 105 ± 12 kg in men and in women from 137 ± 26 to 104 ± 21 kg.

The results of the study are summarized in Table I. Before surgery hyper-triglyceridaemia was found only in men, and after the operation the elevated TG concentrations were normalised. In women, who had considerably lower serum TG concentrations before surgery, no significant change was observed. As expected, the serum cholesterol concentration fell by more than one third. In the serum lipoproteins these overall findings corresponded to the following changes: In men both the serum TG as well as the cholesterol reductions were the results of significant reductions of both VLDL and LDL TG and cholesterol concentrations. The HDL cholesterol concentration was not significantly affected by surgery. In women, the reductions of TG and cholesterol in VLDL just reached statistical significance ($p<0.05$). However, the marked fall of the total serum cholesterol concentration was the result of reductions in the LDL as well as the HDL fractions, although the LDL cholesterol fall by about 40% was most important from the quantitative point of view. The higher the initial LDL cholesterol concentration, the greater was the absolute reduction after surgery.

It is of interest that in both sexes the VLDL TG concentration was reduced after surgery but the HDL cholesterol concentration remained low. Thus after operation there seems to be a dissociation between the well established negative relation between these two parameters[18]. HDL seems to play a role in the efficient removal of VLDL from the circulation. However, the fall in VLDL after surgery seems to be caused by other factors than a high HDL concentration.

LIPOPROTEINS AFTER ILEAL RESECTION IN CROHN'S DISEASE[19]

Serum lipoproteins were determined in 37 patients (18 women) with Crohn's disease, who had been submitted to ileal resections. At the time of this study the patients were in a clinically stable phase and at least 2 years had elapsed since the last operation (average interval 5 years). Only patients in whom the length of the resection could be assessed by peroperative measurements were included. In all cases the diagnosis Crohn's disease was confirmed by histo-pathological examination according to Morson. Six patients on small prednisolone doses were included in the study, whereas patients on cholestyr-amine, oestrogen or supplementation with medium chain triglycerides were ex-cluded. The patients had received instruction by dietician to keep the daily fat intake below 70 g/day and had a caloric intake of about 2500-3000 kcal, containing about 400 mg cholesterol. Total TG concentrations were similar in patients and the matched control groups. In spite of the fact that the mean

TABLE 1.

TG AND CHOLESTEROL CONCENTRATIONS (mmol/l, S.D.) IN WHOLE SERUM AND THE MAJOR LIPOPROTEIN FRACTIONS OF OBESE SUBJECTS BEFORE AND AFTER SHUNT OPERATION:

Statistically significant differences (Student's paired t-test) are indicated as x = $p < 0.05$, xx = $p < 0.01$ and xxx = $p < 0.001$.

		Mean interval in months and (ranges)	Body weight kg	VLDL		LDL		HDL		Total	
n				TG	Chol	TG	Chol	TG	Chol	TG	Chol
Men 10	Before surgery	16(7-28)	145±7	1.90 ±1.10	0.91 ±0.50	0.50 ±0.13	3.78 ±0.75	0.21 ±0.08	1.07 ±0.41	2.69 ±1.19	5.83 ±1.16
	After surgery		105±12	1.06[x] ±0.47	0.46[x] ±0.19	0.32[xx] ±0.11	2.00[xxx] ±0.64	0.20 ±0.07	1.01 ±0.34	1.69[x] ±0.55	3.55[xxx] ±1.03
Women 19	Before surgery	10(5-19)	137±26	0.92 ±0.43	0.44 ±0.18	0.43 ±0.13	3.77 ±0.90	0.21 ±0.07	1.16 ±0.27	1.61 ±0.47	5.44 ±0.93
	After surgery		104±21	0.75[x] ±0.43	0.36[x] ±0.18	0.45 ±0.15	2.19[xx] ±0.54	0.19 ±0.06	1.02[x] ±0.27	1.42 ±0.48	3.63[xxx] ±0.66

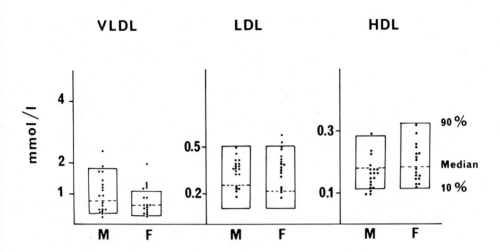

Fig. 1. TG concentrations (mmol/l) in the VLDL, LDL and HDL fractions of male (M) and female (F) patients with Crohn's disease. For comparison, data from a control sample have been included and the 10th and 90th percentile as well as the median value of the controls are shown.

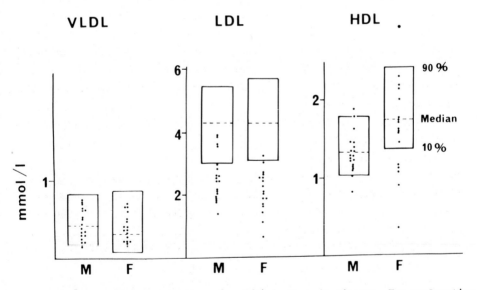

Fig. 2. Cholesterol concentrations (mmol/l) in Crohn's disease. For explanation, see legend to Figure 1.

resection length was 8.6 dm of ileum, Type IV hypertriglyceridaemia was found
in 7 patients (5 males). The distribution of TG and cholesterol are shown in
Figure 1 and 2. The TG concentrations in both sexes were similar to the
corresponding control values. The LDL cholesterol concentration was markedly
reduced in the patients, and in most cases were found far below the 10th percentile of control data. There were significant negative correlations ($p < 0.01$)
between the cholesterol concentrations of both the LDL and the HDL fraction
respectively and the length of the corresponding resected intestinal segment.
This relationship was not observed for any other lipid fraction.

In spite of the chronic disease and the limited fat intake the Crohn
patients maintained their concentrations of circulating TG at normal levels.
No correlations were found between TG in any lipoprotein fraction and the
extent of the resection or faecal fat excretion. This suggests that other
mechanisms may compensate for the limited supply of fat via the intestine. One
such mechanism could be that the adipose tissue by an increased lipolysis
supplies free fatty acids to the liver for subsequent TG synthesis, such as
in situations of catabolism and stress.

Hyperlipoproteinaemia type IV (elevated VLDL-TG) was diagnosed in 7/37
patients, which corresponds to the expected prevalence in a randomly selected
population of the same age. In these 7 patients, the relative body weight was
significantly higher than in the other Crohn patients. The usual association
between hypertriglyceridaemia and obesity therefore seems to exist even after
extensive resection of the small intestine and in patients with considerable
faecal loss of dietary fat.

It is well documented that intestinal surgery is followed by reduced total
serum cholesterol[15]. After resections of the distal ileum the reduction is
considered secondary to the increased loss of bile acids which is proportional
to the length of the resected intestine and a powerful stimulus to hepatic
bile acid synthesis from cholesterol. It is not known whether part of the
reduction is due to decreased intestinal absorption of cholesterol but mechanisms other than bile acid malabsorption should be suspected as a lowering of
the serum cholesterol occurs independent of the site of the intestinal resection
or of the bypassed part of the intestine[5,15].

The low LDL cholesterol led to a LDL-fraction relatively rich in TG compared
to cholesterol. Such a LDL composition could be explained by an increased
elimination of the final LDL-form, the cholesterol rich LDL_2, which should
leave more of the TG-rich LDL_1 fraction in the circulation.

Despite the normal mean HDL cholesterol concentration in Crohn patients

a negative correlation was found between the extent of the resection and HDL
cholesterol.   This finding is an indirect support
of the hypothesis that the intestine secretes HDL particles.

ACKNOWLEDGEMENTS

Supported by Swedish Medical Research Council (19X-204) and Nordisk Insulinfond.

REFERENCES

1. Lewis, B. (1977) in The Hyperlipidaemias clinical and laboratory Practice,
   Blackwell Scientific Publications, Oxford London Edinbourgh Melbourne,
   pp 67-92.

2. Mahley, R.W., Bersot, T.P., Levy, R.I., Windmueller, H.G. and LeQuire, V.S.
   (1970) Fed Proc 29, 629 (Abstract).

3. Windmueller, H.G., Herbert, P.N. and Levy, R.I. (1973) J Lipid Res,14, 215-223.

4. Grundy, S.M., Hofmann, A.F., Davignon, J. and Ahrens, E.H.Jr. (1966) J Clin
   Invest, 115, 1018-1019.

5. Carlson, L.A., Hallberg, D. and Killander, A. (1971) Acta Chir Scand 137,
   757-762.

6. Buchwald, H. and Vasco, R. (1967) Surg Gynec & Obstet, 124, 1231.

7. Moore, R.B., Vasco, R.L. and Buchwald, H. (1973) Am J Cardiol, 31, 148.

8. Payne, J.H. and DeWind, L.T. (1969) Am J Surg, 118, 141-147.

9. Hallberg, D., Backman, L. and Espmark, S. (1975) Prog Surg 14, 46-83.

10. Carlson, K. (1973) J Clin Path Suppl 5, 26, 32.

11. Kessler, G. and Lederer, H. (1965) in Automation in analytical chemistry,
    Skeggs, L.T. ed., Medical Inc., New York, p 341.

12. Block, W.D., Jarrett, K.J.,and Leoine, B. (1965) in Automation in analytical
    chemistry, Skeggs, L.T., ed., Medical Inc., New York, p 345.

13. Carlson, L.A. and Ericsson, M. (1975) Atherosclerosis, 21, 417-433.

14. Nestel, P. and Goldrick, B. (1976) Clin Endocrinol and Metabol,5, 313.

15. Buchwald, H., Moore, R.B., Frantz, I.D., Jr, and Vareo, R.L. (1970) in
    Proceedings of the Second Symposium on Atherosclerosis, Springer Verlag,
    New York, p 464.

16. Rössner, S. and Hallberg, D. (1976) Acta Med Scand,200, 475.

17. Rossner, S. and Hallberg, D. (1978) Acta Med Scand, 204, 103.

18. Olsson, A.G. (1975) Acta Med Scand (Suppl), 581.

19. Johansson, C., Rössner, S., Walldius, G. and Kollberg, B. Digestion,
    in press.

Lipoprotein Metabolism and Endocrine Regulation
L.W. Hessel and H.M.J. Krans editors
© ECSC, EEC, EAEC, Brussels-Luxembourg, 1979
Published by Elsevier/North-Holland Biomedical Press-Amsterdam

EFFECTS OF VARIOUS LOW DOSE CONTRACEPTIVE PILLS ON SERUM LIPOPROTEINS

STEPHAN RÖSSNER, OLLE FRANKMAN AND LARS MARSK

King Gustaf V Research Institute, Departments of Gynecology and Obstetrics
at Karolinska Hospital and South Hospital, Stockholm (Sweden)

ABSTRACT

Triglyceride (TG) and cholesterol concentrations in the major lipoprotein
fractions were determined in 33 young females before and during treatment for
two cycles with three different oral contraceptive agents. These were combinations of ethinyloestradiol and l-norgestrel in the following ($\mu g/\mu g$)
doses: 30/150, 50/150 and 50/250. All drugs affected the lipid concentrations
in similar ways. No significant concentration changes were found for whole
serum TG and cholesterol. However, the LDL-TG concentrations increased from
0.24 to 0.33 mmol/l ($p < 0.001$) and HDL-cholesterol fell from 1.54 to 1.35 mmol/l
($p < 0.001$) in the whole group. The clinical significance of this HDL-cholesterol
reduction in relation to the development of atherosclerotic manifestations
is discussed.

As recently stated by Spellacy et al a review of studies on the effects of
steroid contraception on lipid metabolism is confusing[1]. The designs have been
different, data from women on different types of steroids have been combined,
in many studies the women have not been their own controls and furthermore the
women have been on medication for periods which have varied from weeks to
years. Finally, results from studies of postmenopausal women on hormonal treatment certainly may give other results than studies of young or middle aged
women on oral contraceptives

Medication with oral contraceptives often continues for many years, during
which a woman is exposed to several metabolic abnormalities, associated with
this treatment. However, there has been a rapid development within this research
field, and oral contraceptives of today contain considerably lower concentrations of hormones than some years ago, with less unwanted side effects.

In a study, published in 1971[2] we described the effects of Anconcene[R] (0.1
mg mestranol + 3 mg chlormadinone acetate) on serum lipoproteins. After two
months the serum TG concentration had almost doubled and the serum cholesterol
concentration increased 12%. In the serum lipoproteins, the TG concentration
rose in the VLDL, LDL and HDL fractions and a cholesterol increase was

observed in HDL. When the women continued with a preparation, which only contained chlormadinone acetate, these values were subsequently normalised, but not until after six weeks.

Wynn et al recently demonstrated that after treatment with a low dose preparation containing 30 μg ethinyloestradiol + 150 μg l-norgestrel a different serum lipid pattern emerged[3]. The serum TG concentration was increased by about 10% with a serum cholesterol reduction of the same magnitude. In terms of lipoprotein composition such changes of whole serum lipid concentrations indicate that lipoprotein concentrations of TG and cholesterol must have been significantly affected.

The object of the present study was to analyse serum lipoproteins in women on low dose oral contraceptives. Since combinations of oestrogens and progestagens may have complex effects on lipoprotein metabolism, three different preparations with varying amounts of these two compounds were studied.

PATIENTS AND METHODS

The women studied had all applied to a contraceptive clinic run by the Stockholm County Civil Council and asked for prescriptions of oral contraceptives. They were invited by the gynecologist who examined them to take part in the study and their informed consent was obtained. Conventional criteria for exclusion of women for whom oral contraceptives are not advisable were used as suggested by the Swedish National Board of Health recommendations 1977.

Forty-one women (mean age 22 years, range 17-29 years) were referred to the Lipid Unit, Karolinska Hospital, where a fasting blood specimen was drawn for lipoprotein analysis. The women were then given one of three contraceptive preparations at random for two cycles, and were asked to return after this period for another blood sample. Both samples were drawn during the same parts of the menstrual cycle between the 21st and 26th day. In order to eliminate the possible influence of seasonal variation on lipid concentrations which could possibly play an important role in this group of individuals with presumably low serum lipoprotein concentrations, the patients were evenly recruited to the study throughout one whole year.

For unknown reasons 8 women, who had come to the Lipid Unit for the first visit, did not appear on the second occasion in spite of repeated calls.

The three different oral contraceptive preparations (kindly supplied by AB Kabi, Stockholm) contained ethinyloestradiol/l-norgestrel in the following combinations: Follimin[R] (30 μg/150 μg), code number "5042" (50 μg/150 μg) and Follinett[R] (50 μg/250 μg).

Serum lipoproteins were determined by preparative ultracentrifugation as described in detail by K. Carlson[4]. After centrifugation at d=1.006 the top fraction was harvested and called the very low density lipoprotein (VLDL) fraction. Heparin-manganese chloride was added to the infranatant, which precipitated the B-apoprotein containing low density lipoprotein (LDL) fraction. The remaining lipoprotein in solution was defined as the high density lipoprotein (HDL) fraction. The concentrations of TG and cholesterol in whole serum, VLDL, LDL+HDL and HDL were determined by Technicon Auto Analyzer methods[4,5].

The LDL concentrations of TG and cholesterol were calculated by subtraction. The recovery ranged from 90-110%.

RESULTS

Thirty-three women completed the study. There were no major complaints with regard to drug tolerance. The body weight before and after treatment were respectively: Follimin (30/ug/150/ug) 62.8 ± 2.2 kg (SEM) versus 63.1 ± 2.2 kg ($p > 0.05$), "5042" (50/ug/150/ug) 58.2 ± 2.2 versus 59.4 ± 2.1 kg ($p < 0.05$) and Follinett (50/ug/250/ug) 64.5 ± 2.4 kg versus 64.8 ± 2.4 kg ($p > 0.05$). In all three groups, patients were similar with regard to smoking habits. The lipoprotein concentrations before treatment did not differ significantly between the groups. The results of the serum lipoprotein analyses are shown in Table I. The serum concentrations of total TG and cholesterol did not change during treatment with either preparation, although there was a tendency for TG to rise. All women had low to normal serum lipid concentrations, and no subject developed hyperlipoproteinaemia during treatment. In the VLDL fraction, TG and cholesterol concentrations were not increased by any preparation, and the VLDL cholesterol /TG ratio was not affected. In the LDL fraction the TG concentration increased significantly by about 35% in all three groups. The LDL cholesterol concentration did not change. In the HDL fraction, a slight TG increase was observed after treatment only with the 50/150 preparation. The HDL cholesterol concentration fell by a mean value of 12% in all groups ($p < 0.001$). In the 50/250 and the 30/150 groups significant reductions were found ($p < 0.001$ and $p < 0.05$ respectively), whereas the reduction found in the smaller 50/150 group did not quite reach statistical significance.

DISCUSSION

The advantage of the present study is that the women were their own controls and that three hormone combinations could be studied under identical conditions. One possible disadvantage may be the fact that the follow up period was only

TABLE 1

TG AND CHOLESTEROL CONCENTRATIONS (mmol/l) IN THE LIPOPROTEIN FRACTIONS BEFORE AND DURING TREATMENT WITH ORAL CONTRACEPTIVES OF VARYING HORMONAL COMPOSITION.

Statistically significant differences (Student's paired t-test) are indicated: $x = p < 0.05$, $xxx = p < 0.001$.

Hormonal composition ethinyloestradiol/µg /l-norgestrel/µg	n		VLDL TG	VLDL Chol	LDL TG	LDL Chol	HDL TG	HDL Chol	Total TG	Total Chol
30/150	11	Before	0.43 ± 0.07	0.23 ± 0.05	0.23 ± 0.02	2.73 ± 0.15	0.13 ± 0.02	1.68 ± 0.08	0.83 ± 0.10	4.70 ± 0.21
		During	0.46 ± 0.05	0.28 ± 0.03	0.31 ± 0.02^{x}	2.86 ± 0.31	0.14 ± 0.02	1.44 ± 0.08^{xxx}	0.96 ± 0.07	4.70 ± 0.31
50/150	9	Before	0.61 ± 0.12	0.34 ± 0.05	0.26 ± 0.03	2.94 ± 0.10	0.14 ± 0.03	1.37 ± 0.10	1.05 ± 0.13	4.62 ± 0.15
		During	0.61 ± 0.07	0.36 ± 0.05	0.35 ± 0.02^{x}	2.92 ± 0.10	0.17 ± 0.02^{x}	1.26 ± 0.10	1.17 ± 0.09	4.57 ± 0.21
50/250	13	Before	0.53 ± 0.09	0.31 ± 0.05	0.25 ± 0.04	2.68 ± 0.23	0.15 ± 0.01	1.52 ± 0.10	0.96 ± 0.14	4.52 ± 0.23
		During	0.48 ± 0.06	0.28 ± 0.03	0.33 ± 0.03^{x}	2.81 ± 0.16	0.15 ± 0.01	1.34 ± 0.08^{x}	1.00 ± 0.09	4.41 ± 0.18
All women	33	Before	0.52 ± 0.04	0.28 ± 0.03	0.24 ± 0.02	2.78 ± 0.10	0.14 ± 0.01	1.54 ± 0.06	0.94 ± 0.07	4.59 ± 0.12
		During	0.51 ± 0.04	0.30 ± 0.03	0.33 ± 0.01^{xxx}	2.86 ± 0.12	0.15 ± 0.01	1.35 ± 0.05^{xxx}	1.03 ± 0.05	4.52 ± 0.14

two months. However, it was considered too difficult to ensure that these young and symptom free women would return fasted to a clinic for further blood sampling if the time interval had been further extended.

In spite of different compositions the three drugs, used in this study, gave similar results. Total serum lipid concentrations did not increase although there was a tendency for serum TG to increase, which is in accordance with other studies[3,7,8,9]. However, in contrast to some of these studies, no significant serum cholesterol reduction was observed[3,8,9]. It has been argued that a possible advantage of low dose oral contraceptives of the types, used here, might be the fact that these drugs may even lower the serum cholesterol concentration[3]. This would undoubtedly have been an advantage, had the reduction occurred in a lipoprotein fraction which accelerates the development of atherosclerosis. However, this was not the case with any of our hormone combinations, since the cholesterol concentrations in VLDL and LDL remained unaffected and the only cholesterol reduction was found in HDL. The 35% LDL-TG increase during therapy is a new and uncommon change of the lipid interrelationships in serum lipoproteins. There is a wellknown inverse relationship between the VLDL TG and the HDL cholesterol concentrations. A tendency for such a relationship before medication can also be seen in Figure 1. The HDL reduction would therefore rather have been associated with a VLDL TG increase.

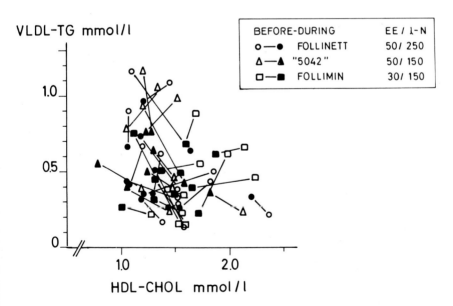

Fig. 1. Relationship between VLDL-TG and HDL-cholesterol in females before and during treatment with oral contraceptives.

The meaning of an isolated increase of the LDL TG concentration is difficult to interpret. In man, LDL is considered to be the endproduct of VLDL after
TG removal from its core and concomitant rearrangement of the surface structures[10]. An isolated LDL-TG increase would rather suggest an impaired clearance
of LDL TG, since in this study the VLDL concentrations remained unaffected.

Oestrogen treatment stimulates hepatic TG secretion[11]. Impaired lipolysis
has also been described, and in a recent study selective impairment of the
hepatic lipase activity could be demonstrated[12]. In contrast to these results,
Kushwaha et al demonstrated that ethinyloestradiol (1 ug/kg body weight and
day) caused a paradoxical normalisation of the type III hyperlipoproteinaemia[13].
The LDL lipids were, however, not affected in any systematic way, and in HDL
both TG and cholesterol concentrations increased.

The oestrogen doses in the study of Kushwaha et al are slightly higher than
used in the present study, and it is obvious that effects on the patients with
type III hyperlipoproteinaemia may differ greatly from the effects on the low
serum lipoprotein concentrations seen in healthy young women. It is possible
that in our study the oestrogenic effects may have been partly counteracted by
the norgestrel component of the oral contraceptives.

Krauss et al have compared lipoprotein levels in 18 users with 19 age-
matched non-users[14]. A significant increase was found only of the HDL fraction.
By detailed fractionation this increase could be located to the denser part of
this fraction, the so-called HDL_3. However, the 18 women studied had used oral
contraceptives of seven different compositions, which makes a critical comparison difficult.

Several epidemiologic studies have compared serum lipid levels of hormone
users to non-users. The results are often quite different. The Lipid Research
Clinic Program found a 48% increase of the plasma TG concentrations in women
on oral contraceptives in the age group 20-24 years[7]. The mean plasma cholesterol
concentration was 5% higher. However, the exact type of hormone medication
was never specifically asked for by these investigators.

In the Leiden population study, the HDL cholesterol concentration was about
10% lower in women on oral contraceptives than in non-users[15]. It is possible
that clinical practice in the Leiden area has led to some degree of conformity
in the prescription of low dose preparations, which might lead to a more uniform
pattern of lipoprotein values.

Only in a recent study (Contraceptive Drug Study, Kaiser Foundation Health
Plan) the importance of the type of oral contraceptive was taken into account
in the lipoprotein data analysis[16]. These 5001 women also supplied information

about smoking, drinking habits and about the brand and dosage of the hormone
preparation they were using. In oestrogen users, the HDL -cholesterol concentrations were significantly higher than in controls, whereas in progestin users,
significantly lower HDL-cholesterol concentrations were found. In women on
combination drugs, the levels varied with the type and dose of the steroids,
but the general pattern was an increase of HDL cholesterol with increasing
oestrogen doses and a decrease with increasing dose or potency of the progestin
component.

The clinical consequence of a reduced HDL cholesterol concentration in this
group of young women is not clear. A low HDL concentration is a strong and
independent risk factor for the development of atherosclerotic manifestations[17].
So far no longitudinal studies have shown whether lower HDL concentrations in
these women after several years of hormonal medication will be the cause of
the increased risks to develop atherosclerotic manifestations that has been
demonstrated in women on oral contraceptives[18]. However, as pointed out by
Arntzenius et al in the Leiden study, their 40 year old women on oral contraceptives had "disturbingly low serum HDL-cholesterol concentrations", which
were similar to the concentrations found in men of the same age group. From
the theoretical point of view, a chronically lowered HDL-cholesterol in
women may be one factor that increases their risk for atherosclerotic manifestations to the same level as in men.

REFERENCES

1. Spellacy, W.N., Newton, R.E., Buhi, W.C. and Birk, S.A. (1976) Fertility
   and Sterility, 27, 157.

2. Rössner, S., Larsson-Cohn, U., Carlson, L.A. and Boberg, J. (1971) Acta
   Med Scand,190, 301-305.

3. Wynn, V., Adams, P., Oakley, N. and Seed, M. (1974) Amsterdam: Excerpta
   Medica, 47-55.

4. Carlson, K. (1973) J Clin Path (Suppl) 26, Ass Clin Pathol,5, 32-37.

5. Kessler, G. and Lederer, H. (1965) in Automation in Clinical Chemistry,
   Skeggs, L.T. ed., Medical Inc., New York, pp 341-344.

6. Block, W.D., Janett, K.J. and Leone, B. (1965) in Automation in Clinical
   Chemistry, Skeggs, L.T.,ed., Medical Inc., New York, pp 345-346.

7. Wallace, R.B., Hoover, J., Sandler, D., Rifkind, B.M. and Tyroler, H.A.
   (1977) Lancet,ii, 11-15.

8. Sutherland, W.H.F. and Nye, E.R. (1976) Proceedings of the University of
   Otago Medical School, 54, 83-84.

9. Magnani, H.N. and Moore, B. (1976) Postgrad Med J, 52(Suppl. 6), 55-58.

10. Olsson, A.G. (1975) Acta Med Scand (Suppl), 581.

11. Glueck, C.J., Fallat, R.W. and Scheel, D. (1975) Metabolism, 24, 537-544.

12. Applebaum, D.M., Goldberg, A.P., Pykälistö, O.J., Brunzell, J.D. and Hazzard, W.R. (1977) J Clin Invest, 59, 601-608.

13. Kushwaha, R.S., Hazzard, W.R., Gagne, C., Chait, A. and Albers, J.J. (1977) Ann Int Med,87, 517-525.

14. Krauss, R.M., Lindgren, F.T., Silvers, A., Jutagir, R. and Bradley, D.D. (1977) Clin Chim Acta, 80, 465-470.

15. Arntzenius, A.C., Van Gent, C.M., Van Der Voort, H., Stegerhoek, C.I. and Styblo, K. (1978) Lancet, i, 1221-1224.

16. Bradley, D.D., Wingerd, J., Petitti, D.B., Krauss, R.M. and Ramcharan, S. (1978) N Eng J Med, 299, 17-20.

17. Miller, C.J. and Miller, N.E. (1975) Lancet, i, 16-19.

18. Wilhelmsen, L. (1978) Epidemiology of coronary heart disease in young women. I: Coronary Heart Disease in Young Women, Oliver, M.F. ed., Churchill Livingstone, Edinburgh London & New York, pp 3-11.

Lipoprotein Metabolism and Endocrine Regulation
L.W. Hessel and H.M.J. Krans editors
© ECSC, EEC, EAEC, Brussels-Luxembourg, 1979
Published by Elsevier/North-Holland Biomedical Press-Amsterdam

HIGH- DENSITY -LIPOPROTEIN -CHOLESTEROL AND TESTOSTERONE.

L.VERSCHOOR, H.JANSEN, A.J.ZONNEVELD, J.D.BARTH AND J.C.BIRKENHÄGER.

Department of Medicine III, Division of Clinical Endocrinology and Metabolism,
University Hospital "Dijkzigt", Erasmus University, Rotterdam, The Netherlands.

INTRODUCTION

While the article by Miller and Miller, written in 1975 [1], focused attention
on the possible importance of HDL for atherosclerosis, by showing an inverse
relationship between HDL-cholesterol concentration and the total body choleste-
rolpool, and on low HDL(-cholesterol) levels in conditions prone to cardiovascular disease with the suggestion that these findings support the role of HDL
in the clearance of cholesterol from the arterial wall [2], it deserves mentio-
ning that the subject has been raised long before [3,4].

Epidemiologic evidence of an inverse relationship between HDL(-cholesterol)
and clinical manifestations of atherosclerosis has accumulated [5-9]. Lower
HDL(-cholesterol) concentrations in males are a constant finding [8,10,11], and
have been related to the presence of androgens, since pharmacologic amounts
of androgens induce a decrease of HDL [12]. However the difference can also be
ascribed to the absence of oestrogens. Pharmacologic [13,14] as well as near
physiologic [11] amounts of oestrogens raise HDL(-cholesterol) concentration.
Reports of the effect of oral contraceptives are contradictory, possibly related to differences in composition [11,15-18]. On the basis of ischaemic heart
disease death rate statistics Heller and Jacobs have suggested that androgens
are a risk factor for coronary heart disease, and that oestrogens are not
protective [19].

Disappearance of the sex difference in HDL-cholesterol concentration has
been reported by Arntzenius et al [17] in cigarette smoking, contraceptive
using women. Calculation of the data of Glueck et al [20] on familial
hyperalphalipoproteinaemia learned us that, although among all family members
the sex difference in HDL-cholesterol was retained, the male and female
patients with the abnormality mentioned, showed no difference in HDL-
cholesterol: 86 and 81 mg/dl, respectively. A third condition characterized
by the disappearance of the sex difference of plasma HDL-cholesterol content,
chronic intermittent heamodialysis, has been presented in preliminary form [21],
and will be discussed more in detail here.

Aim of the present study was to answer two questions:

1. Is the sex difference in HDL(-cholesterol) concentration causally related to androgen levels: are spontaneous differences in plasma testosterone level accompanied by differences in HDL-cholesterol concentration ?

2. Is the sex difference in HDL(-cholesterol) still present in conditions with raised total plasma-cholesterol and/or total plasma-TG ?

PATIENTS AND METHODS

The first question was studied in thirty-four consecutive males, referred to our department for analysis of infertility. None showed any disease known to affect lipid metabolism. Routine physical examination revealed no abnormalities, except for hypogonadistic features in some of them. Routine laboratory investigation showed no abnomalities.

To answer the second question four groups of patients were studied: Group A consisted of four male and four female patients with familial primary hyperlipoproteinaemia type IIA (WHO- classification [22]). These patients had never been treated. Group B: three male and three female patients with untreated primary hypothyroidism. Group C: thirteen male and eleven female patients with chronic renal failure treated with intermittent haemodialysis. Group D: ten women with gross obesity, studied before weight reduction.

All patients were investigated after an overnight fast, except the men examined for infertility: from these patients blood was drawn between 2 and 4 p.m. The patients with chronic renal failure (treated with regular haemodialysis) were examined just before a dialysis session.

Cholesterol was measured using an enzymatic, colorimetric method (Cholesterol Test-Combination, Boehringer Mannheim GmbH, W-Germany). Triglycerides was measured according to Laurell [23]. HDL-cholesterol was measured using the heparin/manganese chloride precipitation technique [24] with slight modifications (final $MnCl_2$ concentration 91 mmol/l). Normal values in our laboratory (mean $\pm$ S.D.): males 1.14 $\pm$ 0.32 mmol/l, females 1.50 $\pm$ 0.34 mmol/l. Plasma testosteron was measured using a radioimmunoassay method [25]. The normal lower limit for males in our laboratory is 17.4 nmol/l.

RESULTS

In table I the lipid concentrations obtained in men with normal and subnormal testosterone levels, respectively, are summarized.

List of abbreviations used: HDL, High-density-lipoprotein; TG, Triglycerides; LPL, Lipoprotein lipase; PHLA, Post-heparin lipolytic activity; HTGL, Hepatic triglyceride lipase.

TABLE 1
LIPID LEVELS (MEAN ± SD) IN TESTOSTERONE-DEFICIENT MEN (T.D.) AND MEN WITH
NORMAL TESTOSTERONE LEVELS (N.T.).

		T.D. n= 17	N.T. n= 17	
plasma testosterone	(nmol/l)	12.34 ± 3.96	22.58 ± 4.68	p < 0.0001
total cholesterol	(mmol/l)	5.40 ± 1.07	5.31 ± 1.15	n.s.
HDL-cholesterol	(mmol/l)	1.27 ± 0.34	1.16 ± 0.18	n.s.
triglycerides	(mmol/l)	1.86 ± 1.17	1.33 ± 0.52	n.s.

No significant differences were observed, although in the testosterone-
deficient group the total plasma-TG concentration tended to be higher than in
the group with normal testosterone levels. When compared to normal male control
values (1.01 ± 0.41 mmol/l; n = 22) the total plasma-TG level was significantly
increased (p < 0.005) in the testosterone-deficient group. No correlation was
found between testosterone levels and HDL-cholesterol concentrations for the
entire group (Fig.1). No correlation was found either between total plasma-TG
and HDL-cholesterol for the entire group, nor for the two subgroups of males

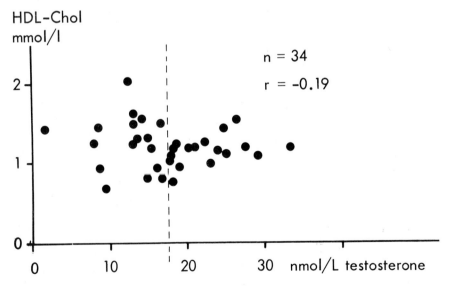

Fig. 1. Plasma testosterone levels are plotted against HDL-cholesterol
concentration. The broken line marks the lower limit of plasma testosterone
in normal men.

102

with and without testosterone-deficiency. Also no correlation existed between
total plasma- and HDL-cholesterol levels.

Figure 2 shows the HDL-cholesterol levels of the patients in the groups
A - D (cf. Patients and Methods), compared with the normal range (mean ± 2 S.D.)
in men and women. The values of all individuals of group A and B and all but
one of group D are within the normal range. However in group D the mean value
is significantly different from normal (p< 0.005), because the levels in all
other patients are in the lower half of the normal range. Most patients in
group C showed decreased HDL-cholesterol levels (seven out of thirteen male and
nine out of eleven female patients), leading to significantly decreased
(p< 0.0001) mean values as compared to normal, for men as well as for women:
0.54 ± 0.21 mmol/l and 0.63 ± 0.15 mmol/l, respectively. In the groups A and B
the sex difference in HDL-cholesterol was maintained, while no sex difference
was present anymore in the patients of group C.

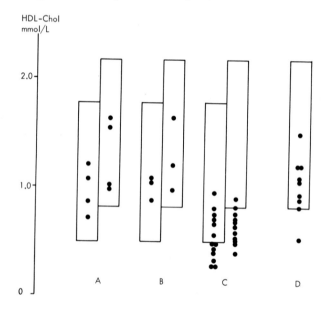

Fig. 2. Individual HDL-cholesterol concentrations of patients in group A
(hyperlipoproteinaemia type IIA), B (primary hypothyroidism before substitu-
tion), C (chronic renal failure, treated with intermittent haemodialysis) and
D (gross obesity) are shown in relation to normal values in men and women
depicted as rectangulars (mean ± 2 S.D.).The left of each pair of rectangulars
denotes the men.

For the four groups the mean values for HDL-cholesterol are given for men and women separately in Table 2, together with other lipid levels.

TABLE 2
LIPID LEVELS (MEAN $\pm$ SD, IN MMOL/L) IN PATIENTS OF GROUP A - D

	group A		group B	
	males (4)[*]	females (4)	males (3)	females (3)
total plasma chol.	15.95 $\pm$ 3.48	10.57 $\pm$ 2.15	8.83 $\pm$ 3.34	9.73 $\pm$ 3.30
total plasma-TG	1.58 $\pm$ 1.12	1.00 $\pm$ 0.43	2.17 $\pm$ 2.09	1.05 $\pm$ 0.35
HDL-cholesterol	0.97 $\pm$ 0.21	1.29 $\pm$ 0.34	1.00 $\pm$ 0.10	1.27 $\pm$ 0.33
HDL-TG	0.05 $\pm$ 0.02[1]	0.06 $\pm$ 0.03[1]	0.12 $\pm$ 0.02	0.12 $\pm$ 0.03

	group C		group D
	males (13)	females (11)	females (10)
total plasma chol.	5.50 $\pm$ 2.01	5.04 $\pm$ 1.38	6.81 $\pm$ 1.49
total plasma-TG	2.21 $\pm$ 1.14	1.89 $\pm$ 0.99	1.14 $\pm$ 0.55
HDL-cholesterol	0.54 $\pm$ 0.21	0.63 $\pm$ 0.15	1.00 $\pm$ 0.26
HDL-TG	0.16 $\pm$ 0.04[2]	0.11 $\pm$ 0.03[3]	0.08 $\pm$ 0.03

* between parentheses number of patients studied
1) n = 3   2) n = 5   3) n = 4

No correlation was found between HDL-cholesterol and total plasma-TG within the groups studied.

DISCUSSION

Although profound effects of pharmacologic amounts of androgens have been described[26], we found no effect of testosterone deficiency on HDL-cholesterol levels, nor a relationship between HDL-cholesterol and plasma testosterone over a range of the latter of 1.7 to 33.3 nmol/l (the entire group studied). Two main possibilities will be discussed to explain the observations. Firstly, the suggestion may be made that oestrogens, and not androgens are responsible for the repeatedly observed normal sex difference in HDL-cholesterol. Comparison can be made with the regulation of LPL activity, the stimulation of which by oestrogens can not be reproduced by orchidectomy[27].

More specificially the regulation of HDL-cholesterol might in part be achieved
by an endocrine regulation of TG metabolism, for which sex difference is primarily located at the removal site: women have a more efficient removal system
than men[28,29]. Higher LPL activity measured as PHLA[30] as well as adipose tissue
activity[31] have been described in women. Further evidence for this possibility
comes from the inverse relationship between HDL-cholesterol and total or VLDL-
TG[32,33]. The fact that we did not find this relationship in this study is probably explained by the rather small sample size. More direct evidence for the
hypothesis comes from the positive correlation between HDL-cholesterol and
adipose tissue LPL activity[31] and PHLA[34]. Secondly the effect of testosterone
deficiency may have been masked by a concomitantly occuring slight increase of
plasma TG concentration,
thereby indicating a more important regulatory role of TG metabolism than of androgens in determining HDL-cholesterol levels. However, matching teststoterone-
deficient males with men having normal testosterone levels for plasma-TG levels
no significant difference in HDL-cholesterol concentration between both groups
was found, although in the first group levels tended to be slightly higher
(Table 3).

TABLE 3
COMPARISON OF HDL-CHOLESTEROL IN PLASMA-TG MATCHED PAIRS (N = 8) OF MEN WITH
(T.D.) AND WITHOUT (N.T.) TESTOSTERONE DEFICIENCY.

N.T.		T.D.	
HDL-cholesterol mmol/l	plasma-TG mmol/l	HDL-cholesterol mmol/l	plasma-TG mmol/l
1.18 ± 0.25	1.49 ± 0.68	1.36 ± 0.35[*)	1.53 ± 0.72

*) n.s.

Decreased HDL-cholesterol levels were found in male patients of group C and
the women of the groups C and D. No sex difference appeared to be present anymore in Group C. That the decrease in the men is less extensive than in women
is very probably not to be explained by the subnormal testosterone levels
described in male patients suffering from renal insufficiency [35,36]. Both male

and female patients showed a decrease of LPL activity to the same level, with no change in the level and the normally observed sex difference in HTGL activity[37]. It is tempting to suggest that the changes in LPL activity could explain the disappearance of the sex difference in HDL-cholesterol concentration.

In conclusion: no important regulatory role for plasma testosterone (below and within the normal range) in determining HDL-cholesterol level has been found. Evidence is presented for regulation of HDL-cholesterol levels by LPL activity. The level of this activity may also be responsible for the difference in the level of HDL-cholesterol between men and women, in health and some pathological conditions.

ACKNOWLEDGEMENTS

Part of this study was supported by the Foundation for Medical Research, FUNGO. We thank Drs. L.D.F.Lameyer and G.Kolsters for giving us the opportunity to study the patients with renal failure, Dr. F.H. de Jong for the plasma testosterone measurements and Mrs. G.A. van Wessen for excellent secretarial help.

REFERENCES

1. Miller, G.J. and Miller, N.E. (1975) Lancet I, 16 - 19.
2. Glomset, J.A. (1968) J.Lipid Res. 9, 155 - 167.
3. Barr, D.P., Russ, E.M. and Eder, H.A. (1951) Amer. J. Med. 11, 480 - 493.
4. Nikkilä, E. (1953) Scand. J.Clin. Lab. Invest. 5, suppl. 8, 1 - 101.
5. Berg, K., Børresen, A-L. and Dahlén, G. (1976) Lancet I, 499 - 501.
6. Rhoads, G.G., Gulbrandsen, C.L. and Kagan, A. (1976) New Engl. J.Med. 294, 293 - 298.
7. Gordon, T., Castelli, W.P., Hjortland, M.C., Kannel, W.B. and Dawber, T.R. (1977) Amer J.Med. 62, 707 - 714.
8. Miller, N.E., Førde, O.H., Thelle, D.S. and Mjøs, O.D. (1977) Lancet I, 965 - 968.
9. Logan, R.L. Riemersma, R.A., Thomson, M., Oliver, M.F., Olsson, A.G., Walldius, G., Rössner, S., Kayser, L., Callmer, E., Carlson, L.A. Lockerbie, L. and Lutz, W. (1978) Lancet I, 949 - 955.
10. Lewis, B., Chait, A., Wrotton, I.D.P., Oakley, C.M., Krikler, D.M., Sigurdsson, G., February, A., Mauer, B. and Birkhead, J. (1974) Lancet I, 141 - 146.
11. Albers, J.J., Wahl, P.W., Cabana, V.C., Hazzard, W.R. and Hoover, J.J. (1976) Metabolism 25, 633 - 644.
12. Solyom, A. (1972) Lipids 7, 100 - 105.

106

13. Gustafson, A. and Svanborg, A. (1972) Endocrinology 35, 203 - 207.

14. Tikkanen, M.J., Nikkilä, E.A. and Vartiainen, E. (1978) Lancet II, 490 - 491.

15. Rössner, S., Larsson-Cohn, H., Carlson, L.A. and Boberg, J. (1971)
    Acta Med. Scand. 190, 301 - 305.

16. Cheung, M.C. and Albers, J.J. (1977) J.Clin. Invest. 60, 43 - 50.

17. Arntzenius, A.C. van Gent, C.M., van der Voort, H., Stegerhoek, C.I. and
    Styblo, K. (1978) Lancet I, 1221 - 1223.

18. Rössner, S. (1978) Lancet II, 269.

19. Heller, R.F., Jacobs, H.S. (1978) Brit. Med. J. 1, 472 - 474.

20. Glueck, C.J., Fallat, R.W., Millett, F., Gartside, P., Elston, R.C. and
    Go, R.C.P. (1975) Metabolism 24, 1243 - 1265.

21. Verschoor, L., Jansen, H., Zonneveld, A.J. and Birkenhäger, J.C. (1977)
    Proc. XXth. International Conference on the Biochemistry of Lipids (ICBL),
    38 (abstract).

22. Beaumont, J.L., Carlson, L.A., Cooper, G.R., Fejfar, Z., Frederickson,
    D.S. and Strasser, T. (1970) Bull. Wld. Hlth. Org. 43, 891 - 915.

23. Laurell, S. (1966) Scand. J. Clin.& Lab. Invest. 18, 668 - 672.

24. Burstein, M., Scholnick, H.R. and Morfin, R. (1970) J.Lipid. Res. 11,
    583 - 595.

25. Verjans, H.L., Cooke, B.A., de Jong, F.H., de Jong, C.M.M. and van der
    Molen, H.J. (1973) J.Steroid Biochem. 4, 665 - 676.

26. Masarei, J.R.L and Lynch, W.J. (1977) Lancet II, 827 - 828.

27. Wilson, D.E., Flowers, C.M., Carlile, S.I. and Udall, K.S. (1976)
    Atherosclerosis 24, 491 - 499.

28. Nikkilä, E.A. and Kekki, M. (1971) Acta Med. Scand. 190, 49 - 59.

29. Olefsky, J., Farquhar, J.W. and Reaven, G.M. (1974) Europ. J.Clin. Invest.
    4, 121 - 127.

30. Huttunen, J.K., Ehnholm, C., Kekki, M. and Nikkilä, E.A. (1976)
    Clin. Sc. Mol. Med. 50, 249 - 260.

31. Nikkilä, E.A., Taskinen, M-R. and Kekki, M. (1978) Atherosclerosis 29,
    497 - 501.

32. Schaefer, E.J., Levy, R.I., Anderson, D.W., Danner, R.N., Brewer, H.B. and
    Blackwelder, W.C. (1978) Lancet II, 391 - 393.

33. Brunzell, J.D., Albers, J.J. Haas, L.B., Goldberg, A.P., Agadoa, L. and
    Sherrard, D.J. (1977) Metabolism 26, 903 - 910.

34. Verschoor, L., Jansen, H., Lamberts, S.W.J. and Wilson, J.H.P. (1978)
    in Diabetes and Obesity, Vague, Ph. ed., Elsevier, Amsterdam (in press).

35. Lim, V.S. and Fang, V.S. (1976) J.Clin. Endocrinol. Metab. 43, 1370 - 1377.

36. Holdsworth, S., Atkins, R.C. and de Kretser, D.M. (1977) New Engl. J. Med.
    296, 1245 - 1249.

37. Verschoor, L., Jansen, H., Zonneveld, A.J. and Birkenhäger, J.C. (1978)
    Proc. Europ. Soc. Clin. Invest., abstract no. 251.

Lipoprotein Metabolism and Endocrine Regulation
L.W. Hessel and H.M.J. Krans editors
© ECSC, EEC, EAEC, Brussels-Luxembourg, 1979
Published by Elsevier/North-Holland Biomedical Press-Amsterdam

RELATIONSHIP BETWEEN THYROID FUNCTION, PLASMA LIPIDS AND CORONARY HEART DISEASE - A REVIEW

L. VANHAELST°, P.A. BASTENIE°°

°Metabolic Unit, Vrije Universiteit Brussel, °°Laboratory of Experimental Medicine, Université Libre de Bruxelles, Brussels, Belgium.

Since a long time it is known that clearcut alterations in thyroid function are associated with marked changes of blood lipid levels, especially cholesterol[1,2]. Usually the hypocholesterolemia of hyperthyroidism is of rather abrupt onset since the disease itself has a short installation period. On the contrary, primary myxoedema in the adult is the end result of a protracted process of immune destruction of the thyroid[3]. The different stages before the definite failure of thyroid function, essentially characterized by humoral and cellular immune reactions against thyroid components may be considered as an evolving premyxoedematous state[4]. In view of the predominant importance of hypercholesterolemia in the etiology of coronary heart disease (CHD), it seems worthwile to assess if this essential feature of established myxoedema plays already a role during the progressive thyroid involution process.

HYPERTHYROIDISM

In the classical Graves' disease, as well as in the solitary toxic nodule and in the toxic multinodular goiter (Plummer's disease) a lowering in serum cholesterol levels is the rule[1,5]. This has been ascribed to an acceleration of the cholesterol degradation and excretion rates overwhelming a simultaneous stimulation of cholesterol biosynthesis[6,7]. Owing to the broad range of normal, the measurement of cholesterol levels is of little diagnostic use. However, the rise of cholesterol following antithyroid therapy can be used as one of the earliest laboratory parameters of response to therapy[8].

   Plasma triglyceride levels have been found either lowered[9], normal[10,11], or moderately elevated[12] in thyrotoxicosis. These discrepant observations may be due to the interaction of different effects of high thyroid hormone levels on triglyceride metabolism : augmented production of triglycerides[12], increased fractional clearance of triglycerides[11], augmented[12] or decreased[10,11] post heparin plasma lipolytic activity (PHLA), reflecting the lipoprotein lipase (LPL) activity. Plasma free fatty acids (FFA) and glycerol levels are increased[12], as a consequence of the enhanced formation of adenylcyclase in the adipose tissue[13]. Data concerning coronary heart disease in thyrotoxicosis are scarce : angina pectoris occurs only occasionally : about fifty cases of myocardial infarction have been reported until now[14]. It has been postulated that the lowering in serum cholesterol might prevent the development of coronary atherosclerosis[15]. It seems however difficult to admit that the long standing evolution of the atherosclerotic process might be favourably influenced by an intercurrent illness of short duration, even if it is cholesterol lowering. Some cases of myocardial infarction in thyrotoxic patients with normal coronary arteries on coronarography[14,16] raise the question of a direct noxious effect of thyroid hormones on the myocardium. Excessive thyroid hormone demanding an increasing cardiac output

might cause a critical imbalance resulting in angina pectoris
and/or myocardial infarction. Further work is obviously war-
ranted to elucidate the reason of the unusual occurrence of CHD
in thyrotoxicosis.

HYPOTHYROIDISM

Blood lipids are markedly deranged in primary hypothyroidism[2].
These changes are mostly characterized by the isolated increase
of blood cholesterol and β lipoproteins, thus suggesting the
picture of a secondary type IIa hyperlipoproteinemia[17]. This
elevation results essentially from a decrease in the rate of
cholesterol catabolism, though cholesterol biosynthesis is also
depressed. Myxoedematous patients show a decreased catabolic
rate of low density lipoproteins (LDL), the principal carriers
of plasma cholesterol[7], a slow disappearance rate of radioactive
cholesterol from the circulation[18] and a lowered incorporation
of ^{14}C-acetate into serum cholesterol[19]. Treatment with thyroid
hormones normalizes these situations and accelerates the rate of
appearance of the end products of cholesterol metabolism, i.e.
fecal cholesterol and bile acids[20]. Some investigators report
that over 80 percent of patients with hypothyroidism have serum
cholesterol levels greater than 300 mg/dl[21], but most clinicians
report a lower frequency. In a recent study[22] where hypothyroid
patients were fitted into four groups of increasing grades of
thyroid failure based on serum TSH levels, only in the two most
severely hypothyroid groups was cholesterol significantly elevated as compared with control levels. Decrease in serum cholesterol may help to follow the response of hypothyroid patients
to thyroid hormone replacement and fall of cholesterol after even

small doses of thyroid hormone has ever been used as a confirmatory diagnostic index.

Plasma triglyceride level is generally moderately elevated in myxoedema[11,12]. This has been ascribed to impaired triglyceride clearance, itself owing to lowered plasma PHLA[10,12]. In all hypothyroid patients, plasma triglyceride levels decrease after thyroid treatment, apparently by reversal to normal of the decreased lipoprotein lipase activity[23], thus allowing a faster triglyceride hydrolysis and storage of long chain fatty acids in tissues.

Thus, whereas type IIa hyperlipoproteinemia appears as the condition usually associated with hypothyroidism[5], a number of myxoedematous subjects present with the IIb type.

Conversely, Hazzard and Bierman[24] have described a case in which primary type III hyperlipoproteinemia was greatly aggravated by hypothyroidism. Moreover, Lasser et al.[25] have published a case of congenital dyslipidemia in which type III pattern was clearly secondary to hypothyroidism which had converted patient's primary type IV to type III. These observations emphasize the possible role of hypothyroidism in the production of hyperlipoproteinemia particularly associated with pre-β and β very low density lipoproteins (VLDL).

In myxoedema plasma FFA levels are usually slightly decreased[12]; this finding conforms with the observations of decreased lipolytic activity in adipose tissue of hypothyroid animals[26].

The association of myxoedema with CHD has been well documented and fits with the presence of hypercholesterolemia and hypertriglyceridemia, both known risk factors of cardiovascular disease. In our study[27] on 87 patients with clinical myxoedema and on 25

necropsies of patients who died with inadequately treated hypothyroidism, independently of sex, age, and associated disorders,
myxoedema clearly favoured the development of CHD. Despite increased atherosclerosis and myocardial ischemia, the incidence
of myocardial infarcts was not increased, except after therapy.
This apparently paradoxical contrast illustrates the protective
effect of hypothyroidism on the cardiac muscle, which benefits
from reduced metabolic needs and reduced activity.

PREMYXOEDEMA

Autoimmune atrophic thyroiditis (AAT), characterized by the
presence of humoral and cellular immune reactions against the
thyroid and anomalies of iodine metabolism, may be considered
as a condition of premyxoedema[28]. In this disorder, thyroid
hormone levels are normal but the frequent slightly elevated TSH
levels and/or the exaggerated TSH secretory response to TRH
suggest that euthyroidism is solely maintained through hyper-
stimulation of thyroid cells by thyrotropin. This is in accordance with the supranormal pituitary TSH content found at
necropsy of patients with AAT[29].

Contradictory results have been obtained in different population studies concerning the prevalence of hyperlipidemia in AAT.
Fowler et al.[30] have considered hypercholesterolemia as an essential, not sex-linked biological feature of premyxoedema. In
our own studies however, only female patients with antithyroid
antibodies had higher cholesterol levels when compared with
paired controls[31]. Other population surveys failed to find any
association between premyxoedema and high cholesterol or triglyceride levels[22,32]. Conversely in one study[33] where hyperlipi-

demic patients of different types were investigated for the presence of premyxoedema, one third, principally men, had high
titers of thyroid antibodies and/or high serum TSH levels.
Similarly an association was found between hyperlipidemia (essentially hypertriglyceridemia) and high TSH levels in women, sur-
vivors of myocardial infarction[34].

The significance of these discrepant findings remains difficult
to explain. The hypothesis, put forward by Baschieri et al.[33],
that latent thyroid failure induces clearcut hyperlipoproteinemia
only in genetically prone subjects might conciliate all the data.
Moreover, it might be extended to myxoedema and partially explain
why only 50 % of true hypothyroid patients are hyperlipidemic[5]
and why type IIa is not the only hyperlipoproteinemia encountered
in this disease. This hypothesis is further strenghtened by a
study in a beagle dog family with hypercholesterolemia, which
showed that overt hypothyroidism was at the origin of the lipid
disturbance. However, beagles with thyroiditis and depressed
thyroid function, but not belonging to this family, showed no
alteration of their cholesterolemia[35].

The existence of an association between CHD and premyxoedema,
independent of the presence of other risk factors, has been
advocated in different studies[31,32,36]. Some authors however
denied its reality[37]. Our first studies in hospitalized patients[31,36] showed that CHD was related to the presence of
thyroid antibodies in females, but not in males; on the contrary,
in necropsies of patients who died with a myocardial infarction,
an increased prevalence of thyroid lymphocytic infiltrates, an
histological feature of thyroiditis, was present in females and
males. Our latest study[38] was conducted on a male population,

aged 50 to 69 years, in West and East Finland. At the initial
survey in 1969, thyroid autoantibodies were found in 5.3 % of
247 men from West Finland and in 5.3 % of 207 men from East
Finland who were free from CHD. In men with evidence of CHD,
the prevalence of thyroid autoantibodies was 18 % (6/32) in
West Finland and 8 % (5/62) in East Finland; the association
was significant in West Finland only. Among the men who were
CHD-free but had thyroid autoantibodies in 1969, CHD developed
by 1974 in 4/13 (31 %) in West Finland and in 5/11 (45 %) in
East Finland. The 5-year incidences of CHD in those without
thyroid autoantibodies were 21 % in West Finland and 24 % in
East Finland. These findings indicate that the presence of
asymptomatic thyroid autoimmunity is a predictor of subsequent
development of CHD in men in their sixth and seventh decades
and that it should be added to the other known risk factors.

The hypothesis first proposed by us[36] that the hypercholesterolemia of premyxoedema could be responsible for the high
prevalence of CHD in this disease is no longer tenable. Indeed,
in our male patients with AAT hypercholesterolemia was not present and in the necropsy material the thyroid focal lymphocytic
infiltrates were often too small to have induced even mild hypothyroidism. Moreover, premyxoedema is a risk factor for the
development of CHD in these age groups where total cholesterol
levels are no longer considered to increase CHD incidence[39,40].
Other possible explanations might involve the action of circulating immune complexes[41], that of high concentrations of TSH[36],
or hypothetical modifications in high-density lipoprotein (HDL)
cholesterol levels. Finally some common factors, of genetic
origin, might be responsible for the development of metabolic

114

disorders leading both to atherosclerosis and to thyroid auto-immune disease.

ACKNOWLEDGMENTS

This work was supported by a grant from the National Research Council of Belgium (FNRS-FGWO).

R e f e r e n c e s

1. Man, E.B., Gildea, E.F. and Peters, J.P. (1940) J. clin. Invest., 19, 43

2. Peters, J.P. and Man, E.B. (1950) J. clin. Invest., 29, 1

3. Bastenie, P.A., Bonnyns, M. and Vanhaelst, L. (1972) In Thyroiditis and thyroid function. Bastenie, P.A. and Ermans, A.M. (eds), Pregamon Press, Oxford, p. 211

4. Bastenie, P.A., Neve, P., Bonnyns, M., Vanhaelst, L. and Chailly, P. (1967) Lancet i, 915

5. Koppers, L.E. and Palumbo, P.J. (1972) Med. Clin. N. Amer., 56, 1013

6. Myant, N.B. (1964) In Lipid Pharmacology. Paoletti, R. (ed), Academic Press Inc., New York, p. 299

7. Walton, K.W., Scott, P.J., Dykes, P.W. and Davies, J.W.L. (1965) Clin. Sci., 29, 217

8. Furth, E.D., Becker, D.V. and Schwartz, M.S. (1963) J. clin. Endocrinol. Metab., 23, 1130

9. Sandhofer, F., Sailer, S. and Braunsteiner, H. (1966) Klin. Wschr., 44, 433

10. Kirkeby, K. (1968) Acta endocrinol., 59, 555

11. Tulloch, B.P., Lewis, B. and Russel Fraser, T. (1973) Lancet i, 391

12. Nikkilä, E.A. and Kekki, M. (1972) J. clin. Invest., 51, 2103

13. Krishna, G., Hynie, S. and Brodie, B.B. (1968) Proc. Nat. Acad. Sci., 59, 884

14. Symmes, J.C., Lenkei, S.S.C. and Berman, N.D. (1977) Canad. Med. Assoc. J., 117, 489

15. Kotler, M.N., Michaelides, K.M. and Bouchard, R.J. (1977) Arch. Intern. Med., 132, 723

16. Proskey, A.J., Saksena, F. and Towne, W.D. (1977) Chest, 72, 109

17. Malmros, H. and Swahn, B. (1953) Acta Med. Scand., 145, 361

18. Kurland, G.S., Lucas, J.L. and Freedberg, A.S. (1961) J. Lab. Clin. Med., 57, 574

19. Lipsky, R.S., Bondy, P.K., Man, E.B. and McGuire, J.S. (1955) J. clin. Invest., 34, 950

20. Miettinen, T.A. (1968) J. Lab. Clin. Med., 71, 737

21. Wayne, E.J. (1960) Brit. Med. J., I, 78

22. Kutty, K.M., Bryant, D.G. and Farid, N.R. (1978) J. clin. Endocrinol. Metab., 46, 55

23. Pykälisto, O., Goldberg, A.P. and Brunzell, J.D. (1976)

24. Hazzard, W.R. and Bierman, E.I. (1972) Arch. Intern. Med., 130, 822

25. Lasser, N.L., Burns, J. and Solar, S. (1974) In Atherosclerosis III. Schettler, G. and Weizel, A. (eds), Springer Verlag, Berlin, p. 621

26. Goodman, H.M. and Bray, G.A. (1966) Amer. J. Physiol., 210, 1053

27. Vanhaelst, L., Neve, P., Chailly, P. and Bastenie, P.A. (1967) Lancet ii, 800

28. Bastenie, P.A., Bonnyns, M., Ermans, A.M., Neve, P. and Van-

haelst, L. (1972) In Thyroiditis and thyroid function. Bastenie, P.A. and Ermans, A.M. (eds), Pergamon Press, Oxford,
p. 229

29. Bonnyns, M., Pasteels, J.L., Herlant, M., Vanhaelst, L. and
Bastenie, P.A. (1972) J. clin. Endocrinol. Metab., 35, 722

30. Fowler, P.B.S., Swale, J. and Andrews, H. (1970) Lancet ii,
488

31. Bastenie, P.A., Vanhaelst, L., Bonnyns, M., Nève, P. and
Staquet, M. (1971) Lancet i, 203

32. Tunbridge, W.G.M., Evered, D.C., Hall, R., Appleton, D.,
Brewis, M., Clark, F., Grimley-Evans, J., Young, E., Bird, T.
and Smith, P.A. (1977) Clin. Endocrinol., 7, 495

33. Baschieri, L., Fellin, R., Martino, E., Crepaldi, G., Pin-
chera, A., Cariferri, R., Macchia, E. and Sardano, G. (1975)
Rev. franç. Endocr. clin., 16, 211

34. Green, W.L., Hazzard, W.R. and Hershman, J.M. (1976) Metabolism, 25, 465

35. Manning, P.J., Corwin, L.A. and Middleton, C.C. (1973) Exp.
Mol. Path., 19, 378

36. Bastenie, P.A., Vanhaelst, L. and Nève, P. (1967) Lancet ii,
1221

37. Heinonen, O.P., Gordin, A., Aho, K., Punsar, S., Pyorala, K.
and Puro, K. (1972) Lancet i, 785

38. Bastenie, P.A., Vanhaelst, L., Golstein, J., Smets, Ph.,
Keys, A., Karvonen, M.J. and Punsar, S. (1977) Lancet ii, 155

39. Gordon, T., Castelli, W.P., Hjortland, M.C., Kannel, W.B. and
Dawber, T.R. (1977) Amer. J. Med., 62, 707

40. Carlson, L.A. and Böttiger, L.E. (1962) Lancet i, 865

41. The Lancet Editorial (1977), Lancet ii, 173

Lipoprotein Metabolism and Endocrine Regulation
L.W. Hessel and H.M.J. Krans editors
© ECSC, EEC, EAEC, Brussels-Luxembourg, 1979
Published by Elsevier/North-Holland Biomedical Press-Amsterdam

THE ROLE OF CORTISOL IN DIRECTION OF SUBSTRATE FLOW

D.G. JOHNSTON, A. POSTLE[*] A.J. BARNES[+] K.G.M.M. ALBERTI[°]

Endocrine Unit, Royal Victoria Infirmary, Newcastle upon Tyne NE1 4LP, U.K.

*Department of Chemical Pathology and Human Metabolism, General Hospital,
 Southampton, SO9 4XY, U.K.

+Department of Medicine, Royal Postgraduate Medical School, Hammersmith
 Hospital, London W12 OHS, U.K.

° Department of Clinical Biochemistry, Royal Victoria Infirmary, Newcastle upon
 Tyne, NE1 4LP, U.K.

ABSTRACT

    Cortisol is a major stress hormone but differs from other catabolic hormones
in that its actions on intermediary metabolism are delayed and sustained.
Chronic excessive cortisol secretion produces fasting hyperglycaemia by effects
on both glucose production and utilisation. Circulating concentrations of the
gluconeogenic precursors, lactate and pyruvate, are increased and probably
derived largely from α-keto acid moities from deaminated amino acids. Circulating concentrations of alanine, the principal glucogenic amino acid, are also
raised as a result of a glucocorticoid-induced increase in muscle free amino
acid pool and release of amino acids into the circulation. In addition to
an increase in precursor supply for glucose production, glucocorticoids cause
induction of several key hepatic gluconeogenic enzymes. Fasting hyperglycaemia
occurs despite a rise in circulating insulin concentrations suggesting insulin
resistance. Cortisol antagonism of peripheral insulin action is particularly
important in the intolerance observed to oral or intravenous glucose and the
hyperglycaemia seen after normal meals.

    The influence of glucocorticoids on fat metabolism is complex and the
effects are dependent on the insulin response. Thus in normal subjects given
ACTH chronically or in patients with Cushing's syndrome, cortisol produces
no appreciable change in plasma NEFA or blood ketone body levels. After an
initial fall in serum triglyceride, chronic hypercortisolaemia results in a
rise in triglyceride concentrations, which correlates with peripheral insulin
levels. In insulin-deprived diabetic subjects, or in normal subjects rendered
insulin deficient by somatostatin infusion, chronic glucocorticoid excess has
little effect on plasma NEFA concentrations. However in the absence of a
normal insulin response, there is an exaggerated rise in blood ketone body

concentrations which is not attributable to increased substrate supply. In
insulin-deficient man, chronic glucocorticoid excess increases channelling of
NEFA metabolism into ketogenic pathways.

INTRODUCTION

An important role for cortisol in intermediary metabolism has been known
for many years since the early descriptions of the clinical syndromes of
cortisol excess and deficiency. Thus Cushing's syndrome is associated with
obesity, premature vascular disease, muscle wasting and glucose intolerance
and Addison's disease with weight loss, fatigue and occasional hypoglycaemia.
Glucocorticoids were, however, labelled merely as "permissive" by Ingle (1951)
on the basis of investigations on their role in the nitrogen loss of experimental injury[1] and this term has subsequently been applied to many of their
metabolic effects. It is only recently that a more active role for cortisol
has again been sought and some of the biochemical mechanisms involved in glucocorticoid-induced effects elucidated.

Hypercortisolaemia in normal subjects is associated with increased insulin
secretion either as a result of hyperglycaemia or a direct pancreatic action[2].
Insulin hypersecretion may modify the response to cortisol, particularly the
effects on adipose tissue and ketone body metabolism. We have therefore
examined some of the metabolic actions of cortisol in both normal and insulin-
deficient man and in patients with Cushing's syndrome.

TABLE 1

EXPERIMENTAL MODELS

Insulin present	Insulin deficient
Normal subjects after tetracosactrin administration	Somatostatin infusion after tetraco-sactrin administration to normal subjects
Cushing's syndrome	Juvenile-onset diabetics after gluco-corticoid administration

In addition, we shall report some preliminary work on hepatic lipogenesis in
rats rendered glucocorticoid deficient by adrenalectomy or hypercortisolaemic
by administration of tetracosactrin-depot.

NORMAL MAN

Administration of tetracosactrin-depot

The metabolic actions of cortisol are dependent on entry of the steroid molecule into the cell with binding by specific cytoplasmic and nuclear proteins and subsequent changes in DNA and RNA synthesis. Thus, unlike glucagon and catecholamines, there is a delay of several hours between an increase in plasma cortisol levels and the onset of metabolic effects. Infusion of cortisol into normal subjects to produce pathophysiological serum levels for 4 h has little effect on circulating metabolites. Similarly, injection of tetracosactrin 250 ug intramuscularly to transiently increase endogenous cortisol secretion has no effect on blood metabolites measured over the succeeding 3 hours. It should be remembered however that in pathological states increased cortisol secretion may persist for hours or days. We have therefore studied the long-term effects of cortisol excess by administration of tetracosactrin-depot, 1 mg daily intramuscularly for 2-3 days in normal subjects. Serum cortisol levels produced were in the upper physiological range, 900-1400 nmol/l.

Two to three days of hypercortisolaemia produced a rise in fasting blood glucose from 5.0 to 7.0 mmol/l, despite a doubling of fasting serum insulin levels. Circulating concentrations of the gluconeogenic precursors, lactate, pyruvate and alanine, were also raised. The rise in lactate and pyruvate may derive from α-keto-acid moieties from deaminated amino acids as well as from glycolysis. Cortisol causes a marked increase in the free amino acid pool in muscle and release of amino acids into the circulation[3,4] and as alanine and glutamate are the principal amino acids released[5,6], the rise in blood alanine concentration is accounted for.

Fasting hyperglycaemia in situations of cortisol excess has several mechanisms. Not only is the supply of gluconeogenic precursors increased but there is increased activity of hepatic aminotransferases and an increase in activity of key gluconeogenic enzymes[7]. Hepatic glucose output is increased but there is in addition a decrease in glucose uptake by peripheral tissues[8] despite peripheral hyperinsulinaemia. This effect on peripheral glucose utilisation has been demonstrated for muscle[9], adipose tissue[10], skin[11] and lymphoid tissue[8].

Plasma NEFA concentrations were unaffected by 2-3 days tetracosactrin administration. Glucocorticoids in vitro have a marked lipolytic action[12] after a long period of 1-2 hours[13] on rat epididymal adipose tissue but enhanced lipolysis is not seen after prolonged glucocorticoid administration

in vivo[14]. The absence of a lipolytic effect in vivo in animals and normal
man is likely to be due to feedback inhibition of lipolysis secondary to
the increase in insulin secretion. No change in ketone body concentrations
was observed after tetracosactrin. Interestingly, fasting serum triglyceride
levels decreased by 50% after 2-3 days hypercortisolaemia. This fall in triglyceride concentration in the first few days of hypercortisolaemia has been
noted previously in rabbits[15] in which the phase persists for 48 h and is
followed in 5 days by development of hyperlipidaemia associated with appearance
in plasma of abnormally large VLDL molecules. The biphasic response has been
noted also in man[16,17] but the mechanism is uncertain. Suppression of
hepatic lipoprotein secretion has been postulated to explain the early fall[18]
although an effect on peripheral triglyceride uptake has not been investigated.
Indeed recent in vitro studies using abdominal wall human adipose tissue
cultures have shown an increase in lipoprotein lipase activity which is
dependent on both hydrocortisone and insulin for its appearance (Cigolini, M.,
personal communication).

CUSHING'S SYNDROME

To investigate the metabolic effects of more prolonged hypercortisolaemia,
we have studied a group of patients with Cushing's syndrome in whom the
clinical history suggested presence of the disease for 6 months to 2 years.
Six patients were compared with ten age and sex matched controls. Basal
fasting samples were obtained from all subjects at 08.30 h and at half
hourly intervals until 20.00 h. Breakfast was consumed at 08.30 h with
lunch at 12.00 h and evening meal at 18.00 h. Snacks were taken at 10.30 h
and 15.00 h and all meals were standard hospital meals containing approximately
45% carbohydrate, 15% protein and 40% fat. Subjects were encouraged to be
mobile during the study period.

Basal blood glucose concentrations were the same in controls and subjects
with Cushing's syndrome (4.8 $\pm$ 0.1 vs 5.1 $\pm$ 0.3 mmol/l respectively) although
fasting serum insulin concentrations were raised (6.7 $\pm$ 0.9 vs 12.6 $\pm$ 2.2 mU/l.
Marked hyperglycaemia however occurred after meals, particularly breakfast
and this was associated with hyperinsulinaemia, in some subjects of gross
degree with levels of up to 460 mU/l. This normal fasting blood glucose in
Cushing's syndrome is perhaps surprising in view of the fasting hyperglycaemia
observed after 2-3 days of cortisol excess in normal subjects. In normal
subjects however, administration of exogenous glucocorticoid results in
diminished glucose tolerance which improves during chronic glucocorticoid

treatment[19,20]. This adaptation to glucocorticoid excess has been observed also in dogs[21], and may be related to changes in insulin receptor binding. Thus administration of prednisone to rats for one week markedly decreases insulin binding to both adipocytes and hepatocytes but after three weeks prednisone administration, insulin binding returns to near normal levels, at least in adipocytes[22]. Decreased insulin binding and consequent insulin resistance may be partially responsible for the initial period of fasting hyperglycaemia in chronic cortisol excess in normal subjects with a return towards normal with more prolonged exposure. In view of the persisting hyperinsulinaemia however, considerable insulin resistance must remain and it is likely that changes in insulin binding are only a part of the adaptation response. This is not surprising in view of the complex actions of cortisol on hepatic gluconeogenesis and effects on peripheral glucose uptake which are independent of insulin[8].

In patients with Cushing's syndrome, concentrations of the gluconeogenic precursors lactate and pyruvate were elevated and the normal rise in concentration of these metabolites with meals was exaggerated. Blood alanine concentrations were also raised throughout the study period. Thus changes in blood concentrations of gluconeogenic precursors were similar with short or long term exposure to hypercortisolaemia.

Basal plasma glucagon concentrations were raised in patients with Cushing's syndrome (15.7 $\pm$ 2.1 vs 11.9 $\pm$ 1.0 pmol/l) and hyperglucagonaemia persisted throughout the day. Administration of tetracosactrin to normal subjects did not produce a significant change in plasma glucagon levels. Basal glucagon concentrations have been found to be increased after three days dexamethasone treatment in normal subjects and the glucagon response to intravenous alanine was exaggerated[4]. The importance of this hyperglucagonaemia in blood glucose homeostasis is uncertain. Although glucagon levels are raised in Cushing's syndrome, insulin is increased relatively more, so that the insulin:glucagon ratio in hypercortisolaemia is consistently higher than controls. However in view of the resistance to insulin action and the known effects of glucocorticoids to sensitise and enhance the hepatic response to the gluconeogenic effects of glucagon[23,24], glucagon may play some role in the observed basal hyperglycaemia. There is only slender evidence that glucagon has a significant effect on disposal of ingested carbohydrate[25] and it is unlikely to be of major importance in the hyperglycaemia after meals in Cushing's syndrome. Glucagon is likely to have little importance in the lipid abnormalities seen in Cushing's syndrome in view of the coexistent hyperinsulinaemia which may antagonise the glucagon effects.

Blood ketone body concentrations did not differ markedly between controls
and patients with Cushing's syndrome. A consistent feature of the normal
diurnal blood ketone body variation is a rise in the late afternoon before
the evening meal. The mechanism of this at present is uncertain but it is
not seen in patients with Cushing's syndrome. Plasma NEFA concentrations
did not differ in the two groups. Similarly, normal fasting NEFA concentrations
have been found by Birkenhäger and colleagues[26] although NEFA turnover was
found to be decreased when expressed in terms of body weight. They attributed
these findings to suppression of lipolysis as a consequence of hyperinsulinaemia.

Fasting serum triglyceride concentration was raised in patients with
Cushing's syndrome (2.2 ± 0.4 vs 0.8 ± 0.3 mmol/l) and hypertriglyceridaemia
persisted throughout the study period. Within the Cushing's group, there
was however a wide scatter of triglyceride levels with two subjects having
values consistently in the normal range and one subject showing marked
hypertriglyceridaemia reaching a peak after the evening meal of 13.8 mmol/l.
There was no correlation between serum triglyceride and plasma glucagon
concentrations, suggesting that the hypotriglyceridaemic effect of glucagon
was of little importance in this situation. Triglyceride values did not
correlate with cortisol but did correlate positively with serum insulin concentrations, suggesting a role for insulin.

The mechanism of hypertriglyceridaemia is likely to be complex. Chronic
glucocorticoid treatment in rats and mice[27] increases serum triglyceride
levels associated with an increase in hepatic VLDL production, although a
decrease in triglyceride clearance has also been demonstrated[28]. A direct
effect of cortisol to stimulate triglyceride release by the isolated perfused
liver has also been shown although this effect is not marked and requires
a critical cortisol concentration in the perfusate[18].

Insulin has opposing effects to increase and decrease serum triglyceride
levels and the outcome must reflect a balance between these actions. Hyperinsulinaemia in non-diabetic subjects may limit corticoid-induced lipolysis
and thus decrease NEFA supply for triglyceride synthesis. In addition,
insulin increases triglyceride uptake from plasma, at least in diabetic subjects, by actions on lipoprotein lipase and also by stimulating reesterification
of fatty acid, a potentially rate limiting event in triglyceride uptake[29,30].
These actions of insulin tend to decrease serum triglyceride levels and are
opposed by the direct hepatic effects of insulin to increase lipogenesis
and triglyceride formation. Thus insulin stimulates fatty acid synthesis

from glucose by liver slices from insulin-deficient rats[31] and isolated
perfused livers from diabetic animals show impaired fatty acid synthesis[32],
impaired triglyceride formation[33] and impaired apolipoprotein production[34].
A hypertriglycerideaemic role for hyperinsulinaemia in non-diabetic states
is however more difficult to find. Thus liver slices from normal rats do
not show increased triglyceride synthesis when insulin is added in vitro[35];
pretreatment of normal rats with insulin increased triglyceride secretion
by the isolated perfused liver in one study, particularly when fructose was
present in the perfusate[36], but other studies have failed to demonstrate
this effect[37,38]. In normal man, insulin administration does not increase
incorporation of labelled palmitate into plasma triglyceride[39,40]. The most
convincing evidence for a role for insulin in increasing triglyceride
concentrations is the substantial fall in triglyceride levels observed after
diazoxide administration to hypertriglyceridaemic patients[41].

Thus the overall effect of chronic glucocorticoid excess, whether a direct
effect of glucocorticoid, insulin or a combination of the two, is increased
triglyceride formation and a possible decrease in triglyceride clearance
resulting in increased serum triglyceride levels. In the presence of a
normal insulin response, hypercortisolaemia has little effect on ketone body
metabolism.

INSULIN DEFICIENCY

Many pathophysiological situations in man associated with increased
cortisol secretion are associated also with an absolute or relative decrease
in insulin secretion. This is evident in development of diabetic ketoacidosis
and also occurs in stress situations, e.g. trauma and surgical operations,
in which insulin secretion is diminished probably as a result of co-existent
catecholamine secretion or increased sympathetic drive.

In view of the importance of increased insulin secretion in modifying
the effects of glucocorticoid excess we have looked further at insulin-
deficient man using two experimental models; firstly, normal subjects were
rendered artificially insulin deficient by infusion of somatostatin before
and after 2-3 days tetracosactrin administration; secondly, hypophysectomised
insulin-dependent diabetics were studied during a 12 h period of insulin
deprivation on two occasions, receiving their normal glucocorticoid replacement therapy on the first occasion and three times their usual replacement
on the second.

Somatostatin infusion

Five normal subjects were studied after an overnight fast. They received an infusion of 0.154 molar saline or synthetic linear somatostatin, 100 ug/h for 3.5 h and each infusion was performed before and after 2-3 days administration of tetracosactrin-depot, 1 mg I.M. daily[42].

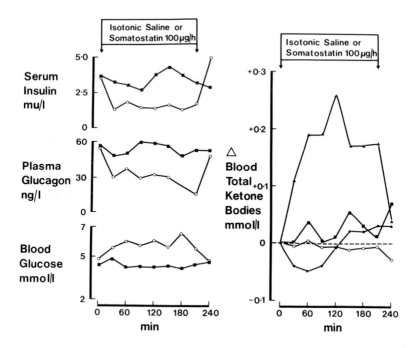

Fig. la. Effect of infusion of 0.154 molar saline (■) or somatostatin 100 ug/h (O) on serum insulin, plasma glucagon and blood glucose concentrations in one normal subject.

Fig. lb. Effect of infusion of 0.154 molar saline before (O) and after (●) 3 days tetracosactrin-depot, 1 mg I.M. daily, and effect of somatostatin infusion 100 ug/h before (■) and after (▲) 3 days tetracosactrin-depot 1 mg I.M. daily, on blood total ketone body concentration, measured as the sum of 3-hydroxybutyrate and acetoacetate.

Somatostatin infusion caused a 50% decrease in circulating insulin levels (Fig.1a) compared with saline both before and after tetracosactrin. Plasma glucagon concentrations showed a similar fall and serum growth hormone levels were below the detection limits of the assay. Somatostatin caused an initial fall in blood glucose in the first 60 min. followed by a rise in glucose compared with saline towards the end of the infusion period, reflecting insulin deficiency. The change in glucose concentration with somatostatin infusion was similar before and after tetracosactrin.

Saline infusion before and after tetracosactrin administration produced no change in ketone body concentrations over the study period (Fig.1b). Somatostatin infusion in untreated subjects produced a small rise in ketone body concentrations but after prior administration of tetracosactrin-depot, blood ketone body concentrations showed a pronounced and sustained rise. NEFA concentrations during somatostatin infusion before and after tetracosactrin-depot were similar, so the increased ketone body levels seen after tetra-cosactrin cannot be explained solely on the basis of increased substrate supply.

Hypophysectomised diabetics

Somatostatin infusion caused suppression of glucagon and growth hormone secretion in addition to insulin in normal man while catabolic states with glucocorticoid hypersecretion are associated with normal or elevated con-centrations of glucagon and growth hormone. Furthermore it is possible that somatostatin exerts a direct effect on ketogenesis in hypercortisolaemia independent of its role in modifying hormone secretion. We have therefore used a further experimental model to investigate the ketogenic effect of cortisol in man.

Insulin-dependent diabetics received a continuous intravenous insulin infusion for 20 h to maintain normoglycaemia prior to study[43]. They were fasted for 12 h and then deprived of insulin for a further 12 h study period during which they remained fasting and blood samples were taken for metabolite estimation. Five patients with normal pituitary function were compared with five diabetics who had previously undergone pituitary ablation for retino-pathy. Pituitary ablated patients were studied on two occasions; on one occasion they received their normal glucocorticoid replacement therapy prior to study and cortisol levels were maintained within the normal range by hydrocortisone infusion during the period of fasting; on a second occasion they received three times their normal glucocorticoid replacement therapy for two days before the study period and plasma cortisol levels were elevated by hydrocortisone infusion in the fasting period to 1000-1500 nmol/l.

Blood glucose rose sharply from 5.2 to 15.5 mmol/l during the 12 h period of insulin deprivation in diabetics with intact pituitary function. The blood glucose rise in pituitary-ablated subjects on "normal" glucocorticoid replacement therapy was delayed and diminished (4.3 to 9.7 mmol/l after 12 h). High-dose glucocorticoid replacement increased the glucose rise in pituitary ablated subjects (4.8 to 13.6 mmol/l) but values remained lower than those obtained in diabetics with intact pituitary function. Growth hormone levels were below the detection limit for the assay in pituitary-ablated subjects and it is likely that growth hormone deficiency was responsible for this difference.

Ketone body levels rose briskly in diabetic subjects with intact pituitary function over the 12 h period of insulin deprivation (0.15 to 4.63 mmol/l). The rise in ketones was diminished in pituitary ablated subjects on "normal" glucocorticoid replacement (0.11 to 1.43 mmol/l). High glucocorticoid dosage increased the ketone response (0.16 to 1.91 mmol/l) but, as for glucose, values did not achieve those found in diabetics with intact pituitary function, again possibly reflecting growth hormone deficiency. NEFA concentrations after insulin deprivation were lower than those obtained in diabetics with intact pituitaries in hypophysectomised subjects, irrespective of glucocorticoid replacement dose (intact pituitary 1.36 mmol/l:normal glucocorticoid replacement 0.75 mmol/l:high glucocorticoid replacement 0.74 mmol/l).

Thus a ketogenic effect of cortisol was evident in this experimental situation as with somatostatin-induced insulin deficiency and in both experimental situations, the effect appeared independent of NEFA substrate supply.

Other evidence for a ketogenic effect of cortisol in insulin-deficiency

Increased cortisol secretion and decreased insulin secretion are of major importance in the stress response and in the early phase after injury, plasma cortisol levels correlate with blood concentrations of ketone bodies, NEFA and gluconeogenic precursors[44]. A ketogenic action of cortisol in diabetes has been suggested on the basis of observations in both man and animals. Thus hypophysectomy[45] or adrenalectomy[46] in rats may retard the development of ketoacidosis in insulin-deprived diabetic animals and administration of corticosterone to adrenalectomised alloxan-diabetic rats restores their ketogenic potential[47]. The development of diabetic ketoacidosis in both rats[47] and man[48] is associated with a progressive rise in plasma corticosterone and cortisol concentrations respectively. Furthermore in insulin-dependent diabetic man maintained on fixed insulin therapy, artificially raising and lowering the plasma cortisol concentration increases and decreases blood ketone body concentrations respectively[49].

Mechanism of cortisol-induced ketogenesis in insulin-deficiency

Control of ketogenesis. An adequate supply of substrate in the form of NEFA of adipose tissue origin is necessary for ketogenesis to progress. In vivo ketogenic states, e.g. starvation, diabetes, are associated with high circulating NEFA concentrations. Hormonal control of lipolysis is thus an important mechanism in control of ketogenesis but entry of fatty acid into the hepatocyte appears to be concentration dependent and is not under hormonal control[50]. After entry, fatty acids are converted to fatty acyl CoA after which two major metabolic pathways are available. Fatty acyl CoA may be converted to triglyceride after esterification to triacylglycerol in the cytosol depending on esterase activity and glycerol-1-phosphate availability. Alternatively fatty acyl CoA may enter the mito-chondria under the influence of carnitine acyl transferases 1 and 11. This transfer of fatty acyl CoA across the mitochondial membrane can be influenced by carnitine acyl transferase activity and total carnitine content[51]. It has recently been reported that carnitine acyl transferase 1 is inhibited by malonyl CoA, the first intermediate specific to fatty acid synthesis[52]. Transfer of fatty acyl-CoA into mitochondria is a major regulatory step in ketogenesis.

Within the mitochondria, fatty acyl CoA is degraded by β-oxidation to acetyl CoA and the rate of β-oxidation is linked to the rate of gluconeo-genesis so that inhibition of gluconeogenesis is associated with inhibition of β-oxidation and hence ketogenesis[53]. The final step in ketogenesis is form-ation of 3-hydroxy -3 methylglutaryl-CoA from acetyl CoA with subsequent cleavage to acetoacetate. Overall, entry of fatty acyl-CoA into the mitochondria is probably more important in the regulation of ketogenesis than the intramitochondrial steps[54].

Effects of insulin-deficiency. Insulin deficiency increases ketogenesis largely through an increase in substrate supply. The effect of insulin on adipose tissue is to suppress lipolysis and increase re-esterification of fatty acids through an increase in glucose entry into the cell with a

consequent increase in glycerol-l-phosphate availability. Adipose tissue
is exquisitely sensitive to small changes in circulating insulin concentrations with an increase of 10 mU/l above the fasting level sharply decreasing
NEFA release[55].

A direct hepatic effect of insulin to decrease ketogenesis is likely but
more difficult to demonstrate in view of the potent effects on lipolysis. A
difference in NEFA disposal in perfused livers from fed animals, compared
with fasted or diabetic, has been demonstrated by numerous workers[56,57,50].
Thus it was observed that livers from fasted or diabetic animals primarily
oxidised fatty acids to ketone bodies while in livers from fed animals the
major metabolic fate was re-esterification. A direct hepatic action of insulin
to produce these effects has been difficult to establish. Thus Haft and
Miller (1958) showed that insulin would inhibit ketogenesis in vitro[58] but
other workers have failed to demonstrate this effect. Insulin may inhibit
the stimulatory effect of glucagon on ketogenesis although no effect could
be shown when plasma NEFA were artificially maintained at an increased
concentration[60]. Postulated mechanisms for an hepatic anti-ketogenic action
of insulin include; stimulation of acetyl CoA carboxylase with increased
formation of malonyl CoA which inhibits carnitine acyl transferase 1;[52]
inhibition of intrahepatic triacyl-glycerol lipases[59]; enhanced glycerol-1-
phosphate formation although the bulk of evidence is against this[51].

Effects of cortisol. Cortisol in vitro has a lipolytic effect and in
insulin-deficiency, may enhance ketogenesis by increasing substrate supply.
That this is not a major factor in ketogenesis however is suggested by the
ketogenic effects of glucocorticoid excess during somatostatin infusion
in normal man and during insulin-deprivation in hypophysectomised diabetics
when plasma NEFA concentrations were similar in normal and hypercortisolaemic
states. This suggests a direct hepatic action.

Shafrir and colleagues have postulated that in normal animals, glucocorticoids divert hepatic metabolism to triglyceride formation and away from
ketogenesis by an insulin-induced increase in acetyl CoA carboxylase activity
and increase in hepatic fatty acid synthesis[61]. This would certainly lead
to an increase in malonyl CoA production with consequent inhibition of
carnitine acyltransferace 1 activity. We have confirmed Shafrir's findings
using a rather different animal model.

Normal rats, adrenalectomised rats and rats treated with tetracosactrin-
depot 50 ug/100 g body weight for 3 days were meal-fed for 2 h/day. In vivo
fatty acid biosynthesis was measured by $3H_2O$ incorporation and acetyl CoA

carboxylase activity measured by $14CO_2$ fixation before and after citrate activation. Rats were sacrificed immediately after feeding. After tetracosactrin, hepatic fatty acid biosynthesis increased from 49 to 64 ug atoms H/g liver/h associated with a rise in acetyl CoA carboxylase activity. This was shown by Shafrir to be insulin dependent[61]. Adrenalectomised animals had low rates of fatty acid synthesis and low enzyme activity. This insulin dependent effect of cortisol to increase hepatic lipogenesis may be of importance in production of the hypertriglyceridaemia of glucocorticoid excess in fed animals, particularly in the rat consuming a high carbohydrate diet. It is very unlikely to be a major factor in the fasting state when hepatic lipogenesis is minimal, the rate of β-oxidation high and triglyceride synthesis is derived almost exclusively from fatty acids of adipose tissue origin. In the fasting state, an effect of cortisol and insulin in diverting acetyl CoA to fatty acid synthesis and hence lipogenesis is therefore unlikely to be a major controlling influence on the rate of ketogenesis. The insulin-dependent effect on acetyl CoA carboxylase with a consequent increase in malonyl CoA production may however be important in decreasing fatty acyl CoA transfer across the mitochondrial membrane and lack of this effect in insulin-deficiency may play some role in the ketogenesis of fasting or diabetes.

It is possible that cortisol may potentiate the actions of glucagon to increase ketogenesis and decrease hepatic lipogenesis. Glucagon has potent ketogenic effects possibly through inhibition of acetyl CoA carboxylase with a consequent decrease in hepatic malonyl CoA concentration[52,62]. In our experiments in fed rats adrenalectomy abolished the action of exogenous glucagon (1 mg/kg body weight, subcutaneously) to decrease hepatic lipogenesis. This was not related to glycogen depletion because although liver glycogen was decreased in adrenalectomised animals, the fall in hepatic glycogen content after glucagon injection was comparable in normal and adrenalectomised animals. Glucocorticoids thus appear to be necessary for the anti-lipogenic actions of glucagon in addition to the known effects of glucagon on gluconeogenesis. Pretreatment with ACTH however did not enhance the antilipogenic action of glucagon suggesting that the role of glucocorticoids may be indeed permissive in this respect. In addition, a decrease in lipogenesis does not necessarily imply an increase in ketogenesis. Further evidence against a role for glucocorticoids potentiating the ketogenic action of glucagon comes from the human studies. Thus stomatostatin infusion suppressed glucagon as well as insulin secretion but the ketogenic effect of cortisol excess was still evident.

CONCLUSIONS

Glucocorticoids play a more direct role in intermediary metabolism than a merely "permissive" function for the action of other controlling factors. They are directly important in mobilisation of fuels of carbohydrate, protein and lipid origin and influence the subsequent metabolic fate of these fuels. The overall metabolic effect of glucocorticoids is dependent on the secretory capacity for other catabolic and the anabolic hormones, with insulin exerting the major modifying influence. Further work on the biochemical mechanisms involved in glucocorticoid effects, particularly the actions on hepatic lipid metabolism, is urgently needed.

ACKNOWLEDGEMENTS

D.G. Johnston was the recipient of a Medical Research Council Fellowship.

REFERENCES

1. Ingle, D.J. (1951) Parameters of metabolic problems, Recent Prog. Horm. Res., 6, 159-194.

2. Malaisse, W.J., Malaisse-Lagae, F., (1967) Insulin secretion in vitro by pancreatic tissue from normal, adrenalectomised and cortisol-treated rats, Proc. Soc. Exp. Biol. Med., 124, 924-928.

3. Kaplin, S.A. and Shimizu, C.S.N. (1963) Effects of cortisol on amino acids in skeletal muscle and plasma, Endocrinology, 72, 267-272.

4. Wise, J.K ., Hendler, R. and Felig,P. (1973) Influence of glucocorticoids on glucagon secretion and plasma amino acid concentrations in man, J. Clin. Invest. 52, 2774-2782.

5. Karl, I.E., Garber, A.I. and Kipnis, D.M. (1976) Alanine and glutamine synthesis and release from skeletal muscle III Dietary and hormonal regulation, J. Biol. Chem., 251, 844-850.

6. Sapir, D.G., Pozefsky, T., Knochel, J.P. and Walser, M. (1977) The role of alanine and glutamine in steroid-induced nitrogen wasting in man, Clin. Sci. Mol. Med., 53, 215-220.

7. Weber, G. (1968) Hormonal control of gluconeogenesis. In The Biological Basis of Medicine, Bittar, E.E. and Bittar, N. Eds., Academic Press, New York, Vol. 2, 263-307.

8. Munck, A. (1971) Glucocorticoid inhibition of glucose uptake by peripheral tissues: old and new evidence, molecular mechanisms, and physiological significance, Perspect. Biol. Med. 14, 265-289.

9. Kipnis, D.M. and Stein, M.G. (1963) Ciba Foundation Colloquia on Endocrinology, Churchill, London, 156-184.

10. Fain, J.M., Scow, R.O. and Chernick, S.S. (1963). Effects of glucocorticoids on metabolism of adipose tissue in vitro, J. Biol. Chem., 238, 54-58.

11. Plager, J.E. and Matsui, N. (1966). An in vitro demonstration of the anti-insulin action of cortisol on glucose metabolism, Endocrinology 78, 1154-1158.

12. Fain, J.N. (1964) Effects of dexamethasome and 2-deoxy-D-glucose on fructose and glucose metabolism by incubated adipose tissue, J. Biol. Chem., 239, 958-962.

13. Fain, J.N. and Czech, M.P. (1975) Glucocorticoid effects on lipid mobilisation and adipose tissue metabolism, In Handbook of Physiology, Section 7, Endocrinology 6, Adrenal Gland, Greep, R.O. and Astwood, E.B. Eds., American Physiological Society, Washington, 169-178.

14. Krotkiewski, M., Krotkiewska, J. and Björntorp, P. (1970) Effects of dexamethasone on lipid mobilisation in the rat, Acta Endocrinol., 63, 185-192.

15. Mahley, R.W., Gray, M.E., Hamilton, R.L. and Le Quire, V.S. (1968) Lipid transport in liver II Electronmicroscopic and biochemical studies of alterations of lipoprotein transport induced by cortisone in the rabbit, Lab. Invest., 19, 358-369.

16. Nayak, R.Y., Feldman, E.B. and Carter, A.C. (1962) Adipokinetic effect of intravenous cortisol in human subjects, Proc. Soc. Exper. Biol. Med., 111, 682-686.

17. Bagdade, J.D., Porte, D. Jnr. and Bierman, E.L. (1970) Steroid-induced lipaemia. A complication of high dosage corticosteroid therapy, Arch. Int. Med., 125, 129-134.

18. Klausner, H. and Heimberg, M. (1967) Effect of adrenalcortical hormones on release of triglycerides and glucose by liver, Amer. J. Physiol., 212, 1236-1246.

19. Conn, J.W. and Fajans, S.S. (1956) Influence of adrenal cortical steroids on carbohydrate metabolism in man, Metabolism, 5, 114-127.

20. McKiddie, M.T., Jasani, M.K. and Buchanan, J.D. (1968) The relationship between glucose tolerance, plasma insulin and corticosteroid therapy in patients with rheumatoid arthritis, Metabolism, 17, 730-739.

21. Campbell, J. and Rastogi, J.S. (1968) Elevation in serum insulin, albumin and FFA with gains in liver lipid and protein, induced by glucocorticoid treatment in dogs, Cand. J. Physiol. Pharmacol., 46, 421-429.

22. Olefsky, J.M. and Kimmerling, G. (1976) Effects of glucocorticoids on carbohydrate metabolism, Amer. J. Med. Sci., 271, 202-210.

23. Issekutz, B. and Borkow, I. (1973) Effect of glucagon and glucose load on glucose kinetics, plasma FFA and insulin in dogs treated with methylprednisolone, Metabolism, 22, 39-49.

24. Exton, J.H., Friedmann, N. and Wond, E.H. (1972) Interaction of glucocorticoids with glucagon and epinephrine in the control of gluconeogenesis and glycogenolysis in liver and of lipolysis in adipose tissue, J. Biol. Chem., 247, 3579-3588.

25. Levine, R. (1976) Glucagon and the regulation of blood sugar, New Engl. J. Med., 494-495.

26. Birkenhager, J.C., Timmermans, H.A.T. and Lamberts, S.W.J. (1976) Depressed plasma FFA turnover rate in Cushing's syndrome, J. Clin. Endocrinol. Metab., 42, 28-32.

27. Reaven, E.P., Kolterman, D.G. and Reaven, G.M. (1974) Ultrastructural and physiological evidence for cortico-steroid induced alterations in hepatic production of very low density lipoprotein particles, J. Lipid Res., 15, 74-83.

28. Bagdade, J.D., Yee, E., Albers, J. and Pykalisto, O.J. (1976) Gluco-corticoids and triglyceride transport: effects on triglyceride secretion rates, lipoprotein lipase and plasma lipoproteins in the rat, Metabolism, 25, 533-542.

29. Bagdade, J.D., Porte, D. Jnr. and Bierman, E.L. (1967) Diabetic lipaemia: a form of acquired fat-induced lipaemia., New Engl. J. Med., 276, 427-433.

30. Björntorp, P. (1966) Studies on adipose tissue from obese patients with or without diabetes mellitus, II, Acta Med. Scand., 179, 229-234.

31. Goldman, J.K. and Cahill, G.F. (1964) Insulin effect on glucose-C^{14} incorporation into rat liver and adipose tissue in vivo, Metabolism, 13, 572-578.

32. Haft, D.E. (1968) Studies of the metabolism of isolated livers of normal and alloxan-diabetic rats perfused with insulin, Diabetes, 17, 244-250.

33. Van Harken, D.R., Brown, T.O. and Heimberg, M. (1967) Hepatic lipid metabolism in experimental diabetes, III Synthesis and utilisation of triglycerides, Lipids, 2, 231-238.

34. Wilcox, H.G., Dishmon, G. and Heimberg, M. (1968) Hepatic lipid metabolism in experimental diabetes, IV Incorporation of amino acid ^{14}C into lipoprotein-protein and triglyceride, J. Biol. Chem., 243, 666-675.

35. Rubenstein, B. and Rubenstein, D. (1966) The effect of fasting on esterification of palmitate by rat liver in vitro, Canad. J. Biochem., 44, 129-140.

36. Topping, D.L. and Mayes, P.A. (1972) The immediate effects of fructose and insulin on the metabolism of the perfused liver, Changes in lipo-protein secretion, fatty acid oxidation and esterification, lipogenesis and carbohydrate metabolism, Biochem. J., 126, 295-311.

37. Heimberg, M., Dunkerley, A. and Brown, T.O. (1966) Hepatic lipid meta-bolism in experimental diabetes, Release and uptake of triglycerides by perfused livers from normal and alloxan-diabetic rats, Biochim. Biophys. Acta, 125, 252-264.

38. Boden, G. and Wilms, B. (1966) Einfluss von Insulin auf Kohlenhydrat und fettstoffwechsel der perfundierten leber bei normalen und alloxan-diabetischen ratten, Klin. Woch., 44, 579-588.

39. Csorba, T.R., Matsude, I. and Kalant, N. (1966) Effects of insulin and diabetes on flux rates of plasma glucose and free fatty acids, Metabolism, 15, 262-270.

40. Nestel, P.J. (1967) Relationship between FFA flux and TGFA influx in plasma before and during the infusion of insulin, Metabolism, 16, 1123-1132.

41. Eaton, R.P. and Nye, W.H.R. (1973) The relationship between insulin secretion and triglyceride concentration in endogenous lipaemia, J. Lab. Clin. Med., 81, 682-695.

42. Johnston, D.G., Gill, A., Hanson, R., Alberti, K.G.M.M., Batstone, G. and Orskov, H. (1978) Somatostatin: a tool for investigation of the metabolic effects of cortisol and glucagon, Metabolism, 27, Suppl. 1, 1445-1447.

43. Barnes, A.J., Kohner, E.M., Bloom, S.R., Johnston, D.G., Alberti, K.G.M.M. and Smythe, P. (1978) Importance of pituitary hormones in aetiology of diabetic ketoacidosis, Lancet, 1, 1171-1174.

44. Batstone, G.F., Alberti, K.G.M.M., Hinks, L., Smythe, P., Laing, J.E., Ward, C.M., Ely, D.K. and Bloom, S.R. (1976) Metabolic studies in subjects following thermal injury, Intermediary metabolites, hormones and tissue oxygenation, Burns, 2, 207-225.

45. Chernick, S.S., Clark, C.M., Gardiner, R.J. and Scow, R.O. (1972) Role of lipolytic and glucocorticoid hormones in the development of diabetic ketosis, Diabetes, 21, 946-954.

46. Scow, R.O., Chernick, S.S. and Guarco, B.A. (1958) Ketogenic action of pituitary and adrenal hormones in pancreatectomised rats, Diabetes, 8, 132-142.

47. L'Age, M., Fechner, W., Langholz, J. and Salzmann, H. (1974) Relationship between plasma corticosterone and the development of ketoacidosis in the alloxan diabetic rat, Diabetologia, 10, 131-134.

48. Alberti, K.G.M.M., Christensen, N.J., Wersen, J. and Orskov, H. (1975) The role of glucagon and other hormones in the development of diabetic ketoacidosis, Lancet, 1, 1307-1311.

49. Schade, D.S., Eaton, R.P. and Standefer, J. (1978) The modulation of basal ketone body concentration by cortisol in diabetic man, J. Clin. Endocrinol. Metab., in press.

50. Woodside, W.F. and Heimberg, M. (1972), Hepatic metabolism of free fatty acids in experimental diabetes, Isr. J. Med. Sci., 8, 309-316.

51. McGarry, J.D. and Foster, D.W. (1977) Hormonal control of ketogenesis, Arch. Int. Med., 137, 495-501.

52. McGarry, J.D., Mannaerts, G.P. and Foster, D.W. (1977) A possible role for malonyl-CoA in the regulation of hepatic fatty acid oxidation and ketogenesis, J. Clin. Invest, 60, 265-270.

53. Blackshear, P.J., Holloway, P.A.H. and Alberti, K.G.M.M. (1975) The effects of inhibition of gluconeogenesis on ketogenesis in starved and diabetic rats, Biochem. J., 148, 353-362.

54. Di Marco, J.P. and Hoppel, C. (1975) Hepatic mitochondrial function in ketogenic states, Diabetes, starvation and after growth hormone administration, J. Clin. Invest., 55, 1237-1244.

134

55. Zierler, K.L. and Rabinowitz, D. (1963) Roles of insulin and growth hormone, based on studies of forearm metabolism in man, Medicine (Balt), 42, 385-402.

56. McGarry, J.D. and Foster, D.W. (1971) The regulation of ketogenesis from oleic acid and the influence of antiketogenic agents, J. Biol. Chem., 246, 6247-6253.

57. Ontko, J.A. (1972) Metabolism of free fatty acids in isolated liver cells, J. Biol. Chem. 247, 1788-1800.

58. Haft, D.E. and Miller, L.L. (1958) Alloxan diabetes and demonstrated direct action of insulin on metabolism of isolated perfused rat liver, Am. J. Physiol., 192, 33-42.

59. Söling, H.D. and Seufert, C.D. (1975) Handbook of Experimental Pharmacology, New Series (Hasselblatt, A. and v. Bruchausen, F., Eds), 32/2, Springer, Berlin, 413-434.

60. Menahan, L.A. and Wieland, O. (1969) Interactions of glucagon and insulin on the metabolism of perfused livers from fasted rats, Europ. J. Biochem., 9, 55-62.

61. Diamant, S. and Shafrir, E. (1975) Modulation of the activity of insulin-dependent enzymes of lipogenesis by glucocorticoids, Europ. J. Biochem., 53, 541-546.

62. Cook, G.A., Nielsen, R.C., Hawkins, R.A., Mehlman, M.A., Lakshmanan, M.R and Veech, R.L. (1977) Effect of glucagon on hepatic malonyl Coenzyme A concentration and on lipid synthesis, J. Biol. Chem., 252, 4421-4424.

Lipoprotein Metabolism and Endocrine Regulation
L.W. Hessel and H.M.J. Krans editors
© ECSC, EEC, EAEC, Brussels-Luxembourg, 1979
Published by Elsevier/North-Holland Biomedical Press-Amsterdam

A SHORT REVIEW OF THE EFFECTS OF GLUCOCORTICOIDS ON FAT METABOLISM, ESPECIALLY ON LIPOLYSIS IN VITRO AND IN VIVO

J.C. BIRKENHAEGER AND S.W.J. LAMBERTS.

Department of Internal Medicine III, Division of Clinical Endocrinology and Metabolism, University Hospital "Dijkzigt", Erasmus University, Rotterdam, The Netherlands.

In man an intravenous bolus or infusion of hydrocortisone induces on increase of plasma FFA over at least the next 2 hours[1-3]. The last group observed that a rather low dose of insulin is able to block this effect. This is paralleled by the results of in vitro experiments of Jeanrenaud and Renold[4] and of Fain and coworkers[5], who found that prolonged incubation of rat epididymal or parametrial adipose tissue with hydrocortisone or dexamethasone leads to a stimulation of basal lipolysis and an inhibition of glucose uptake and utilisation by adipose and other tissues and that these effects may be reversed by low concentrations (4 uU/l) of insulin. Other workers found that pretreatment or incubation with excess glucocorticoid hormone does not stimulate basal lipolysis in vitro but potentiates the lipolytic effect of epinephrine and glucagon[6,7]. As to lipogenesis mainly data obtained in experimental animals are available. In rats treated with high doses of glucocorticoids for days an increase of fatty acid synthesis, of acetyl-CoA carboxylase and fatty acid synthetase activity in liver(dependent on the presence of a normal insulin reserve) and a decrease of these activities in epididymal adipose tissue have been found [8]. This last finding confirms that of Jeanrenaud and Renold[4] with regard to the inhibition of lipogenesis in rat epididymal adipose tissue by excess glucocorticoid hormone, probably by way of the inhibition of glucose uptake. The depression of glucose uptake and utilisation by glucocorticoids has been surmised for muscle and demonstrated for adipose and other tissues[9,10].

In acute hypercortisolism the initial increase of liver glycogen by way of activation of glycogen synthetase is well-known[11]. Under these circumstances the glucose output by the liver is depressed[12]. Prolonged hypercortisolism may be accompanied by an increase of the glucose output by the liver. Gluconeogenesis is known to be activated by fasting, insulin-deficiency and excess glucocortoid hormone. In the last mentioned situation increased substrate influx into the liver (mainly in the form of alanine[13]) from increased muscle proteolysis, as well as increased activity of key enzymes of liver gluconeogenesis, especially phosphoenolpyuvate carboxykinase[14] are responsible. This last effect, however, is rapidly neutralized by insulin, so that in _vivo_ the stimulation of gluconeogenesis by glucocorticoids is mainly effected by the sustained increase of substrate flux to the liver. Still, it has been postulated that the hyperglycaemia of hypercortisolism is caused by the decrease of peripheral glucose uptake rather than by an increase of glucose introduction[15].

While the acute effect (after 4 hours) of a moderately high dose of dexamethasone (5 ug per rat subcutaneously) consisted of a substantial increase of the rate of release of glycerol from isolated epididymal adipose tissue, led treatment with 3-5 ug dexamethasone, daily for 14 days to a secondary decrease to subnormal of the lipolysis rate as measured in vitro [16]. This phenomenon was ascribed to the reactive hyperinsulinism that could be demonstrated in the second group of rats. Perley and Kipnis showed that in normal people and non-insulin-dependent diabetics the insulin response to an oral glucose load may be increased upto five times after dexamethasone treatment (8 mg daily for 2-3 days), whereas the glucose curve is raised much less or not at all[17]. The stimulation of insulin secretion in this situation may be mediated by hyperglycaemia, the increased secretion of glucagon (see below), the elevated plasma level of alanine[13] and/or sensitization of the beta cell to glucose[18]. According to the data of Karam et al.[19] hyperinsulinism in patients with hypercortisolism is especially associated with overweight. In line with the abovementioned experimental data of Krotkiewski et al.[16] and of importance for the explanation of our own data in patients with hypercortisolism (see below) are the data of Owen and Cahill, who in fasting obese people showed that the catabolic effects of prolonged administration of cortisone (200 mg i.m. daily for 6 days), i.e. on plasma FFA, glycerol and aminoacids and on urinary nitrogen, are rapidly neutralized by endogenous insulin[15].

The secretion of glucagon (basal levels and responses to arginine or alanine) is stimulated by repeated administration of prednisone or dexamethasone[13,20] (40 mg daily for 4 days and 2 mg daily for 3 days, resp.), as well as in patients with Cushing's syndrome[13], in whom it appeared to be accompanied by an elevation of the basal plasma alanine level. In contrast, in obesity the glucagon secretion rate appears to be subnormal, basally as well as after administration of alanine[21]. This finding has been challenged by Gossain et al.[22] In the light of these findings peripheral glucagon/insulin ratios may assumed to be higher in hypercortisolism that in simple obesity.

Looking for an explanation of the centripetal distribution of body fat mass in Cushing's syndrome we found, using the 40 K-counting and tritiated water

dilution methods for the determination of the lean bone body mass, that most
patients with pituitary dependent Cushing's syndrome have an increased body
fat mass[23]. We further studied comparatively the turnover rate of plasma FFA in
normal people (n = 6), patients with simple obesity (n = 7) and patients with
Cushing's syndrome (n = 16; 12 of them pituitary dependent)[24]. With constant
rate infusion of $1-^{14}C$-palmitic acid complexed to human serum albumin in the
fasting state we found a high absolute plasma FFA turnover rate in obesity
(as had been reported before by Nestel and Whyte[25]). When the turnover rate in
this condition is related to body weight a normal average is obtained, while
expressing it per kg body fat ends up in a subnormal value. Surprisingly, the
absolute plasma FFA turnover rate in our Cushing patients was significantly
lower than normal. This difference with the control group as well as with the
simple obese group persisted when the turnover rate was expressed per kg body
weight. Seven of the 16 patients with Cushing's syndrome were restudied at
least 3 months after correction of the hypercortisolism. The average FFA turnover rate (absolute as well as per kg body weight) had returned to normal.
Although the fasting plasma FFA levels in the 4 groups were not statistically
different a definite positive relationship was observed by us between the absolute plasma FFA turnover rate and the fasting plasma FFA level. This applied to
the Cushing's patients separately as well as to all individuals studied together (r = 0.77 and 0.52, p   0.01 for both; n = 16 and 36, resp.).
No correlation between the plasma FFA turnover rate and the estimated total
body fat was found in the patients with hypercortisolism or in all patients
together. In 10 patients with Cushing's syndrome the FFA turnover rate did not
correlate with the fasting plasma insulin level, which in most cases was not
elevated. The depressed FFA turnover rate in hypercortisolism is not easily
explained. In the light of the data reviewed from the literature it might be
postulated that in hypercortisolism most of the adipose tissue mass is not
insulin-resistant to the degree that occurs in simple obesity. In this connection it is of importance to note that there may be regional differences, not
only in fat cell size, for instance when patients with Cushing's syndrome are
compared to normal people[26], but also in metabolic activity, for instance when
omental and subcutaneous adipose tissue in normal people are compared[27].
The centripetal distribution of body fat in hypercortisolism may, of course
also be causally related to regional differences in the activity of adipose
tissue lipoprotein lipase (LPL). Data on the influence of glucocorticoid
hormone on LPL of various tissues are rather conflicting. Stimulation of rat
heart and epididymal adipose tissue LPL after a single injection of

138

glucocorticoid hormone has been found by de Gasquet et al.[28], while Bagdade and coworkers [29] and Krotkiewski et al.[30] reported that prolonged administration of dexamethasone to rats lowered epididymal and perirenal adipose tissue LPL.

REFERENCES

1. Dreiling, D.A., Bierman, E.L., Debons, A.F., Elsbach, P. and Schwartz, I.L. (1962) Metabolism 11, 572.

2. Nayak, R.V., Feldman, E.B. and Carter, A.C. (1962) Proc. Soc. Exp. Biol. Med. 111, 682.

3. Mischke , W.J., Ebers, S., Boisch, K.H. and Tamm, J. (1974) Acta Endocr. (Kbh), Supp. 186, 1.

4. Jeanrenaud, B. and Renold, A.E. (1960) J. biol. Chem. 235, 2217.

5. Fain, J.N., Scow, R.O. and Chernick, S.S. (1963) J. biol. Chem. 238, 54.

6. Reshef, L. and Shapiro, B. (1960) Metabolism 9, 551.

7. Lamberts, S.W.J., Timmermans, H.A.T., Kramer-Blankenstijn, M. and Birkenhäger, J.C. (1975) Metabolism 24, 681.

8. Diamant, S. and Shafrir, E. (1975) Eur. J. Biochem. 53, 541.

9. Munck, A. (1971) Perspectives in Biology and Medicine, p. 265.

10. Randle, P.J., Garland, P.B., Hales, C.N. and Newsholme, E.A. (1963) The Lancet I, 785.

11. Mersmann, H.J. and Segal, H.L. (1969) J. biol. Chem. 244, 1701.

12. Lecocq, F.R., Mebane, D. and Madison, L.L. (1964) J. clin. Invest. 43, 237.

13. Wise, J.K., Hendler, R. and Felig, Ph. (1973) J. clin. Invest. 52, 2774.

14. Weber, G. (1968) In: The Biological Basis of Medicine. Ed. E.E. Bittar and N. Bittar, Acad. Press, New York. Vol. 2, p. 263.

15. Owen, O.E. and Cahill, G.F. Jr. (1973) J. clin. Invest. 52, 2596.

16. Krotkiewski, M., Krotkiewska, J. and Björntorp, P. (1970) Acta Endocr. (Kbh) 63, 185.

17. Perley, M. and Kipnis, D.M. (1966) New Engl. J. Med. 274, 1237.

18. Malaisse, W.J., Malaisse-Lagae, F., McCraw, E.F. and Wright, P.H. (1967) Proc. Soc. Exp. Biol. Med. 124, 924.

19. Karam, J.H., Grodsky, G.M. and Forsham, P.H. (1965) Ann. N.Y. Acad. Sci. 131, 374.

20. Marco, J., Calle, C., Roman, D., Diaz-Fierros, M., Vilanueva, M.L. and Valverde, I. (1973) New Engl. J. Med. 288, 128.

21. Wise, J.K., Hendler, R. and Felig, Ph. (1973) New Engl. J. Med. 288, 487

22. Gossain, V.V., Matute, M.L. and Kalkhoff, R.K. (1974) J. Clin. Endocrinol. Metab. 38, 238.

23. Lamberts, S.W.J. and Birkenhäger, J.C. (1976) J. Clin. Endocrinol. Metab. 42, 864.

24. Birkenhäger, J.C., Timmermans, H.A.T. and Lamberts, S.W.J. (1976) J. Clin. Endocrinol. Metab. 42, 28.

25. Nestel, P.J. and Whyte, H.M. (1968) Metabolism 17, 1122.

26. Krotkiewski, M., Blohmé, B., Lindholm, N. and Björntorp, P. (1976) J. Clin. Endocrinol. Metab. 42, 91.

27. Hamosh, M., Hamosh, P., Bar-Maor, J.A. and Cohen, H. (1963) J. Clin. Invest. 42, 1648.

28. Gasquet, P. de, Pequignot-Planche, E., Tonnu, N.T. and Diaby, F.A. (1975) Horm. Metab. Res. 7, 152.

29. Bagdade, J.D., Yee, E., Albers, J. and Pykalisto, O.J. (1976) Metabolism 25, 533.

30. Krotkiewski, M., Björntorp, P. and Smith, U. (1976) Horm. Metab. Res. 8, 245.

Lipoprotein Metabolism and Endocrine Regulation
L.W. Hessel and H.M.J. Krans editors
© ECSC, EEC, EAEC, Brussels-Luxembourg, 1979
Published by Elsevier/North-Holland Biomedical Press-Amsterdam

THE REGULATION OF STEROL SYNTHESIS IN HUMAN LEUCOCYTES

W. KRONE, D. J. BETTERIDGE AND D. J. GALTON
Diabetes and Lipid Research Laboratory, St. Bartholomew's Hospital,
London, E.C.1. (United Kingdom)

INTRODUCTION

Several metabolic diseases may be associated with defects in the regulation of rate-determining enzymes in metabolic pathways[1, 2]. Three types of defects have been identified: (i) disorders of short-term modulation of enzymes e.g. defective allosteric inhibition of phosphofructokinase by citrate in lipomatosis[3] and defective modulation of lipoprotein lipase by very low density lipoprotein in apoprotein C-II deficiency[4]; (ii) defects in the covalent activation of enzymes e.g. defective activation of triglyceride lipase by catecholamines in triglyceride storage disease[5]; and (iii) defects in the induction/repression of enzymes e.g. defective regulation of 3-hydroxy-3-methylglutaryl coenzyme A reductase in familial hypercholesterolaemia[6, 7] (summarized in Fig. 1).

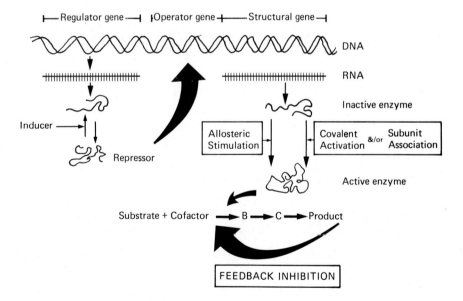

Fig. 1. Scheme for the regulation of enzyme activity illustrating mechanisms for: (i) induction or repression, (ii) covalent modification and (iii) allosteric modulation.

Demonstration of these types of enzyme disorder requires more than basal enzyme assays as activities in cells from affected individuals may be similar to those in normal subjects. However, defects in the regulatory properties of enzymes may be revealed by assay of the enzyme before and after incubation of cells under conditions which modify the activity of the enzyme. A good example of this is the defect in the regulation of the enzyme 3-hydroxy-3-methylglutaryl-coenzyme A reductase (HMG-CoA reductase) in cells from patients with familial hypercholesterolaemia, (F.H.).

Normal cells incubated in medium containing lipid-depleted serum show increased activity of HMG-CoA reductase leading to increased sterol synthesis. If these cells are then transferred to medium containing low density lipo-protein (LDL), activity of the enzyme is suppressed with parallel reduction of sterol synthesis. However, in cells from patients homozygous for F.H. addition of LDL to the medium fails to suppress HMG-CoA reductase activity, while cells from heterozygous individuals show an intermediary defect. Such defects have been identified in cultured fibroblasts[8], freshly isolated mixed leucocytes[9] and cultured lymphocytes[10]. These findings have been explained by the absence in F.H. cells of specific high-affinity receptors for LDL. As a result these cells are unable to take up and degrade LDL and therefore do not suppress HMG-CoA reductase activity in the presence of LDL[8]. One family with F.H. has been described in which the defect appears to be on the LDL; in that LDL from affected individuals failed to regulate HMG-CoA reductase activity in both normal and patients' cells[11].

An alternative explanation of the genetic defect in F.H. has been proposed from the observation that mutant cells release more endogenously synthesized sterols into a lipid-free incubation medium than normal cells. This suggests that the abnormality in F.H. could be accounted for by a mutation resulting in a weaker binding of a repressor to a steroid metabolite[7].

In this chapter we wish to report some of our recent results on the regulation of sterol synthesis in leucocytes with particular reference to:-

(i)   the possible mechanism for the regulation of sterol synthesis by LDL-derived cholesterol.

(ii)   the specificity of the regulatory defect of sterol synthesis described in F.H., and

(iii) the heterogeneity of the response of sterol synthesis to LDL in a family with F.H.

PATIENTS AND METHODS

Subjects. Normal subjects were healthy individuals who had total plasma cholesterol concentrations of less than 5.5 mM and no family history of ischaemic heart disease. Subjects with F.H. were diagnosed by the presence of hypercholesterolaemia (> 7.5 mM), xanthomata, together with a strong family history of premature vascular disease. Details of individual patients are given in the text and legends. Patients with acute myeloblastic leukaemia were diagnosed by the presence of typical blast cells in the peripheral blood and on bone marrow aspirate. All patients were studied prior to the commencement of cytotoxic therapy.

Isolation and incubation of leucocytes. Peripheral blood lymphocytes were isolated under sterile conditions by the method of Böyum[12] and mixed leucocytes (approximately 65% granulocytes, 30% lymphocytes and 5% monocytes) by a modification of the method of Coulson and Chalmers[13]. Cells were washed with Krebs-Ringer phosphate buffer, containing 15 mM glucose, pH 7.4. The washed cell pellet was resuspended and transferred into plastic culture flasks. Each flask contained $3-5 \times 10^6$ lymphocytes or $1-2 \times 10^7$ leucocytes suspended in Krebs-Ringer phosphate buffer, pH 7.4, fortified with 15 mM glucose, aminoacids and vitamins according to a MEM buffer, 100 units of penicillin/ml, 100 μg of streptomycin/ml ,0.5 mM Na acetate or 0.5 mM mevalonate and 40% full or lipid-depleted serum. Cell viability, as assessed by trypan blue exclusion, was routinely determined and was greater than 90% under all experimental conditions. The morphology of the cells was assessed in fixed and stained preparations.

Incorporation of $\left[2^{-14}C\right]$ acetate into sterols by intact cells. The flasks containing either lymphocytes or leucocytes were incubated in a shaking water bath at $37^{\circ}C$ for the appropriate time when the volume of the incubation was made up to 2 ml by the addition of 50 μl of $\left[2^{-14}C\right]$ acetate and the incubation continued for 2 hours. The incubations were terminated by the addition of chloroform/methanol and 10^5 cpm of $\left[1,2^{-3}H\right]$ cholesterol were added as an internal standard. Lipids were extracted by the method of Bligh and Dyer[14] and saponified by methanolic potassium hydroxide (2 M) for 6 hours at $70^{\circ}C$. The non-saponifiable fraction was extracted with hexane and counted in a Packard Tri-Carb scintillation spectrometer (model 2425) using a toluene based scintillant. The recovery of $\left[^3H\right]$ cholesterol was used to correct for procedural losses of $\left[^{14}C\right]$ acetate incorporated into non-saponifiable lipids.

Assay of HMG–CoA reductase. HMG–CoA was synthesized from HMG–anhydride by the method of Goldfarb and Pitot[15]. The rate of conversion of $\begin{bmatrix}14C\end{bmatrix}$ HMG–CoA to $\begin{bmatrix}14C\end{bmatrix}$ mevalonate was measured in leucocyte extracts as previously described[16]. HMG–CoA reductase activity is expressed as picomoles of $\begin{bmatrix}14C\end{bmatrix}$ mevalonate formed per hour per mg of cell protein.

Preparation of lipid-depleted serum. Lipid-depleted serum was prepared according to the method of McFarlane[17] from pooled AB-negative, complement-inactivated serum.

Extraction of RNA and isolation of Poly (A) – containing RNA. Lymphocytes (2×10^6) were labelled with $\begin{bmatrix}3H\end{bmatrix}$ adenosine (100 μ Ci; 23 Ci/mmol) for 40 min. Ribosomal RNA synthesis and mitochondrial RNA synthesis were first suppressed with 0.04 μg/ml of actinomycin D[18] and 1 μg/ml ethidium bromide[19], respectively. Actinomycin D, ethidium bromide and cordycepin were added 30 min prior to labelling.

Cytoplasmic extracts were prepared by harvesting, washing and resuspending cells in 2 ml of hypotonic buffer (10 mM NaCl, 1.5 mM $MgCl_2$, 10 mM Tris, pH 7.4), adding the detergent Nonidet (NP 40) to a final concentration of 0.5% and agitating with a vortex mixer for 30 sec; nuclei were removed by centrifugation at 800 g for 2 min[20].

The supernatant was adjusted to a final concentration of 100 mM NaCl, 10 mM EDTA, 50 mM, Tris-HCl, 1.5 mM $MgCl_2$, 0.5% SDS (W/V). The cytoplasmic RNA was extracted by a conventional phenol/chloroform procedure[21].

Poly (A) – containing RNA was isolated by binding to oligo (dT) – cellulose[22]. The bound RNA (poly (A)$^+$ RNA) and the unbound RNA (poly (A)$^-$ RNA) were precipitated with 2 volumes of ethanol at -20°C for 18 hours. The precipitates were dissolved in water and radioactivity in both types of RNA was measured by scintillation spectrometry using a toluene based scintillant. The recovery of $\begin{bmatrix}32P\end{bmatrix}$ – labelled ribosomal RNA was used to correct for procedural losses of $\begin{bmatrix}3H\end{bmatrix}$ RNA.

RESULTS

Mechanism of regulation of sterol synthesis by LDL – derived cholesterol. It is well established that high concentrations of blood cholesterol and in particular LDL levels are related to an increased risk of developing ischaemic heart disease. Attention has therefore focused on the regulation of endogenous cholesterol synthesis, the rate of which is determined by the activity of the enzyme HMG–CoA reductase in a variety of human cells[23]. The activity of this enzyme is regulated primarily by LDL. Thus when freshly isolated human lymphocytes are incubated in the presence of LDL the activity of HMG–CoA reductase remains suppressed. However, removal of lipoprotein from the medium leads to a substantial increase in the activity of the enzyme, while subsequent exposure to LDL is followed by a suppression of enzyme activity. Since under these conditions sterol synthesis is strictly proportional to the activity of HMG–CoA reductase, the incorporation of $[^{14}C]$ -acetate into sterols can be taken as a measure of the enzyme activity[7,16]. There is evidence that the rise in HMG–CoA reductase activity of cells in medium containing lipid-depleted serum is due to a stimulation of de novo synthesis of the enzyme since the effect of lipid-depleted serum on the increase in HMG–CoA reductase activity is relatively slow, requiring at least 4-6 hours; and the increase is prevented by cycloheximide, a translational inhibitor of protein synthesis[24].

Since actinomycin D, a transcriptional inhibitor, has been found to block totally the subsequent rise in HMG–CoA reductase activity in fibroblasts following incubation in lipid-depleted serum[24], it has been suggested that gene transcription is involved in the regulation of the enzyme by LDL. It should however be noted that this antibiotic may produce side-effects such as the inhibition of initiation of protein synthesis[25].

We have therefore studied the effect of cordycepin (3'-deoxyadenosine), another RNA inhibitor, on sterol synthesis in human lymphocytes. Although the mechanism by which cordycepin acts at the molecular level is still in dispute[26,27], an effect of the drug in HeLa cells[20], mouse sarcoma 180 cells[28] and cultured fibroblasts[29] is an inhibition of mRNA synthesis. The results shown in Fig. 2(A) demonstrate that cordycepin added to freshly isolated lymphocytes 30 minutes prior to the addition of $[^3H]$ -adenosine inhibited the appearance of the tracer in the cytoplasmic poly (A) - containing RNA. However, the incorporation of label into cytoplasmic RNA containing no poly (A)- sequences was unaffected by the drug. As most of the mammalian mRNA is present as poly (A) - containing RNA[30] our data indicate that cordycepin can substantially inhibit mRNA synthesis in lymphocytes.

Although cordycepin, at a concentration of 50 µg/ml, blocked mRNA synthesis in lymphocytes by more than 50% the drug had no inhibitory effect on the four-fold increase in sterol synthesis from $[^{14}C]$ -acetate in cells incubated in lipid-depleted medium for 16 hours (Fig. 2(B)).

146

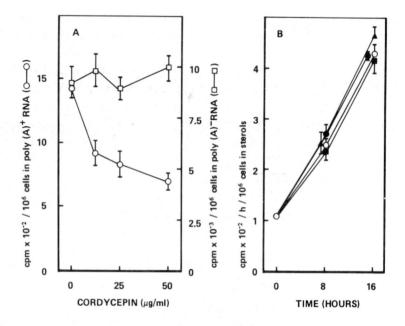

Fig. 2(A). The effect of cordycepin on the incorporation of $[^3H]$ -adenosine into cytoplasmic poly (A) - containing RNA (○—○) and into RNA without poly (A)-sequences (□—□) in human lymphocytes. Points are means $\pm$ S.E. for 3 to 4 experiments.

Fig. 2(B). The effect of cordycepin on the induction of sterol synthesis from $[^{14}C]$ -acetate by lipid-depleted serum in human lymphocytes. After the indicated intervals cells were pulse-labelled with $[^{14}C]$ -acetate for 2 hours. Controls without cordycepin (○—○); cordycepin 12.5 µg/ml (●—●); 25 µg/ml (▲-▲) and 50 µg/ml (■-■). Points are means $\pm$ S.E. for 3 to 4 observations.

When lymphocytes were pre-incubated with full serum for up to 40 hours in the presence of cordycepin (50 µg/ml), by which time the pool of mRNA with a short half-life might be expected to be greatly reduced, the subsequent rise in sterol synthesis after removal of LDL from the medium was the same as in cells pre-incubated without the drug (Fig. 3).

Assuming that cordycepin inhibits mRNA synthesis for HMG-CoA reductase to a similar extent to that of total mRNA synthesis it may be concluded that new mRNA synthesis is not required for the effect of lipid-depleted serum on the induction of sterol synthesis in lymphocytes. This suggests that HMG-CoA reductase is regulated by LDL-derived cholesterol at a post-transcriptional level, at a point between the inhibitory sites of cordycepin and cycloheximide.

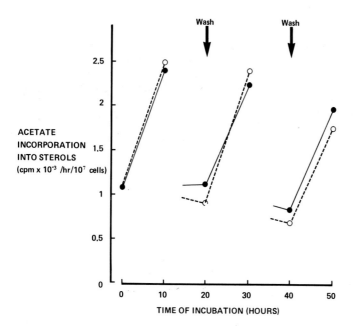

Fig. 3. Effect of pre-incubation with cordycepin on the induction of sterol synthesis from [^{14}C] -acetate in human lymphocytes following transfer of cells from full serum to lipid-depleted serum. Cells were pre-incubated in full serum with or without cordycepin (50 µg/ml) for 0, 20 and 40 hours. At the end of pre-indubation cells were washed, resuspended in medium containing lipid-depleted serum plus cordycepin (50 µg/ml) and incubated for 10 hours. After the indicated times cells were pulse-labelled with [^{14}C] -acetate for 2 hours. Pre-incubation without drug (O—O), and with drug (●—●). Points are means of duplicate incubation.

Inhibition of sterol synthesis by compactin.

Current therapeutic measures for the treatment of hypercholesterolaemia are not satisfactory and new types of hypocholesterolaemic drugs are needed. Recently ML-236 B and compactin, which are identical fungal metabolites, have been isolated from strains of Penicillium citrinum[31] and Penicillium brevi-compactum[32]. ML-236 B and compactin have been shown to be potent competitive inhibitors of HMG-CoA reductase activity in rat liver[33] and in extracts of cultured human fibroblasts, respectively[34].

We have measured the effect of compactin (a gift of Dr. R. B. Fears of Beecham Pharmaceuticals) on sterol synthesis from [^{14}C] -acetate in freshly isolated human lymphocytes of normal subjects and patients heterozygous for F.H. As can be seen in Fig. 4(A) compactin inhibited sterol synthesis from [^{14}C] -acetate by 65% at a concentration of 2×10^{-7} M, inhibition being almost complete at a concentration of 2×10^{-6} M.

In contrast to the incorporation of $\left[^{14}C\right]$ -acetate into sterols, compactin did not affect the incorporation of $\left[^{14}C\right]$ -mevalonate indicating that the drug may be specifically inhibiting the activity of the enzyme HMG-CoA reductase. Cells from patients heterozygous for F.H. also show inhibition of sterol synthesis from $\left[^{14}C\right]$ -acetate (Fig. 4(B)). Since the dose-response curves are similar this provides additional evidence that HMG-CoA reductase in normal and mutant cells have similar properties. Although compactin has been shown to lower blood cholesterol in animals[31], it remains to be seen whether it will prove of use in human subjects.

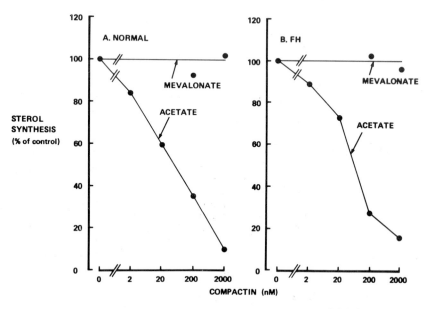

Fig. 4(A). Effect of compactin on sterol synthesis from $\left[^{14}C\right]$ -acetate or $\left[^{14}C\right]$ -mevalonate in lymphocytes from two normal subjects (A) and two patients with heterozygous F.H. (B). Cells were incubated in medium containing lipid-depleted serum for 10 hours. Compactin was then added 30 min. prior to the addition of $\left[^{14}C\right]$ -acetate or $\left[^{14}C\right]$ -mevalonate. Sterol synthesis of cells incubated in lipid-depleted serum for 10 hours is expressed at 100%. Points are means of duplicate incubations.

Is the defect in sterol biosynthesis specific for familial hypercholestero-laemia?

The defect in the regulation of HMG-CoA reductase and sterol biosynthesis in fibroblasts and leucocytes has been considered as a specific defect in F.H. However, we have recently observed that peripheral blast cells from patients with acute myeloblastic leukaemia failed to regulate sterol synthesis by

LDL[35]. It can be seen in Fig. 5 that leukaemic blast cells incubated in
lipid-depleted serum show increased sterol synthesis from $[^{14}C]$ -acetate.
After transfer of these cells to medium containing full serum as a source of
LDL there was failure of suppression of sterol synthesis. This is possibly due
to a defect in the LDL pathway resulting in a failure of internalisation of
LDL-derived cholesterol with consequent failure of suppression of HMG–CoA
reductase. This is supported by the finding that exogenous cholesterol
(100 µg/ml) administered in ethanol normally suppressed sterol synthesis in
leukaemic cells (Fig. 5(B)) indicating that the intracellular mechanisms for
the regulation of sterol synthesis are intact.

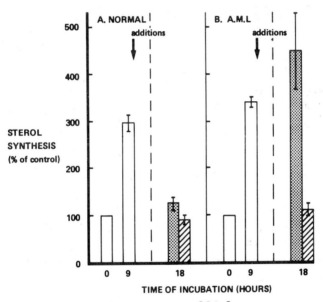

Fig. 5. Regulation of sterol synthesis from $[^{14}C]$ -acetate in leucocytes from
normal subjects (A) and patients with acute myeloblastic leukaemia (B) after
incubation in lipid-depleted serum. Leucocytes were pre-incubated for 9 hours
in medium containing lipid-depleted serum and then transferred to a medium
containing complete serum (stippled bars) or cholesterol (100 µg/ml) in ethanol
(hatched bars) and incubated for a further 9 hours. After indicated intervals
cells were pulse-labelled with $[^{14}C]$ -acetate for 2 hours. Activities of
freshly isolated cells are expressed as 100%. Mean activity in freshly isolated normal cells : 148 c.p.m. / 10^6 cells / h; in leukaemic cells 287 c.p.m.
/ 10^6 cells / h.

Heterogeneity of the regulation of HMG–CoA reductase in a family with
Familial Hypercholesterolaemia.

Most patients with F.H. whom we have studied show a defect in the regulation
of HMG–CoA reductase and sterol synthesis in their leucocytes (Fig. 6).

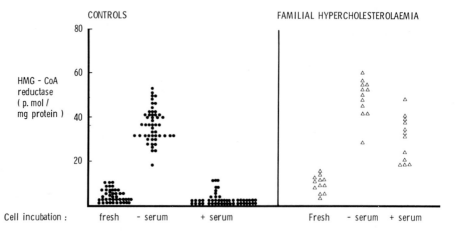

CONTROLS   FAMILIAL HYPERCHOLESTEROLAEMIA

Fig. 6. Regulation of the activity of HMG–CoA reductase in leucocytes from normal subjects and patients heterozygous for F.H. Leucocytes were isolated and an aliquot taken for enzyme assay. The remaining cells were incubated in a medium containing lipid-depleted serum (- serum) for 8 hours and an aliquot taken for enzyme assay. A further aliquot of the cells were then transferred to a medium containing full serum (+ serum) and incubated for a further 8 hours and then assayed for enzyme activity. Controls   , F.H.

However, we have observed an interesting exception to this in a patient homozygous for F.H.

The proband (M.Y.) whose family tree is shown in Fig. 7 was noted to have gross tendon xanthomata and hypercholesterolaemia (15.8 mmol/l) in early childhood. He developed ischaemic heart disease in late teenage life and died of acute myocardial infarction at the age of 23 years. Autopsy showed extensive and severe arterial disease with supravalvar atheroma typical of homozygous F.H.

FAMILY TREE OF M.Y.

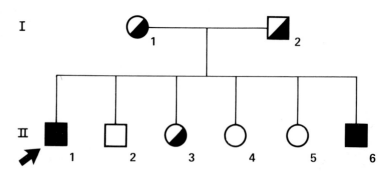

Fig. 7. The family tree of M.Y.
Clinically affected members of the family are designated by either half-filled symbols (heterozygous) or filled symbols (homozygous for F.H.).

Leucocytes from this patient following isolation and pre-incubation in
medium containing lipid-depleted serum showed normal suppression of HMG–CoA
reductase activity when increasing concentrations of LDL were added to the
medium (Fig. 8). A dose-response curve for a patient (B.N.) heterozygous for
F.H. from another kindred is shown for comparison in Fig. 8. Other family
members were examined (Fig. 9). A sister (II,3) with serum cholesterol of
8.6 mmol/l and clinically a heterozygote showed a partial suppression with LDL.
Whereas the youngest brother (II,6) aged ll years and clinically a homozygote
with severe hypercholesterolaemia (19.0 mmol/l) and extensive tendon xanthomata,
showed failure of suppression of HMG–CoA reductase activity in leucocytes incubated with LDL (100 µg/ml).

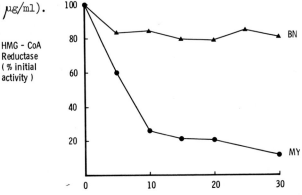

Fig. 8. The regulation of the activity of HMG–CoA reductase by LDL in leucocytes from the proband M.Y. (Fig. 7; II,1) with homozygous F.H. (●—●) and a
patient B.N. with heterozygous F.H. (▲—▲) from another kindred. B.N. with
tendon xanthomata, serum cholesterol of 11.5 mM, triglyceride of 1.5 mM and
five affected first-degree relatives, died aged 37 years from myocardial
infarction.
Leucocytes were incubated for 8 hours in a medium containing lipid-depleted
serum and aliquots of cells were taken for enzyme activities (expressed as 100%)
Remaining cells were then transferred to medium containing the LDL concentrations indicated in the figure, incubated for a further 8 hours and enzyme
assays performed.

It is of interest to note that in leucocytes of the mother (I,1) although
clinically heterozygous for F.H. HMG–CoA reductase activity was normally
suppressed by LDL (Fig. 9).

The genetic disorder in F.H. may be transmitted by an autosomal mutant allele
at a single gene locus[36]. One would therefore expect to see the same biochemical abnormality in all the clinically affected members of the same
kindred. Because we have demonstrated differences in the regulation of HMG–CoA
reductase in affected members from one kindred, it is clear that the regulation

152

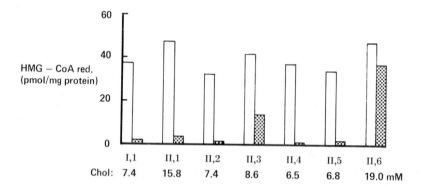

Fig. 9. Regulation of HMG—CoA reductase by LDL in leucocytes from members of the family with F.H. (Fig. 7). Leucocytes were incubated for 8 hours in a medium containing lipid-depleted serum and aliquots were taken for enzyme assay (open bars). The remaining cells were then transferred to a medium containing LDL (100 µg/ml) incubated for a further 8 hours and enzyme assays performed (stippled bars). Numbers refer to family tree of Fig. 7.

of reductase does not invariably reflect the genetic defect. This is probably due to the complex reaction sequence between LDL-cell interaction and consequent suppression of HMG—CoA reductase. This complex reaction sequence may allow many environmental factors to intervene and may explain the variability of enzyme suppression within the kindred.

SUMMARY

We have described experiments on the regulation of HMG—CoA reductase activity and sterol synthesis in freshly isolated leucocytes. We have found that:-

(1) Cordycepin, an inhibitor of mRNA synthesis, had no effect on the induction of sterol synthesis in lymphocytes incubated in medium containing lipid-depleted serum although the drug inhibited mRNA synthesis by more than 50%. This suggests that LDL-derived cholesterol may regulate HMG—CoA reductase at a post-transcriptional level.

(2) Compactin, at similar concentrations, inhibited sterol synthesis in both normal and F.H. lymphocytes from $[^{14}C]$ -acetate but not from $[^{14}C]$ -mevalonate suggesting that the drug is specifically inhibiting the activity of HMG—CoA reductase and providing additional evidence that the properties of the enzyme in normal and mutant cells are similar.

(3) Blast cells from patients with acute myeloblastic leukaemia showed a similar regulatory defect in sterol synthesis as patients with F.H. in that cells previously incubated in medium containing lipid-depleted serum failed to

suppress sterol synthesis from $\left[{}^{14}C \right]$-acetate following transfer to medium containing LDL.

(4) In one kindred with F.H., two members clinically homozygous for F.H. showed differences in the regulation of HMG—CoA reductase by LDL. Leucocytes from one member of the family failed to suppress HMG—CoA reductase by LDL whilst the other member's cells behaved as normal cells suggesting that the regulation of the enzyme does not invariably reflect the genetic defect.

ACKNOWLEDGEMENTS

D. J. Betteridge is a R. D. Lawrence Research Fellow of The British Diabetic Association.

W. Krone is in receipt of a grant from the Deutsche Forschungsgemeinschaft

REFERENCES

1. Galton, D.J., Higgins, M.J.P. and Reckless, J.P.D. (1975) Lancet, 1, 1224-1226.

2. Galton, D.J., Betteridge, D.J., Taylor, K.G., Holdsworth, G. and Stocks, J. (1977) Clin. Sci. and Mol. Med, 53, 197-203.

3. Galton, D.J. and Wilson, J.P.D. (1970) Clin. Sci, 38, 649-660.

4. Breckenridge, W.C., Little, J.A., Steiner, G., Chow, A. and Poapst, M. (1978) N. Engl. J. Med, 298, 1265-1273.

5. Galton, D.J., Reckless, J.P.D. and Taitz, L.S. (1976) Acta. Paediatr. Scand, 65, 761-768.

6. Brown, M.S., Dana, S.E. and Goldstein, J.L. (1974) J. Biol. Chem, 249, 789-796.

7. Fogelman, A.M., Edmond, J., Seager, J. and Popjak, G. (1975), J. Biol. Chem, 250, 2045-2055.

8. Brown, M.S. and Goldstein, J.L. (1976) Science, 191, 150-155.

9. Betteridge, D.J., Higgins, M.J.P. and Galton, D.J. (1975) Brit. Med. J, 4, 500-502.

10. Kayden, H.J., Hatam, L. and Beratis, N.G. (1976) Biochemistry, 15, 521-528.

11. Higgins, M.J.P., Lecamwasam, D.S. and Galton, D.J. (1975) Lancet 2, 737-740.

12. Bøyum, A. (1968) Scand J. Clin. Lab. Invest, 97, (Suppl. 21) 77-89.

13. Coulson, A.S. and Chalmers, D.G. (1969) Lancet 1, 468-469.

14. Bligh, E.G. and Dyer, W.J. (1959) Can. J. Biochem. Physiol, 37, 911-917.

15. Goldfarb, S. and Pitot, H.C. (1974) J. Lipid Res, 12, 512-514.

16. Higgins, M.J.P. and Galton, D.J. (1977) Eur. J. Clin. Invest, 7, 301-305.

17. McFarlane, A.S. (1942) Nature, 149, 439.

18. Perry, R.P. (1963) Exp. Cell. Res, 29, 400-406.

154

19. Zylber, E., Vesco, C. and Penman, S. (1969) J. Mol. Biol, 44, 195-204.

20. Penman, S., Rosbach, M. and Penman, M. (1970) Proc. Nat. Acad. Sci, 67, 1878-1885.

21. Rudland, P.S., Weil, S. and Hunter, A.R. (1975) J. Mol. Biol, 96, 745-766.

22. Iynedjian, P.B. and Hanson, R.W. (1977) J. Biol. Chem, 252, 655-662.

23. Rodwell, V.W., Nordstrom, J.L. and Mitschelen, J.J. (1976) Adv. Lipid Res, 14, 1-74.

24. Brown, M.S., Dana, S.E. and Goldstein, J.L. (1973) J. Biol. Chem, 70, 2162-2166.

25. Singer, R.H. and Penman, S. (1972) Nature, 240, 100-102.

26. Maale, G., Stein, G. and Mans, R. (1975) Nature, 255, 80-82.

27. Horowitz, B., Goldfinger, B.A. and Marmur, J. (1976) Arch. Biochem. Biophys, 172, 143-148.

28. Mendecki, J., Lee, S.Y. and Brawerman, G. (1972) Biochemistry, 11, 792-798.

29. Cholon, J.J. and Studzinski, G.P. (1974) Science, 184, 160-161.

30. Lewin, B. (1975) Cell, 4, 11-20.

31. Endo, A., Kuroda, M. and Tsujita, Y. (1976) J. Antibiot, 29, 1346-1348.

32. Brown, A.G., Smale, T.C., King, T.J., Hasenkamp, R. and Thompson, R.H. (1976) J. Chem. Soc. Perkin, 1, 1165-1170.

33. Endo, A., Kuroda, M. and Tanzawa, K. (1976) FEBS Lett, 72, 323-326.

34. Brown, M.S., Faust, J.R. and Goldstein, J.L., Kaneko, I. and Endo, A. (1978) J. Biol. Chem, 253, 1121-1128.

35. Betteridge, D.J. and Galton, D.J. (1976) Clin. Sci. and Mol. Med, 52, 32P.

36. Fredrickson, D.S., Goldstein, J.L. and Brown, M.S. (1978) in The Metabolic Basis of Inherited Disease, Stanbury, J.B., Wyngaarden, J.B. and Fredrickson, D.S. eds., McGraw-Hill, New York, pp 604-655.

Lipoprotein Metabolism and Endocrine Regulation
L.W. Hessel and H.M.J. Krans editors
© ECSC, EEC, EAEC, Brussels-Luxembourg, 1979
Published by Elsevier/North-Holland Biomedical Press-Amsterdam

DISCUSSIONS ON LIPOPROTEIN TRANSPORT AND HORMONE LEVELS

Paraphrased and annotated by L.W. Hessel, Gaubius Institute, Health Research
Organization TNO, Herenstrat 5d, 2313 AD Leiden (The Netherlands)

Galton: Dr. Assmann, if HDL is as important for atherosclerosis as
epidemiologists suggest, then why do we not find in Tangier disease cholesterol
ester (CE) accumulation in the arterial wall?

Assmann: The cells in which CE accumulates in Tangier patients are histio
cytes, Schwann cells and intestinal smooth muscle cells and as far as we know
there is no CE accumulation in any other cell such as the fibroblast or other
smooth muscle cells. Thus it seems as if HDL is only important for cholesterol
removal from cells which do not regulate their cholesterol balance on the level
of the LDL receptor. There are, however, two reasons why one should be careful
in drawing conclucions: 1. there are only 25 Tangier patients known of whom
there are autopsy reports of only three (see e.g. S.S. Katz et al., J. Clin.
Invest. 59, 1045, 1977. Ed.), and 2. Tangier patients have low serum total
cholesterol levels (50-100 mg/dl) which may mean a low cholesterol influx into
cells.

The HDL issue may be confounded by the effect of elevated TG levels. In
thousands of patients which we investigated we found hardly any with low HDL
cholesterol and normal TG levels. So the excess morbidity associated with low
HDL could very well be due to elevated TG levels and the role of HDL in the
pathogenesis of atherosclerosis may be overestimated.

Hessel: The function of HDL as shuttle of cholesterol from peripheral tissues
to the liver seems to have been proved in the bile fistula patient of Halloran
and Schwartz (cited in Dr. Magill's paper).

Brunzell: Yes, but they were able to account for only 30% of cholesterol
transport. It could have been more, but they could no demonstrate this because
of the speed of cholesterol exchange.

Hessel: Are there data on bile metabolism in Tangier patients?

Assmann: One patient has been investigated, no abnormality was found.

Hessel: Is there a way in which heterozygous Tangier patients could be
identified in epidemiological studies; what is the estimated incidence?

Assmann: The incidence is not known. The segregation of heterozygotes on the basis of lipoprotein determinations is difficult. Their HDL cholesterol and apo A_1 and A_2 levels are reduced by 50% as compared to normals (cf Assmann, J. Clin. Invest. 60, 1025, 1977), but these persons are clinically normal and similar reductions may be due to carbohydrate feeding and/or hypertriglycerid emic disorders. The finding of cholesterol ester accumulation in rectal mucosa may be a useful index for identifying heterozygotes.

Brunzell: Hormonal control of the LDL receptor in tissue culture has been recently investigated by Chait and Bierman. They showed that T_3 levels regulate synthesis of the LDL receptor so that one can titrate the number of LDL receptors (i.e. the high affinity receptors, Ed.) up and down by the amount of T_3 in the system. Similarly with insulin (Chait et al., Clin. Res. 26, 303, 1978 and Biochim. Biophys. Acta 529, 292, 1978. Ed.). So reductions of LDL levels in hyperinsulinemic obese patients may very well be related to increased LDL removal due to increased receptor numbers.

Hessel: If LDL receptors are reduced in hypothyroidism one would expect elevations of LDL rather than IDL levels?

Brunzell: In hypothyroidism almost all metabolic functions are slowed down: VLDL synthesis, lipoprotein lipase activity, conversion of the VLDL remnant to IDL (perhaps by some receptor in the liver), and finally also LDL removal.

Hülsmann: Could the actions of insulin and thyroxin have a common denominator in the effect of both these hormones on membrane fluidity (cf Hülsmann, Biochem. Biophys. Res. Commun. 79, 784, 1977. Ed.).

Brunzell: Some influence on the internalization of the LDL particle seems likely; effects on the binding of LDL to its receptor seem more difficult to conceive.

Galton: Dr. Brunzell, like you we found a defect in adipose tissue lipoprotein lipase (LPL) in insulin independent diabetics, and we were puzzled to find after one week of insulin therapy the total acetone-extractable lipase increased but not the heparin-releasable lipase.

Brunzell: When we studied our patients in the metabolic ward and biopsied them every two weeks, we did not find increased LPL activities at all until the 4th week after institution of therapy. Then both lipase fractions went up, probably at the same time.

Brindley: One of the factors which regulates LPL is the diet. Diets rich in polyunsaturated fatty acids increase lipase activities in rats.

Brunzell: I do not think anybody has done such studies in humans.
Further, as was summarized some time ago by Pykälistö, the rat is a most un-
suitable model for studying human LPL physiology. Although in true insulin
deficiency LPL is decreased in man as well as in rats, in vitro incubation of
diabetic adipose tissue of rats results in restoration of LPL activity but this
is not so in adipose tissue of diabetic man. Estrogen therapy decreases LPL
activity in rats, but not in man; conversely adipose LDL is increased in
severely hypothyroid rats and decreased in hypothyroid man. Finally, LPL is low
in uremic man and normal or elevated in uremic rats; the rat has no cholesterol
ester transport protein, no LDL_2, a different relation of HDL to LCAT and
there are many other differences as well.

Jeanrenaud: Is the release of lipoprotein lipase a true secretory process?

Brunzell: Yes; investigations by Chajek and O. and Y. Stein suggest that it is
under control of the microtubular system (e.g. Chajek et al., Biochim. Biophys.
Acta 488, 270, 1977. Ed.).

Rössner: Dr. Mancini, it seems as if the inverse relation between TG level and
HDL cholesterol level is disturbed during fasting: both go down at the same
time. Is there a restoration of HDL cholesterol when fasting is continued for a
longer time?

Mancini: We did not continue our experiment for longer than 6 weeks; there was
only a slight decrease in HDL cholesterol in the beginning and then it remained
constant for the rest of the time. The gut receives no substrate and no chylomicrons are formed, so HDL production at the gut level is interfered with and
this may explain the difference with the normal, that is not starved,
condition.

Assmann: One should distinguish between total lipoprotein mass and the mass of
particular components. The inverse relation between VLDL and HDL can often be
observed by monitoring only TG in VLDL and cholesterol in HDL, but this is not
always the case. There is a clearcut need to study changes in the other HDL
components, especially the apoproteins alongside with the HDL cholesterol
level. Radioimmunoassays and Laurell techniques have been developed for this
but these are somewhat cumbersome for large scale application. We find
nephelometry a very easy and accurate method for following Apo A_1 and A_2
levels.

Hessel: Do you object to using Mancini assays for this purpose?

Assmann: The Mancini technique has a rather high coefficient of variation and its application for A_1 gives problems.

Galton: Dr. Mancini, I was struck by the appearance of a TG-rich LDL in your fasting subjects. It seems that the VLDL was improperly catabolized; I would be interested to know what the hepatic lipase levels were in these sujects after four or six weeks of fasting. Do these account for the appearance of IDL-like particles?

Mancini: As you know, dr. Nikkilä has studied this (ref 15 in Dr. Mancini's paper. Ed.), and he found a decrease of both adipose tissue and hepatic lipase. We did measure the removal rate of intralipid and this did not change very much. (In contrast to Nikkilä who found a 15% increase in fasting hyper-triglyceridemics. Ed.).

Brunzell: An alternative explanation for the TG-rich LDL would be that during fasting, when there is no need to transport excess TG from meals, the VLDL which is secreted is TG-depleted. If this is true than what you measure as LDL would in fact be the end of the VLDL spectrum, i.e. there would be newly secreted TG-poor lipoprotein in the LDL density fraction.

Marco: I would like to mention another hormone which increases it concentration during prolonged fasting; this is Pancreatic Polypeptide (J.A. Hedo, M.L. Villanueva and J. Marco, 12th Ann. Meeting Eur. Soc. Clin. Invest., Rotterdam, 1978, Abstr. 85. Ed.). However, this hormone has a rather bad reputation for being inactive in intermediary metabolism.

Johnston: Yes, we have infused Pancreatic Polypeptide in normals and found no changes in FFA, ketones, glycerol, cholesterol, etc.

Hessel: A further and more serious candidate for a regulatory function during fasting seems to be T_3 (Triiodothyronine). There was a recent paper (A. Balsam et al., J. Clin. Invest., 62, 415, 1978) showing a redirection in the liver of the monodeiodination of T_4 from the generation of T_3 (active) to the generation of reverse T_3 (inactive) during starvation.

Marco: Dr. Luyckx, how could there be an inhibitory effect of FFA levels on glucagon secretion when during fasting as well as during physical exercise FFA levels and glucagon levels both increase?

Luyckx: The parallel increase of FFA and glucagon is usually ascribed to a lipolytic effect of glucagon or to a parallel adrenergic stimulation of both lipolysis and glucagon secretion. On the other hand, the glucagon response to arginine or hypoglycemia can be suppressed by raising FFA levels to about 1300 ueq/l (A.S. Luyckx et al., Metabolism 27, 1033, 1978. Ed.). This is in the high physiological range and it shows that FFA can modulate the glucagon response to other secretagogues.

Galton: Is glucagon really lipolytic? We tried very hard to find a lipolytic effect in human adipocytes but we could not find it.

Luyckx: The lipolytic effect of glucagon emerges only under conditions of complete insulin deficiency, and in man it is very weak.

Johnston: When we infused glucagon in man there was a fall in FFA levels, probably due to glucagon induced insulin secretion. When we infused somatostatin at the same time, there was no change in FFA level. (D.G. Johnston et al., Metabolism 27, Suppl. 1, 1445, 1978. Ed.).

(Editor's comment: Strong indirect evidence for a lipolytic action of glucagon in fasting man was reported recently by Merimee (J. Clin. Endocrine Metabol., 46, 414, 1978)).

Galton: The importance of glucagon for lipoprotein metabolism should show it-self in patients with glucagonoma.

Luyckx: We have had no opportunity to study lipoproteins in such a patient and I would not know of any other reports.

Johnston: Dr Marco, glucagon has a well established role in the maintenance of basal blood glucose concentration; you are postulating that in addition to this excess secretion of glucagon would contribute to glucose intolerance. But when glucagon is infused in normal persons during the consumption of a meal, there is no additional increase in glucose levels as a result of artifical hyper-glucagonemia. What is the evidence that glucagon does play a role in glucose tolerance?

Marco: There is no direct evidence but the absence of a glucagon effect on glucose tolerance in young persons as reported by the New Haven group (e.g. R.S. Sherwin, New Engl. J. Med., 294, 455, 1976. Ed.), does not necessarily mean that there is no such effect in the elderly.

Jeanrenaud: We have worked with an animal model where glucagon seems to play an important role in glucose tolerance. Rats with hypothalamic lesions are severe-ly hyperinsulinemic, yet they are normoglycemic. Their glucagon levels are strongly elevated and this may be the reason why they have a normal glucose tolerance test in the face of hyperinsulinemia.

Michell: Dr. Buchanan, the difference in insulin response to a glucose load between Edinburgh and Stockholm seems quite dramatic. What would the most likely explanation be?

Buchanan: Clinically one would think cf obesity but the Edinburgh men were not really obese. Their body weight was comparable to that in Stockholm but they were a few cm's shorter.

Michell: Knowing that, one might compare samples from the two cities of men with the same basic dimensions and fatness and see whether the metabolic differences hold up as a difference between the cities or are a difference in fatness.

Rössner: The Edinburgh men were also considerably less fit; a large proportion of them were not able to carry out an ordinary 6 min exercise load.

Galton: Is it worthwhile to process all these epidemiologic data without any hypothesis to start with? Some correlations may be misleading.

Buchanan: A very philosophical question. As long as we do not know the physiological role in fat metabolism of some parameters we measure, such as for example glucagon, we do not know whether they are misleading or not. We may be able to interpret the data at some later date when our physiological insight has become better. The study is very well designed and yields information which cannot be obtained in any other way.

Jeanrenaud: Dr. Ebert, could the elevation in GIP levels seen after meals be due to rapid GIP synthesis rather than to release of stored GIP? I would like to refer to Dr. Felber's paper (Felber et al., Lancet ii, 185, 1974. Ed.) in which he showed that gut mucosal homogenates of rats given glucose or arginine strongly stimulate insulin secretion on injection in receptor rats.

Ebert: When rats are given a glucose load corresponding to 100 g in man the amount of GIP in the duodenum decreases by 30%. We have no data on the rate of synthesis.

Brunzell: On TG ingestion TG in plasma increases and GIP increases; would Dr. Ebert care to speculate on GIP's action in this condition; does it act on TG catabolism?

Ebert: No such effect has been found sofar, and till now nothing is known about GIP and liver metabolism.

Brunzell: We were involved in studies with Dr. J.C. Brown to see whether there was some effect of GIP on lipoprotein lipase in rats, but we found no influence at all.

Ebert: In rat fat cells there is a weak lipolytic and strong antilipolytic effect with respect to glucagon (R. Ebert et al., Eur. J. Clin. Invest., 6,

327, 1976. Ed.).

Jeanrenaud: Did you find a good correlation between GIP release and degree of hyperinsulinism and between GIP release and degree of obesity?

Ebert: No, we failed to find these correlations. Probably the critical point is the nutrition behaviour, not the obesity per se. For example after 5 days of food restriction there is a minor change in body weight but a clear decrease in GIP response.

Marco: Do you have data on GIP in insulinoma patients?

Ebert: Yes, GIP levels are slightly elevated. Strongly elevated levels are found in gastrinomas and this is probably due to the hypersecretion of acid which reaches the duodenum and releases GIP.

Magill: Dr. Rössner, are there any plans to reconnect some of your bypasses? HDL cholesterol should then show a rise.

Rössner: This is not likely; the few patients who were reconnected for other reasons put on weight very rapidly. We are trying a modification of the surgical procedure by connecting the gall bladder to the blind loop. In this way there is an intact gall secretion which is not lost in the stools and patients have less diarrhea. In the few patients we have investigated so far we did not find much difference in the lipoproteins.

Michell: To what extent could the decrease in serum cholesterol be due to decreased intestinal synthesis when part of the intestine is eliminated?

Rössner: This is difficult to estimate because there is also an increased loss of cholesterol and decreased cholesterol absorption.

Michell: What is the contribution of the gut to total cholesterol synthesis in man?

Kempen: Estimates vary from 5 to 20%, depending on the diet.

Hessel: Dr. Rössner, is it necessary to standardize the time of blood sampling with respect to the day of the month; does the lipoprotein pattern change during the menstrual cycle?

Rössner: We sampled only between the 21st and 26th day of the cycle. (Changes in lipoproteins during the cycle are considered to be negligible by Glueck (J. Am. Med. Assoc., 226, 1127, (1973) but there are reports with a different outcome. Discussed by: S. Lussier-Cacan, Proc. Soc. Exp. Biol. Med., 154, 471, 1977. Ed.).

Galton: Dr. Birkenhäger, in our laboratory Dr. Reckless did find a correlation

162

between HDL cholesterol and testosterone level in about 50 males; this seems
to be at variance with your results.

Birkenhäger: It might be a matter of small sample size; we had only 17 persons
in each group. But in any case the correlation must be very weak.

Galton: Yes, the correlation coefficient was about 0.3.

Buchanan: Dr. Vanhaelst, to what extent are the auto-antibodies found in your
patients organ-specific? Do you not find antibodies to other endocrine organs
and could there not be another, more general factor rather than the thyroid to
explain the clinical data?

Vanhaelst: This does not seem very likely because if in some population we find
a frequency of 20% of antithyroid antibodies, we find antibodies against e.g.
betacells or against adrenal cells in less than 1% of the subjects.

Brunzell: As regards the frequency of hypercholesterolemia in thyroid disorders
part of the confusion is caused by the arbitrariness of cut-off levels. This
holds also for lipid elevations in patients in general. Ideally, each person
should be considered as his own control. If this is done one sees, with almost
no exception, that treatment with thyroxin lowers cholesterol and triglyceride
levels; this also happens in control groups of normal persons.

Assmann: Type III hyperlipoproteinemia is known to be especially susceptible to
aggravation by hypothyroidism. Are there data about the apo E levels or shifts
in the apo E_2-E_3 polymorphism in premyxedema patients?

Brunzell: In the studies of Hazzard in which we were involved total apo E went
up in hypothyroidism. This is however difficult to evaluate as any increase of
VLDL or IDL causes apo E levels to rise. It would be surprising if thyroxin
affected E_2/E_3 ratios as these are probably genetically determined.

(Editor's comment: The hypothesis of a frequent interaction of latent thyroid
failure with a genetic predisposition to hyperlipidemia is strengthened by the
high estimated frequency of primary dyslipoproteinemia in the general (German)
population (1% homozygous, 15% heterozygous for the apo E^d allele, related to
type III hyperlipoproteinemia. (Utermann, Nature 269, 604, 1977). The high
frequency of antithyroid antibodies in the general population is also reported
by other groups, e.g. by Tunbridge et al. (Clin. Endocrin., 7, 495, 1977):
these authors note their presence in 3% of males and 12% of females of mean age
47 years.

The lack of association with hypercholesterolemia seems not quite settled, as
in a recent paper from Fowler's group it was again reported that in their

premyxedema patients (of mean age 58 years) cholesterol levels were clearly elevated, even in those with normal TSH levels or without an exaggerated response to TRH (Alaghbad-Zadeh, Lancet ii, 998, 1977).

Possible correlations with HDL cholesterol levels, taking into account inter-actions with diet, smoking, obesity, and alcohol consumption might be of value in evaluating premyxedema as a risk factor. Data on HDL cholesterol levels in these persons seem to be lacking.).

Hülsmann: Diet may be very important in hypothyroid persons prone to coronary heart disease. Heparin releasable liver lipase is reduced in diabetes and in hypothyroidism and one of the reasons may be a decreased membrane fluidity due to desaturase deficiency. Indeed, acylCoA desaturases can be increased by insulin and thyroxin and the low liver lipase activity in diabetic and hypo-thyroid rats can be restored to normal by feeding a diet rich in polyunsaturat-ed fatty acids (Hülsmann, Biochem. Biophys. Res. Commun., 79, 784, 1977. Ed.). Thus, dietary effects may interfere with the relation between lipid metabolism (and coronary vascular disease) and thyroid status in a different way in West Finland than in East Finland, where more butter is consumed.

Luyckx: Dr. Johnston, does ACTH have a lipolytic effect by itself?

Johnston: Only in animal tissues, not in man. We gave ACTH for diagnostic purposes to 2 patients with Addison's disease who had no glucocorticoid response. We found no change in any of the lipid parameters.

Brindley: With regard to the cortisol effect there is a tendency to think that the beta oxidation and ketogenic pathways are antagonistic to TG synthesis in the liver. Yet, this holds only when there is a limited availability of free fatty acids, but if the supply of fatty acids increases the capacity to synthesize TG is not decreased at all. So there can be high ketogenesis and high TG synthesis at the same time, TG synthesis simply mopping up excess free fatty acid.

Tomasi: Dr. Birkenhäger, it has been shown that anti-inflammatory sterols like cortisol and dexamethasone inhibit phospholipase A_2 (cf S. Hammarström, Science 197, 994, 1977, Ed.). Could this explain the depressed FFA turnover you found in the Cushing patients?

Birkenhäger: Not very likely; in adipose tissue release of prostaglandins can be inhibited by glucocorticoids while at the same time lipolysis is unaffected.

Assmann: Phospholipase A_2 has a specificity for unsaturated fatty acids in the 2-position; how accurate is the determination of total FFA turnover when you monitor only one specific acid, i.e. palmitic acid?

Birkenhäger: Palmitic acid has been shown to be a good representative (P.J. Nestel et al., e.g. Metabolism 27, 589, 1978. Ed.). Polyunsaturated fatty acids can certainly not be used for this purpose.

Michell: A clear distinction should be made between the "systemic fatty acids" as studied in the kinetics of the plasma fatty acid pool and the local activation of phospholipase which produces fatty acids which are probably rapidly metabolized by prostaglandin synthetase. (Compare for example differences in arachidonic and oleic acids, reported by Hagenfeldt, Horm. Metabol. Res., 7, 467, 1975. Ed.).

Rössner: Patients are usually treated with corticosteroids for conditions where it is known that lipoprotein metabolism is affected, such as in serious collagen diseases, and then the results are difficult to interpret. Are there data where the effects of corticosteroids on lipid metabolism have been studied in isolation?

Brunzell: We have seen a patient with the monogenic form of familial type IV whose triglyceride increased from 400 to 3000 mg/dl on cortisone but most persons do not respond in that way; the reason is not known and the difference in response between acute and long-term treatment is very important.

Brindley: Dr. Galton, to what extent may the change in HMGCoA Reductase be considered as a measure for a change in sterol synthesis? Modulation of this regulatory enzyme may not be expressed unless the need arises. During the diurnal cycle changes in enzyme content are not reflected by changes in sterol synthesis.

Galton: Under our conditions there is a good parallelism. (Ref 16 in Dr. Galton's paper. A further case where HMGCoA Reductase activity was not parallelled by, but inversely related to sterol synthesis was reported by W.K. Cavenee et al., Proc. Nat. Acad. Sci. USA, 75, 2103, 1978, Ed.).

Michell: The HMGCoA Reductase circadian rhythm in liver is assumed to be a gene activation-repression cycle; yet, your data point to a very long-lived messenger at least in lymphocytes; is this a tissue difference?

Galton: Yes, most probably, because in the circulating cells sterol synthesis is almost completely suppressed at all times by circulating LDL.

Brunzell: Dr. Siperstein showed many years ago, that in hepatoma tissue the feedback regulation of cholesterol on HMGCoA Reductase is lacking (M.D. Siperstein, J. Clin. Invest., 39, 642, 1960. Ed.) and works at the moment at some other malignant tissues (e.g. M.S. Brown, Fed. Proc. 32, 2168, 1973, Ed.).

Are these patients hypercholesterolemic? Did your patient with myeloblastic leukemia have high cholesterol levels?

Galton: Cholesterol levels in our patient were certainly not excessively high. (Siperstein reported cholesterol levels of 463 mg/dl (Cancer Res., 24, 1108, 1964) and 555 mg/dl (Cancer Res., 26, 7, 1966) in two elderly hepatoma patients. Ed.).

Kempen: According to Kandutsch cholesterol is necessary for cell division and when cholesterol synthesis is blocked by hydroxylated cholesterol derivatives division can be stopped and cells die, unless the medium is supplemented by cholesterol (e.g. A.A. Kandutsch, J. Cell Physiol., 85, 415, 1975. Ed.). Does this also hold for myeloma cells?

Galton: It is said that in fastly dividing cells cholesterol synthesis inhibition is lost because all the cholesterol taken up from the medium is utilized in the new membranes. We are studying this in dividing cells from the other leucocyte series because this could be the reason why we did not find suppression in our patient with myeloblastic leukemia.

Hülsmann: In villous microsomes one sometimes does not find HMGCoA Reductase activity, yet on delipidation the activity appears. It might be possible that in the presence of cholesterol there is a kind of latency so that the enzyme is not exposed to its substrate.

Galton: Yes, Dr. Mitropoulos believes that an increased concentration of free cholesterol on endoplasmic reticulum results in a more direct feedback modulation of HMGCoA Reductase activity as compared to the long term modulation by enzyme synthesis. (K.A. Mitropoulos et al., Eur. J. Biochem., 82, 419, 1978. Ed.).

Also Dr. Higgins found that in cycling rats when HMGCoA Reductase protein goes up, the enzyme activity goes down. So there is a direct modulation at the microsome level but it is not allosteric. It could be a phosphorylation- -dephosphorylation sequence.

-/-/-/-/-/-

CHANGES IN HORMONE RECEPTORS
AND RESPONSIVENESS

Lipoprotein Metabolism and Endocrine Regulation
L.W. Hessel and H.M.J. Krans editors
© ECSC, EEC, EAEC, Brussels-Luxembourg, 1979
Published by Elsevier/North-Holland Biomedical Press-Amsterdam

WHAT HAPPENS TO INSULIN AFTER BINDING TO ADIPOCYTES?
HOW DOES INSULIN INCREASE GLUCOSE TRANSPORT?

JØRGEN GLIEMANN, OLE SONNE and RICHARD R. WHITESELL
Institute of Medical Physiology C, University of Copenhagen, Panum
Institute, Blegdamsvej 3C, DK-2200 Copenhagen N, Denmark.

ABSTRACT

A near-steady state of binding of ^{125}I-labelled insulin to rat
adipocytes can be maintained for 10 h at 37^0C. About 95% of the
cell-associated radioactivity is iodoinsulin and 5% is iodotyrosine.
About half of the bound iodoinsulin is degraded in (or on) the cell
and the radioactivity dissociates as iodotyrosine. 3-O-methylglucose
is taken up with a half-time of about 3 s (22^0C substrate concentrations << K_m, insulin present). The hexose transport system
appears quite symmetric and K_m for glucose is about 7 mM.

INTRODUCTION

Lipoprotein lipase(s) is the rate-limiting enzyme for tissue uptake of plasma triglycerides[1]. It is synthesized mainly in adipocytes and can be released from these cells[2,3]. Insulin and glucose
appear to be important regulators of lipoprotein lipase activity[4];
thus, elevated concentrations of insulin in blood are associated
with increased activity whereas defects in insulin secretion are
associated with decreased activity[5]. It is therefore appropriate
in this symposium to summarize our present knowledge with respect
to the questions raised in the title.

Fate of bound insulin. Insulin and [125I]iodoinsulin are degraded
in a suspension of rat adipocytes. Under the incubation conditions
usually employed, this degradation is mainly accounted for by en-
zyme(s) released from the cells or adsorbed to the cell surface[6,7].
This non-receptor mediated degradation of insulin can be decreased
markedly by including 5% albumin and bacitracin (0.5 mg/ml) in the
medium[7]. It has been claimed that a steady state of binding is not
obtained at 37^0C in rat[8] or human[9] adipocytes. However, we have
found that a steady state of binding can be maintained for several
hours at 37^0C[7,10]. We think that other workers have failed to demonstrate a steady state either because the total rate of degrada-

tion of insulin has been high (most pronounced in rat adipocytes) or because the cells have ruptured during incubation (most pronounced in human adipocytes). Fig. 1 illustrates that the steady state is obtained after 30-40 min and that it is maintained for 180 min both with a receptor occupancy of about 1.5% and with an occupancy of about 85%. The results suggest that the number of receptors remains constant for at least 3 h. These findings are extended in the experiment shown in Fig. 2 where the cells were preincubated for 0-10.5 h without insulin or in the presence of 3 nM insulin followed by a 40 min incubation with tracer alone or with tracer plus 3 nM insulin. Surprisingly, preincubation of the cells for 6-10.5 h in the absence of insulin caused a small increase in the binding of tracer. The continuous presence of 3 nM insulin did not change the binding as compared to the binding obtained when 3 nM insulin was added together with the tracer. Finally, binding of the tracer decreased after preincubation for 23 h. It is concluded that a near-steady state can be maintained for at least 10.5 h although a small increase in the number of receptors (or in the affinity) may occur after preincubation for 5-10 h in the absence of insulin. No marked "down regulation" is observed as a result of incubation with 3 nM insulin (occupancy about 60%) for a period corresponding to 70 half times of dissociation (see Fig. 4). This means that if the insulin-receptor complex is internalized in some analogy to the epidermal growth factor-receptor complex[11] or the low density lipoprotein-receptor complex[12] then the receptors return very efficiently to their original sites or they are replaced by new receptors. "Down regulation" of insulin receptors in vitro was suggested by Gavin et al. who found that binding of "tracer" ^{125}I-insulin decreased 30% when cultured lymphocytes of the IM-9 line were preincubated with 10^{-8} M insulin for 5 h followed by extensive wash in order to remove the bound insulin.

We have previously found that at steady state (30-180 min) more than 90% of the radioactivity extracted from the cells was iodoinsulin whereas 5% coeluted with iodotyrosine on Sephadex G50[7]. This pattern is seen in Fig. 3, bottom right panel. The other panels show the nature of the radioactivity extracted from cells incubated with ^{125}I-labelled insulin for 30 s to 16 min. It is seen that practically all extracted radioactivity coelutes with insulin for up to 4 min of incubation whereafter there is a progressive in-

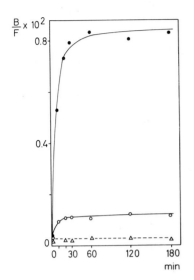

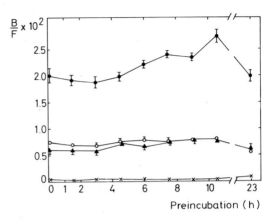

Fig. 1 (left). <u>Steady state of insulin binding</u>. 1 ml of suspended
rat adipocytes (2% packed cell volume in 15 ml roundbottom tubes)
were incubated at 37°C, pH 7.4 in medium containing albumin 5% and
bacitracin 0.5 mg/ml. At the appropriate times 10 ml saline (10°C)
and 1.2 ml silicone oil (D~0.99) was added, the tubes were centrifuged, the cells were recovered from the oil phase and assayed for
radioactivity. 50 pM ^{125}I-insulin alone (●-●), <u>plus</u> 10 nM insulin
(o-o), <u>plus</u> 1 μM insulin (Δ-Δ). For details of the method, ref. 7.
Fig. 2 (right). Incubation medium as described above with the following changes. The medium contained in addition penicillin 100
U/ml, streptomyosin 100 μg/ml and mycostatin 50 U/ml; the cell concentration was 3.4% v/v. The preincubation time is indicated on
the abscissa and during this period there was either no additions
or insulin 3 nM (▲-▲) or 1 μM (x-x) was present. Following the pre-
incubation period 50 pM ^{125}I-insulin was added either alone (●-●)
or with 3 nM insulin (o-o) and the incubation terminated after 40
min. Degradation of ^{125}I-insulin was constant and 4.0% x h^{-1}. Thus,
by 5 h the insulin concentration was 82% and by 10 h 66% of the
initial concentration. The points represent the mean values of 4
incubations ± SD.

crease in the small peak which coelutes with iodotyrosine. In contrast, Kahn and Baird[8] found that 20% of the radioactivity associated with the cells after incubation for 2 min was non-insulin (35%
after 7 min). They used the previously described oil technique[14]
and centrifuged the cells for 30 s. During this process the receptor bound insulin will be degraded (Sonne and Gliemann, unpublished
observation). We have used a technique which stops degradation of

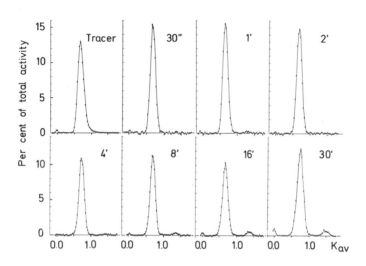

Fig. 3. <u>Nature of radioactivity in the cell pellet</u>. The cells were recovered after incubation for 30 s to 30 min, extracted in urea 6 M, acetic acid 3 M (see ref. 7) and the extract was gel filtered on Sephadex G50, Fine.

receptor-bound insulin immediately[7] and the results will therefore probably be a better reflection of the nature of the radioactivity associated with the cells in the suspension.

It has previously been shown that about half of the bound iodo-insulin dissociates from the cells as iodotyrosine and about half as iodoinsulin[7]. Fig. 4 shows the dissociation of radioactivity from cells incubated with ^{125}I-labelled insulin to steady state. One curve represents cells incubated in wash-out medium with no insulin and the other curve represents cells incubated in medium with 50 nM insulin. The presence of insulin causes a small acceleration of the dissociation of radioactivity, i.e. negative co-operativity among insulin receptors[15] probably exists in adipocytes, although it is not an important phenomenon at 37°C, pH 7.4[16]. By 60 min 96% of the radioactivity had dissociated from the cells and about 50% of that is iodotyrosine (Fig. 4). It should be added that the fraction of bound insulin, which is degraded, is independent of the receptor occupancy[7].

Fig. 5 summarizes how insulin is handled in adipocytes at 37°C. Some insulin is degraded by protease(s) unrelated to receptor binding; however, the contribution of this process to the total degradation is markedly reduced in medium with albumin 5% and bacitracin 0.5 mg/ml. Some insulin is adsorbed to the cell surface but

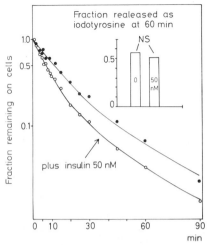

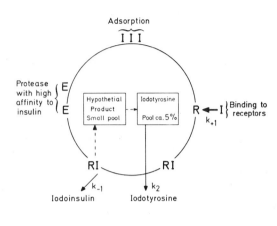

Fig. 4 (left). <u>Dissociation of bound ^{125}I-insulin</u>. The cells (5%
v/v) were incubated for 40 min with 50 pM ^{125}I-insulin and the infranatant medium was then removed to make the cell suspension 40%.
Half of the cell suspension was squirted into 25 fold larger volume of medium (37°C, pH 7.4) without additions (●-●) and the
other half into medium containing 50 nM insulin (o-o). All points
have been corrected for the amount of cell associated radioactivity at 180 min. In a parallel incubation cells were recovered above
oil after the initial 40 min incubation with tracer and resuspended in medium with or without 50 nM insulin. With this technique
nearly all transferred radioactivity is specifically bound insulin
(cf. Fig. 1). By 60 min 96% of the radioactivity had dissociated
from the cells, and, as shown by the bars, about half of that was
iodotyrosine. Degradation of ^{125}I-insulin added to resuspended
non-radioactive cells was 6% x h^{-1}.
Fig. 5 (right). <u>Model</u>. For explanation, see text.

the contribution of this to the total binding is negligible with
the present technique. Half of the (iodo)insulin bound at steady
state dissociates from the cells as iodotyrosine and the pool size
within the cells is about 5% of the total radioactivity. The pool
size of any hypothetical initial labelled cleavage product is very
small.

It should be pointed out that this is basically the same mechanism as that described by Terris and Steiner in hepatocytes[17]. They
found that the total rate of degradation in the cell suspension at
steady state was proportional to the receptor occupancy. This is
not the case in adipocytes due to the presence of insulin degrad-
ing protease. However, the fate of the bound insulin is probably
similar in the two cell types.

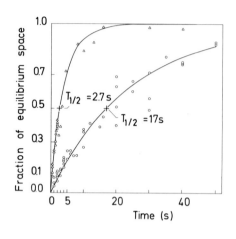

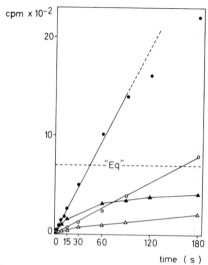

Fig. 6 (left). <u>Uptake of 50 μM 3-O-[¹⁴C]methylglucose</u>. 40 μl of 40%
(v/v) cell suspension was squirted on to 12 μl [¹⁴C]methylglucose
containing buffer placed in a 4 ml roundbottom tube. The incubation was terminated by the addition of 3 ml stopping solutions
(0.3 mM phloretin) and 0.5 ml silicone oil, the tubes were centrifuged and the cells were recovered from the oil phase. Timing was
carried out using a metronome. The distribution space at equilibrium was 1.8 μl per 100 μl packed cells and the mean cell diameter was about 60 μm. pH was 7.4 and the temperature in this and
the following experiments was 22°C. For details of the method see
ref. 24 and 25. No insulin (o-o). Insulin 1 μM (Δ-Δ).
Fig. 7 (right). <u>Uptake of 2-desoxy[¹⁴C]glucose. Effect of glucose</u>.
The incubation conditions were as described in the legend to Fig.6.
Open symbols: No insulin. Closed symbols: Insulin 1 μM. Circles:
50 μM 2-desoxyglucose. Triangles: <u>Plus</u> 7 mM D-glucose. The dashed
line indicates the number of counts which would have been present
in the cells if [¹⁴C]desoxyglucose was uniformly distributed in
the intracellular aqueous phase.

<u>Glucose transport</u>. Transport of glucose has until now not been
measured directly in adipocytes. The problem has been approached
in various indirect ways, e.g. by measuring the rate of conversion
of glucose to metabolic products, mainly lipids and CO_2. However,
whereas transport of glucose across the membrane probably is the
major rate-determining factor when the extracellular concentration
of glucose is low, this is almost certainly not the case when the
glucose concentration is high, particularly not in the presence of
insulin[18,19]. Some workers have measured glucose uptake after
"short term" incubations (45 s) followed by centrifugation through
oil in order to get a better measure of the transport[20]. However,

it can be calculated from the abundant data on the rate of conversion of glucose at 37^0C and the intracellular waterspace in adipocytes (cf. Fig. 4 of ref. 20) that the number of molecules converted to products within less than 10 s exceeds that which would be distributed in the intracellular water if glucose was not metabolized (insulin present, low glucose concentration). Therefore, incubation for 45 s at 37^0C is of little advantage as compared to incubation for 1-3 h.

2-desoxyglucose has been used quite widely[21,22] because it is phosphorylated and not further metabolized. 2-desoxyglucose phosphate is accumulated in the cells and is conveniently measured after incubation for a few min. However, we are left with the question: What is the rate determining factor under various conditions? It may not always be transport.

We have previously characterized equilibrium exchange of the non-metabolizable sugar analogue 3-O-methylglucose using an efflux method[19] and found a half time of about 3 s when the permeability to $[^{14}C]$methylglucose was maximal. Insulin increased V_{max} without causing major changes in K_m[19]. An efflux method is not suitable for analysis of transport of metabolizable sugars. Czech published a method for measuring the initial velocity of methylglucose uptake[23] and reported that it could be measured after incubation for 30 s under conditions where we found a half time of 3 s. We were therefore forced to believe that the initial velocity was markedly underestimated when measured as described by Czech and we designed a new method[24,25].

The principle of this method is to squirt a drop of rather concentrated cell suspension (40 µl, 40% packed cell volume) on to a drop (12 µl) of buffer containing isotope, incubate for an appropriate time period (1-3 s or more), stop influx and dilute extracellular $[^{14}C]$methylglucose by the addition of a large volume of 0.3 mM phloretin in buffer, add oil to the same tube, centrifuge and recover the cells above the oil. We have used the method to evaluate the transport system and we have found that it is largely symmetrical, at least in the insulin stimulated state, i.e. K_m for net uptake is about the same as K_m for equilibrium exchange. Non-mediated diffusion of methylglucose or glucose is negligible. In this communication we shall focus on the evaluation of transport of D-glucose.

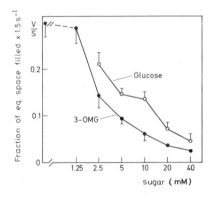 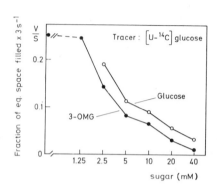

Fig. 8 (left). <u>Inhibition of the initial velocity of [^{14}C]methyl-glucose uptake by methylglucose and glucose</u>. The incubation time was 1.5 s. The points represent the mean of 4 values ± SD.
Fig. 9 (right). <u>Inhibition of the initial velocity of [^{14}C]glucose uptake by methylglucose and glucose</u>. The incubation time was 3 s. The ordinate refers to the distribution space at equilibrium for methylglucose.

Fig. 6 shows the uptake of 50 µM [^{14}C]methylglucose in the absence and the presence of 1 µM insulin at 22°C. It appears that the incubation time must be 2 s or less if a reasonable estimate of the initial velocity of uptake is to be obtained in the presence of insulin. K_m for methylglucose equilibrium exchange is about 3.5 mM at 22°C both in the absence and in the presence of insulin (data not shown). Fig. 7 shows the uptake of 50 µM [^{14}C]desoxyglucose at 22°C. Surprisingly, this analogue is taken up at a much slower rate than methylglucose. However, the main point of Fig. 7 is that the uptake of [^{14}C]desoxyglucose in the presence of 7 mM glucose is markedly non-linear. This implies that the K_i for glucose on the 3 min uptake of desoxyglucose is not a measure of K_m for glucose transport. The value will be too low, probably because the intracellular concentration of glucose increases enough to cause a marked inhibition of the rate of phosphorylation of [^{14}C]desoxyglucose. Olefsky has reported K_i-values of 1.9 mM for glucose and 6.1 for methylglucose using incubation for 3 min[26].

Fig. 8 shows the inhibition of the initial velocity of [^{14}C]methylglucose uptake by methylglucose or glucose. It should be pointed out that the initial velocity will tend to be underestimated

with increasing concentrations of sugar because the net uptake
curve (intracellular sugar concentration initially zero) become
increasingly non-exponential ("flat") with increasing sugar concentrations[25]. This will cause a small bias (decrease) in the estimate of K_i. However, the main point of Fig. 8 is that K_i for glucose is about twice as high as that for methylglucose, i.e. about
7 mM. Fig. 9 shows that the apparent initial rate of uptake of
[^{14}C]methylglucose. Again, methylglucose is a better inhibitor
than glucose.

We have previously estimated K_m for methylglucose exchange, as
about 5 mM at 37°C and the smaller value reported here (3.5 mM) is
probably due to the lower temperature (22°C). Since K_i for glucose
on methylglucose uptake was about 7 mM at 22°C one would predict a
K_i of about 10 mM at 37°C. Loten et al.[27] found a K_i of about 13
mM for glucose inhibition of uptake of D-allose in adipocytes at
37°C. D-allose has a low affinity to the transport system and is
therefore taken up slowly with a half-time of about 5 min in the
presence of insulin[27]. The inhibitor, glucose, will be distributed
asymmetrically on the two sides of the adipocyte membrane within a
few seconds. However, since we have found the transport system to
be largely symmetrical, K_i for glucose on allose uptake should be
the same as K_i on methylglucose uptake. The combined evidence suggests that K_m for the glucose transport system is 2-3 times the
plasma glucose concentration in fasting animals.

Is degradation of receptor-bound insulin necessary for induction
of the increased permeability to glucose? We have attempted to
answer this question by incubating the cells under conditions which
are known to change the binding or which we suspected would block
degradation. Insulin binding is increased about 3 fold at pH 7.6
as compared to pH 7.1; at the same time the insulin dose-response
relationship with respect to uptake of methylglucose is displaced
to the left. However, the same fraction of the bound insulin is
degraded in the pH range 6.8-8.6[28]. Therefore, it is impossible to
say whether the increased effect is due to the increased binding
per se or due to the increased receptor-mediated degradation.

Chloroquin (0.1 mM) and NH_4Cl (10 mM) block degradation of protein by lysosomes in hepatocytes[29]. In fibroblasts they block degradation and increase binding of epidermal growth factor[11]. These
agents do not cause important changes in receptor-mediated insulin

degradation in adipocytes[28]. This is also true for dinitrophenol
(0.5 mM), azide (10 mM) and cyanide (0.5 mM) which block the effect
of insulin on hexose transport in adipocytes[30]. These metabolic inhibitors, which deplete the cells for ATP, also block the transformation of insulin bound to the adipocyte plasma membrane to the
"peak II" described by Kono et al.[30]. The results show that receptor-mediated insulin degradation is not sufficient to induce an
increase in the permeability to glucose. They also suggest that
Kono's "peak II" is not the pathway to degradation of bound insulin. Finally, it seems unlikely that receptor bound insulin is degraded by lysosomal enzymes. However, the link between the insulin-
receptor-(enzyme?) complex and the increase in V_{max} for hexose
transport still remains unidentified.

REFERENCES

1. Robinson, D.S. (1970) Compr.Biochem. 18, 51-116.
2. Pokrajac, N., Lossow, W.J. & Chaikoff, I.L. (1967) Biochim.Biophys.Acta 139, 123-132.
3. Stewart, J.E. & Schotz, M.C. (1971) J.Biol.Chem. 246, 5749-5753.
4. Patten, R.L. (1970) J.Biol.Chem. 245, 5577-5584.
5. Pykälistö, O.J., Smith, P.H. & Brunzell, J.D. (1975) J.clin.Invest. 56, 1108 -1117.
6. Gammeltoft, S. & Gliemann, J. (1973) Biochim.Biophys.Acta 320, 16-32.
7. Gliemann, J. & Sonne, O. (1978) J.Biol.Chem. in print.
8. Kahn, C.R. & Baird, K. (1978) J.Biol.Chem. 253, 4900-4906.
9. Olefsky, J.M., Jen, P. & Reaven, G.M. (1974) Diabetes 23, 565-571.
10. Andersen, O., Gliemann, J. & Gammeltoft, S. (1977) Diabetologia 13, 589-594.
11. Carpenter, G. & Cohen, S. (1976) J.Cell Biol. 71, 159-171.
12. Goldstein, J.L. & Brown, M.S. (1974) J.Biol.Chem. 249, 5153-5162.
13. Gavin III, J.R., Roth, J., Neville, D.M., DeMeyts, P. & Buell, D.N. (1974) Proc.Nat.Acad.Sci.US 71, 84-88.
14. Gliemann, J., Østerlind, K., Vinten, J. & Gammeltoft, S. (1972) 286, 1-9.
15. DeMeyts, P., Bianco, A.R. & Roth, J. (1976) J.Biol.Chem. 251, 1877-1888.
16. Gliemann, J. & Sonne, O. (1977) Clin.Endocrinol. 7, 405-415.
17. Terris, S. & Steiner, D.F. (1975) J.Biol.Chem. 250, 8389-8398.
18. Gliemann, J. (1968) Acta physiol.scand. 72, 481-491.
19. Vinten, J., Gliemann, J. & Østerlind, K. (1976) J.Biol.Chem. 251, 794-800.
20. Livingston, J.N.& Lockwood, D.H. (1975) J.Biol.Chem. 250, 8353-8360.
21. Olefsky, J.M. (1976) J.clin.Invest. 58, 1450-1460.
22. Wieringa, T. & Krans, H.M.J. (1978) Biochim.Biophys.Acta 538, 563-570.
23. Czech, M.P. (1976) Molecul.Cell.Biochem. 11, 51-63.
24. Gliemann, J. & Whitesell, R.R. (1977) Diabetologia 13, 396 (abstract)
25. Whitesell, R.R. & Gliemann, J., manuscript in preparation.
26. Olefsky, J.M. (1978) Biochem.J. 172, 137-145.
27. Loten, E.G., Regen, D.M. & Park, C.R. (1976) J.Cell.Physiol. 89, 651-660.
28. Sonne, O. & Gliemann, J. (1978) 14th Meeting of the Europ.Diabetes Assoc. abstract.
29. Seglen, P.O. (1975) Biochem.Biophys.Res.Commun. 66, 44-52.
30. Kono, T., Robinson, F.W., Sarver, J.A., Vega, F.V. & Pointer, A.H. (1977) J.Biol.Chem. 252, 2226-2233.

Lipoprotein Metabolism and Endocrine Regulation
L.W. Hessel and H.M.J. Krans editors
© ECSC, EEC, EAEC, Brussels-Luxembourg, 1979
Published by Elsevier/North-Holland Biomedical Press-Amsterdam

THE EFFECT OF DIABETES AND PHOSPHOLIPASE TREATMENT ON BINDING
OF INSULIN AND GLUCOSE TRANSPORT IN ISOLATED ADIPOCYTES.

H.M.J. KRANS and TJ. WIERINGA

Department Endocrinology and Metabolic Diseases, University
Hospital, Rijnsburgerweg 10, Leiden (The Netherlands)

ABSTRACT

Low insulin levels in acute diabetes change the affinity for
insulin without rise of the total number of binding sites. The
increased occupancy of insulin receptors is reflected in greater
sensitivity of glucose transport for insulin, but both the basal
glucose transport and the maximal stimulatory effect of insulin
on glucose transport are greatly reduced. These changes are partly
induced by changes in the membrane.

Treatment of fat cells with highly purified phospholipase-A_2
induced a rise in number of binding sites, a greater sensitivity
for insulin, an increase in basal glucose transport and a reduced
maximal insulin effect. Phospholipase treatment mimics the
changes seen in diabetes only partially. Diabetes may induce
changes in phospholipid content. This may be a consequence of
changed intracellular metabolism or the changed external environment, as the rigidity of the membrane can be affected by the
cholesterol/phospholipid ratio and fatty acid structure.

INTRODUCTION

In general an inversed relationship between insulin levels and
binding sites is seen[1]. In non-regulated diabetes mellitus the
effectiveness of insulin is reduced. Reduction of insulin levels
in the blood increases binding with a delay of at least 12 hours
indicating that changes on the membrane level are not a direct
reflection of the insulin levels.

We centered our investigations around the question: How does
diabetes with low insulin levels influence the effect of insulin
in adipocytes? Do changes in the membrane phospholipids cause
identical changes in glucose transport and insulin binding?

METHODS AND MATERIALS

Rats were made diabetic by streptozotocin 90 mg/kg. After three days fat cells were prepared from the epidydymal fat pad. We compared these cells with cells of normal animals of the same age and weight. For experimental details about the preparation of cells, binding experiments, measurements of CO_2 production and 2-deoxyglucose transport see reference 2. Highly purified phospholipase A_2 (PHL-A_2) from Crotalus Adamanteus and from Bee venom was kindly supplied by Dr. R.F.A. Zwaal, (Department of Biochemistry, Utrecht). After preparation and washing cells were incubated with PHL-A_2 for 60 minutes in Krebs Ringer medium containing 5 mM Ca. The reaction was stopped by the addition of 10 mM EDTA. Fresh medium was used for the transport and binding studies. Control cells were incubated during the same time in the same medium without PHL-A_2.

RESULTS

The first step in the action of many polypeptide hormones is binding to the outside of the cell membrane. The specific binding of insulin in normal and diabetic cells is presented in the form of a Scatchard analysis (fig. 1). The binding is not linear. The affinity is increased without a change in total receptor number. This is at variance with the findings in hyperinsulinaemic states, in which both total number of binding sites and affinity are reduced[3,4]. Changes in affinity may be the first effect of a permanent reduction of insulin levels since longer standing insulin depreviation changes the total number of binding sites too[5,6].

Binding must be related with a secondary action, which is elicited by the binding[7,8]. The best effect of insulin to measure in adipocytes is glucose transport[9]. CO_2 production, the endproduct of a cascade of metabolic processes is decreased in diabetic cells in both the basal state and after stimulation with insulin. 2-Deoxyglucose, a glucose analogue which is transported through the cell wall and phosphorylated but not metabolized further inside the cell, gives more precise information about transmembranal transport. We measured the uptake during 3 minutes (linear for at least 5 minutes)[2].

In diabetic cells basal transport is decreased and the maximal
stimulatory effect of insulin is reduced (fig. 2).

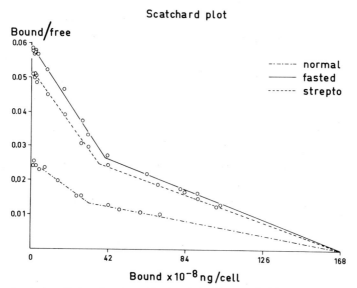

Fig. 1. Scatchard analysis of the binding of insulin to adipocytes
from fasted and diabetic rats.
Note that the insulin levels in the blood never exceed 20 ng/ml
presented on the left side of the X-axis.

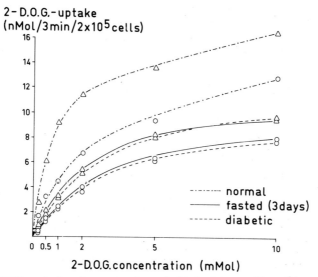

Fig. 2. 2 DOG-uptake in normal and diabetic cells. ● basal ▲ with
10 ng/ml insulin. The data are not corrected for passive diffusion.

The stimulatory effect of lower concentrations of insulin is
relatively less reduced. The stimulation curve of insulin has
shifted towards lower insulin concentrations (fig. 3).

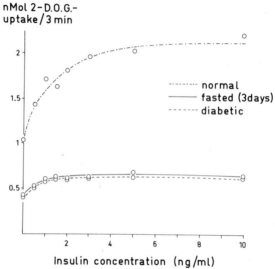

Fig. 3.
In diabetic cells the stimulation of the uptake of 2 DOG by insulin
is decreased but the K_m of the insulin effect is reduced.

The greater sensitivity for insulin is reflected in an increase
in binding although the maximal effect of insulin is reduced. This
may be a compensatory mechanism of diabetic cells for the lower
insulin levels.

These findings indicate that diabetes has an effect on the
membrane. Membrane transport is related with the structure of the
membrane. Physical and biochemical data are in accordance with the
fluid mosaic membrane model of Singer[10]. They are mostly obtained
from studies in the erythrocyt and may be extended to fat cells.

Cellular membranes are composed of a fluid lipid bilayer. The
fluidity allows lateral movement through a rather viscous environment. The membrane components are highly asymmetric with regard to
the cytoplasmatic and the outer side. This asymmetry may regulate
differences in membrane fluidity in each monolayer of the bilayer.
The outer monolayer is less fluid than the inner one[11]. The outer
monolayer may therefore act as the principal barrier between

cytoplasma and extracellular space.

We have seen in the electronmicroscope with the freeze-etch technique that in fat cells of diabetic animals the number of membrane particles which represent integral protein structure intercalating the lipid bilayer has not changed per cell. When our studies were in progress Carpentier et al published his more extensive study[12], which was in accordance with our findings. It may be presumed that the protein particles of the membrane are related to the specific receptors for the hormone. The receptor proteins are glycoproteins. But phospholipids may also be involved in the effect of insulin on glucose transport:

a) Changes in phospholipid components or in charge distribution may interfere with the exposure of the receptor to insulin.

b) They may influence the transport unit for glucose. Changes in fluidity of the membrane may be a contributing factor for the regulation of facilitated glucose transport.

The properties of the bilayer are dependend on the various phospholipid components, the structure of their fatty acids in the membrane, which contributes to the transition temperature. A change in cholesterol/ phospholipid ratio may contribute to the rigidity in the membranes.

In the diabetic fat cell the following changes may be related to changes in the membrane: a) increased binding, b) reduced glucose transport, c) increased insulin sensitivity, but reduced maximal effect of insulin, d) reduced diameter of the cell. Modification of phospholipids by phospholipase has been studied for glucose transport in fat cells[13,14] and for binding to fat cell membranes[15]. But these studies were performed with phospholipases with a high proteolytic activity. We used phospholipases which have a 1600 times higher purity. Highly purified PHL-A$_2$ hydrolyses specifically the fatty acids from the two position. PHL-A$_2$ of Bee venom hydrolyses 50% of the PC content without causing lysis of the cell. PHL-A$_2$ of the Crotalus Adamenteus has no effect (phospholipids may be a contributing factor). After treatment of isolated fat cells with 3.6 IU/ml PHL-A$_2$ $\pm$ 50% of the phospholipids are hydrolysed without causing lysis of the cells[16].

Cells treated in this way show the following characteristics:

a) The diameter of the cell has not changed.

b) The binding of insulin has increased. This is a result of a change in affinity and a rise in total number of binding sites. The latter factor is in contrast to what is seen in the diabetic state.

c) The basal 2-DOG transport is higher. The maximal stimulatory effect of insulin is slightly increased compared to normal cells. Related to the higher basal uptake the insulin effect is slightly decreased (fig. 4).

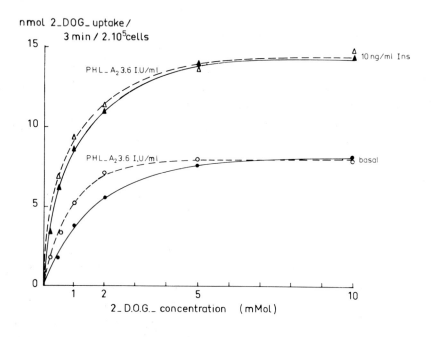

Fig. 4.
Treatment of adipocytes with PHL-A2, 3.6 IU/ml (- - -) increases basal uptake and the stimulatory effect of insulin at lower 2 DOG concentrations. The data are corrected for passive diffusion.

d) Looking at lower concentrations of insulin the PHL-A$_2$ treated cells show an increased sensitivity for insulin (shift towards left) (fig. 5). The findings for glucose transport and insulin effect are summarized in the next table.

TABLE 1

SUMMARY OF THE CHANGES IN 2-DOG TRANSPORT IN DIABETIC AND PHL-A$_2$
TREATED ADIPOCYTES COMPARED TO NORMAL ADIPOCYTES.

	Diabetic cells	PHL-A$_2$ treated cells
Insulin binding	increased by change in affinity only	increased by change in affinity and total receptor number
effect of insulin	shifted to lower insulin concentration	shifted to lower insulin concentration
basal glucose	decreased $K_m\uparrow V_{max}\downarrow$	increased $K_m\downarrow V_{max}$ unchanged
glucose transport with 10 ng/ml insulin	decreased $K_m\uparrow V_{max}\downarrow$	slightly decreased (both in K_m and V_{max})

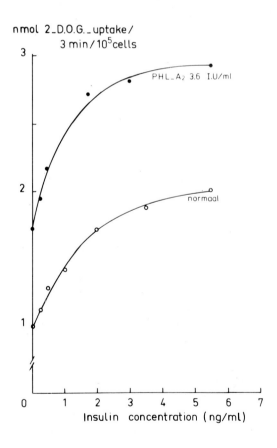

Fig. 5
PHL-A2 (. .) treated
adipocytes show an in-
creased sensitivity for
insulin.

DISCUSSION

Many questions regarding the mechanism of action of the effect of insulin on glucose transport remain undissolved. We provided evidence for an involvement of the membrane in the changes seen in diabetes. Changes in binding are reflected in a greater sensitivity for insulin. If the kinetic data for glucose transport are analyzed, K_m may be seen as a measure for the functional rate of transport and V_{max} as indicative for the total number of transport units provided that the K_m is identical. Insulin lowers K_m in normal cells (accelerates glucose uptake) and rises V_{max}. In diabetic cells the K_m is almost doubled compared to normal cells but insulin has a very small effect on the K_m. The V_{max} values are decreased in diabetic cells both in the basal state and when maximally stimulating concentrations of insulin are used[2]. Phospholipase decreases K_m but it has no effect on V_{max}[17]. It is not clear which factors are responsible for the changes in membrane composition. In diabetes it may be a consequence of intracellular lipolysis due to lack of glucose. But extracellular factors may be a contributing factor to the changes (in fluidity) in the membrane too.

ACKNOWLEDGEMENTS

We acknowledge the secretarial assistence of Miss C. v.d. Haak. The investigation was supported by the Foundation for medical Research FUNGO, which is subsidized by the Netherlands Organization for the Advancement of Pure Research ZWO.

REFERENCES

1. Olefsky, J.M. and Reaven, G.M. (1977) Diabetes, 26, 680-688.
2. Wieringa, Tj. and Krans, H.M.J. (1978) Biochim. Biophys. Acta, 538, 563-570.
3. Soll, H.A., Kahn, C.R., Neville, Jr., D.M. and Roth, J. (1975) J. Clin. Invest., 56, 769-780.
4. Olefsky, J.M. (1976) J. Clin. Invest., 57, 1165-1172.
5. v. Slooten, H., Wieringa, Tj., Jansen, M. and Krans, H.M.J. (1977) J. Endocrinol., 72, 48^p-49^p.
6. Olefsky, J.M. and Kobayashi, M. (1978) J. Clin. Invest., 61, 329-338.
7. Birnbaumer, L. (1973) Biochim. Biophys. Acta, 300, 129-158.

8. Krans, H.M.J., (1976) in Eukaryotic Cell Function and Growth, Dumont, J.E., Brown, B.L. and Marshall, N.J. eds., Plenum Press, New York and London, pp. 67-96.

9. Gliemann, J. and Sonne, O. (1977) Clin. Endocrinol., 7, 405-415.

10. Singer, S.J. and Nicolson, G.L. (1972) Science, 175, 720-731.

11. Emmelot, P. and van der Hoeven, R.D. (1975) Chemistry and Physics of Lipids, 14, 236-246.

12. Carpentier, J.L., Perrelet, A. and Orci, L. (1977) J. Cell Biol., 72, 104-117.

13. Rodbell, M. (1966) J. Biol. Chem., 241, 130-139.

14. Blecher, M. (1967) Biochim. Biophys. Acta, 137, 557-571.

15. Cuatrecasas, P. (1971) J. Biol. Chem., 246, 6532-6542.

16. Wieringa, Tj. and Krans, H.M.J. (1978) Diabetologia, 15, 376.

17. Wieringa, Tj. and Krans, H.M.J., manuscript in preparation.

Lipoprotein Metabolism and Endocrine Regulation
L.W. Hessel and H.M.J. Krans editors
© ECSC, EEC, EAEC, Brussels-Luxembourg, 1979
Published by Elsevier/North-Holland Biomedical Press-Amsterdam

HUMAN FAT CELL ADENYLATE CYCLASE: RESPONSIVENESS TOWARDS CATECHOLAMINES,
PEPTIDE HORMONES AND PROSTAGLANDINS.

HORST KATHER   and   BERND SIMON

Klinisches Institut für Herzinfarktforschung an der Medizinischen Universitätsklinik Heidelberg, Bergheimerstraße 58, D-69 Heidelberg, F.R.G.

ABSTRACT

The responsiveness of the human fat cell adenylate cyclase towards catecholamines, peptide hormones and prostaglandins was studied. The adrenergic agonists adrenaline, noradrenaline, isoproterenol and the β_2-selective agents salbutamol and terbutalin caused a dose-dependent increase of enzymic activity which was competetively inhibited by β-blocking agents. The order of potency of the adrenergic agonists supports the contention that the adrenergic receptors mediating the stimulatory effects of catecholamines are of the β_1-type.

Upon complete β-adrenergic blockade, the naturally occuring catecholamines, adrenaline and noradrenaline, caused an inhibition of enzymic activity below basal values with a maximum of about 40%, indicating that the human fat cell adenylate cyclase is coupled to alpha- as well as beta-adrenergic receptor sites mediating antagonistic catecholamine effects.

Of the peptide hormones tested only parathyroid hormone, which is the only peptide hormone known to activate lipolysis in adipose tissue of adult human beings, was found to stimulate the human fat cell adenylate cyclase.

Prostaglandins of the E- and F-series, which inhibit lipolysis in intact fat cells, were potent activators of the human fat cell adenylate cyclase.

The results suggest that the human fat cell adenylate cyclase might present a useful tool for sreening changes of hormone-responsiveness induced by drugs, diet, metabolic disorders or those related to age.

INTRODUCTION

The mobilization of stored triglycerides from adipose tissue is strictly controlled by lipolytic hormones. The first step in hormone-activated lipolysis is the activation of the receptor-coupled adenylate cyclase catalyzing the formation of cyclic 3,5-adenosine monophosphate (cAMP) from ATP[1]. cAMP activates a protein kinase which converts the hormone-sensitive triglyceride lipase from a state of low activity to an active form[2]. In this sequence of enzymes, the adenylate cyclase is the only step sensitive to the action of *lipolytic hormones. This membrane-bound effector system of hormone action, therefore, plays a central role in hormone-stimulated lipolysis.*

The rat fat cell adenylate cyclase reacts to at least six hormonal acti- vators including catecholamines and peptide hormones such as ACTH, LH, TSH, secretin and glucagon[1]. Human adipose tissue differs from rat adipose tissue in several aspects[3]. Studies on the rat fat cell adenylate cyclase revealed that this effector system of hormone action reflects the responsiveness of the intact tissue including changes of hormone-sensitivity related to age or in- duced by diet or drugs[4,5]. The rat fat cell adenylate cyclase has been thoroughly studied during the past few years. However, little information was available about the properties and hormone-sensitivity of the human fat cell adenylate cyclase. In order to get more detailed insight in the hormonal regulation of human fat cell function we, therefore, studied the properties and the hormone-sensitivity of the human fat cell enzyme. The results suggest that this enzyme system might present a useful tool for gaining more detailed insight in the mechanisms underlying the hormonal control of lipid mobilization under physiological and pathological conditions.

MATERIALS AND METHODS

Experimental procedures were the same as described previously[6,7]. Briefly: biopsies of subcutaneous adipose tissue were obtained from surgical patients not selected on the basis of age, sex, weight, or disease. The subjects were operated after an overnight fast. The biopsies were usually obtained after the skin incision at the start of the operation.

Rat epididymal adipose tissue was obtained from male rats (Sprague-Dawley; Süddeutsche Versuchstierfarm, Tuttlingen, F.R.G.), 150-200g in weight, and maintained on a standard laboratory chow (Altromin[R]). The animals were killed by decapitation.

Fat cells and fat cell ghosts were prepared according to Rodbell[8]. The adenylate cylase activity was determined by the method of Salomon et al.[9] at $30^{o}C$. The assay mixture contained 25 mmol/l tris-HCL, pH 8.0, 5 mmol/l $MgCl_2$, 20 mmol/l creatine phosphate, 100 U/ml creatine phosphokinase, 1 mmol/l cAMP, 1 mmol/l ATP containing 40-50 cpm/pmol $\alpha-^{32}P$ ATP and, when present, GTP as indicated in the legends to figures and tables. The protein content of the samples was measured according to Lowry et al.[10] Data are given as nmol cAMP per mg protein per 15 min. Statistical analysis was by the Wilcoxon test for paired observations.

$\alpha-^{32}P$ ATP (2-6 Ci/mmol) and ^{3}H cAMP (21 Ci/mmol) were from the Radio-

chemical Centre Amersham, Bucks, U.K. L-Adrenaline-bitartrate was from Merck AG, Darmstadt, F.R.G. Isoproterenol and propranolol were from Böhringer Ingelheim, Ingelheim, F.R.G.; methypranol was from Böhringer Mannheim, Mannheim, F.R.G.; prindolol was from Sandoz AG, Nürnberg, F.R.G.; bupranolol was from Pharma Schwarz, Monheim, F.R.G.; alprenolol and atenolol were from Pharma-Stern, Wedel, F.R.G. and from ICI-Pharma, Planckstadt, F.R.G. respectively. Prostaglandin E_1 was a gift of Dr. Brunnberg, Upjohn GmbH, Heppenheim, F.R.G. Synthetic 1-34 parathyroid hormone (PTH) was from Beckman Instruments, Fullerton, California.

RESULTS

The properties of the human fat cell adenylate cyclase are similar to those reported from the rat fat cell enzyme[11]. The pH-optimum in the presence of adrenaline is about pH 8.0. Magnesium in excess of ATP has a stimulatory effect mainly on basal enzyme activity[6]. The naturally occuring guanine nucleotide GTP inhibited basal enzyme activity but had no significant effects on hormone-activated rates of cAMP-formation[12]. The synthetic GTP-analogue 5'-guanylyl imidodiphosphate, on the other hand, caused a marked increase of basal as well as hormone-stimulated rates of cAMP-formation[13]. Similar results were reported by others[14-16].

Table 1 compares the effects of various hormones on the adenylate cyclase from rat epididymal adipose tissue and from membrane preparations of adult human fat cells. The enzyme system of rats reacted to all hormones tested, i.e. adrenaline (0.5 mmol/l), ACTH, glucagon and parathyroid hormone. However, only adrenaline and parathyroid hormone could increase the activity of the human fat cell enzyme, indicating that the species differences in the lipolytic response to hormones are reflected by the hormone-sensitivity of the adenylate cyclases of rats and adult human beings.

Figure 1 shows the effects of ascending concentrations of different adrenergic agonists on the human fat cell adenylate cyclase. Maximally effective concentrations of isoproterenol (5×10^{-5} mol/l) induced about a 6-fold increase of enzymic activity. The ß-adrenergic antagonist propranolol at concentrations of 5×10^{-7} mol/l and 5×10^{-8} mol/l caused a dose-dependent parallel rightward shift of the dose-response curve of the almost pure ß-adrenergic agonist isoproterenol[17,18]; indicating that the receptors mediating the stimulatory effects of catecholamines are of the ß-adrenergic type. The naturally occuring mixed agonists, adrenaline and noadrenaline, by causing a maximal activation of 400% and 300% respectively had lower intrinsic activity than

TABLE 1

EFFECTS OF VARIOUS HORMONES ON THE FAT CELL ADENYLATE CYCLASE OF RATS AND ADULT HUMAN BEINGS

Hormone[b]	Adenylate cyclase activity (nmol cAMP/mg protein/15 min.)[a]	
	Human[c]	Rat[d]
–	1.0 ± 0.2	0.7 ± 0.1
Adrenaline	4.2 ± 0.3	3.3 ± 0.3
PTH	2.3 ± 0.2	1.7 ± 0.1
ACTH	1.0 ± 0.2	2.1 ± 0.2
Glucagon	1.1 ± 0.1	3.0 ± 0.3

[a] *Values are mean ± SEM of six separate experiments carried out in triplicate. The assay mixture contained 0.01 mmol/l GTP.*
[b] *The concentration of adrenaline was 0.5 mmol/l; the concentrations of the peptide hormones were 0.01 mg/ml.*
[c] *Human adipose tissue was from random surgical patients in the age range of 30-60 years.*
[d] *The weight of the rats was 150-200g.*

isoproterenol. These latter hormones were considerably more effective in stimulating the human fat cell adenylate cyclase than the β_2-selective agents salbutamol and terbutalin (Figure 1).

Isoproterenol showed a characteristic higher affinity than adrenaline and noradrenaline. Half-maximal effects were observed at an isoproterenol concentration of 10^{-6} mol/l whereas the corresponding concentrations of adrenaline and noadrenaline were found to be 10-30-times higher. Taken together with the low affinity of the β_2-selective agonists terbutalin and salbutamol, these results suggest, that the β-adrenergic receptor sites mediating the stimulatory effects of catecholamines are of the β_1-subtype. The stimulatory effect of adrenaline depended on the source of the biopsies. Membrane preparations of gluteal adipose tissue were considerably less responsive towards the hormone than abdominal preparations[19] (Figure 5).

However, besides their stimulatory effects the naturally occuring mixed agonists, adrenaline and noradrenaline, - but not isoproterenol - had also inhibitory effects which became apparent upon β-adrenergic blockade. Figure 2 shows a typical dose-response curve for adrenaline in the presence and ab-

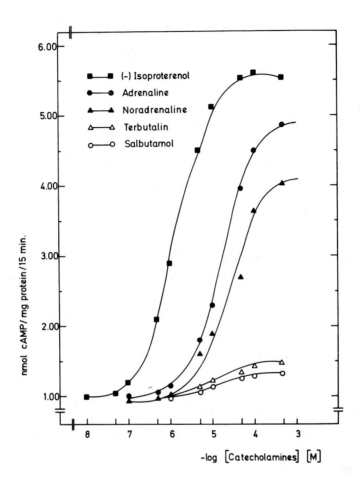

Fig. 1. Dose-Response Curves for various adrenergic Agonists

sence of $5x10^{-5}$ mol/l propranolol. In the presence of this ß-adrenergic antagonist the catecholamine caused a dose-dependent inhibition of basal enzyme
activity with a maximum of about 40%, indicating that the human fat cell
adenylate cyclase is coupled to alpha- and beta adrenergic receptor sites
mediating antagonistic catecholamine effects. This concept is further supported
by the fact that alpha-blocking agents like dihydroergotamine tend to aug-
ment the stimulatory effect of adrenaline (not shown) whereas alpha-adrenergic
excitation by phenylephrine results in an inhibition of isoproterenol-stimulated adenylate cyclase activity[20].

In order to establish the usefulness of the human fat cell adenylate
cyclase in estimating the effects of drugs affecting the mobilization of

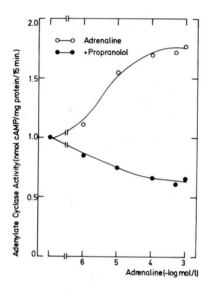

Fig. 2.   Effects of Adrenaline in the Presence and Absence of 5×10^{-5} mol/l
Propranolol.

A representative experiment out of 5 is shown. Values are means
of triplicate determinations.

triglycerides from adipose tissue, the inhibitory effects of various ß-blocking
agents used in the therapy of cardiovascular disease and hypertension on
isoproterenol-stimulated enzyme activity were compared (Figure 3). None of
the drugs had significant effects on basal enzyme activity over the whole
concentration range tested (1×10^{-8} mol/l to 5×10^{-4} mol/l)[21]. The non-selective
ß-blocking agents propranolol, bupranolol, prindolol and oxyprenol were of
comparable potency in inhibiting the stimulatory effect of isoproterenol.
Half-maximal inhibition occured at concentrations between 3×10^{-7} mol/l and
3×10^{-6} mol/l. The cardioselective ß-adrenergic antagonist atenolol, however,
was about 1000-times less effective than the non selectiv drugs, indicating
that the $ß_1$-receptors coupled to the human fat cell adenylate cyclase differ
from those of other organs such as heart.

Prostaglandins are potent inhibitors of hormone-stimulated lipolysis in human and rat adipose tissue[22]. As opposed to their antilipolytic effects in
intact cell preparations prostaglandins of the E- and F-type were potent
activators of the human fat cell adenylate cyclase[23]. This is illustrated
in Figure 4 showing the mutual interrelationship of various concentrations
of prostaglandin E_1 and of adrenaline. Maximally effective concentrations

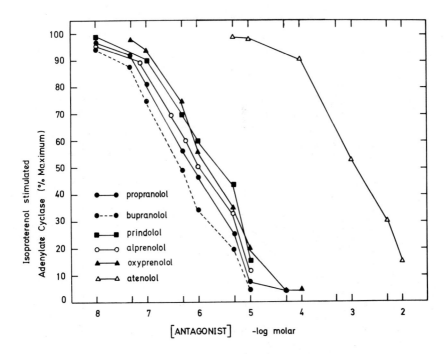

Fig. 3. *Effects of various ß-adrenergic Antagonists on Isoproterenol-stimu-*
lated Adenylate Cyclase Activity.

A representative experiment out of 4 is shown. Values are means of
triplicate determinations. The concentration of isoproterenol was
50 μmol/l.

of prostaglandin E_1 induced about a 4-fold increase of enzyme activity.
Half-maximal effects occured at a prostaglandin E_1 concentration of about
10^{-5} mol/l, indicating that prostaglandin E_1 and adrenaline are of comparable
potency in activating the human fat cell adenylate cyclase. In addition, the
combined effects of adrenaline and prostaglandin E1, although less than
completely additive, were higher than those of each agonist alone.

DISCUSSION

An intriguing feature of hormone-stimulated lipolysis in adipose tissue
is its species specificity. Our studies show that catecholamines and parathyroid hormone, which are the only known activators of lipolysis in adipose
tissue of adult human beings are activators of the human fat cell adenylate
cyclase[3,24]. Glucagon and ACTH which are effective in the rat, but not in
human beings had no stimulatory effects on the enzyme system of adult human

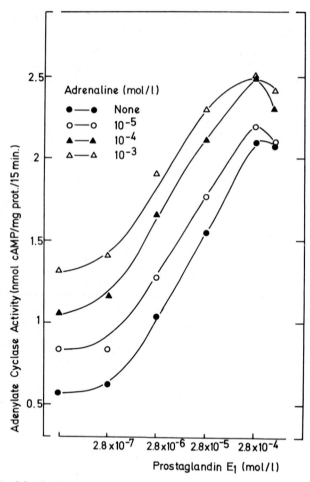

Fig. 4. *Combined Effects of various Concentrations of Adrenaline and Prostaglandin E_1.*

A representative experiment out of 4 is shown. Values are means of triplicate determinations. The assay mixture contained 0.01 mmol/l GTP.

beings. Our results thus support the view that species differences in the response to lipolytic hormones are reflected by differences in the hormone-sensitivity of human and rat fat cell adenylate cyclases. It should be noted, however, that increasing weight and senescence are accompanied by an impaired response of the adenylate cyclase of rat adipose tissue towards peptide hormones such as ACTH and glucagon[4,5]. Our observations about the lacking effects of peptide hormones other than parathyroid hormone may, therefore, be a result of the use of fat from adults. Metabolic studies concerning age-related

*changes of hormone-sensitivity are severely restricted by the small quantities
of adipose tissue obtainable from children. The determination of adenylate
cyclase activity requires considerably less material than metabolic studies
thus providing an opportunity for conducting systematic studies on age-related or diet-induced changes of hormone-sensitivity. Studies currently
underway in our laboratory suggest that the human fat cell adenylate cyclase
is in fact subject to age-related changes of hormone-sensitivity.*

*Adrenergic receptors are generally classified into alpha- and beta-types.
The latter class is divided into β_1- and β_2-subtypes[25]. We have demonstrated
that the human fat cell enzyme reacts to β_1- and β_2-adrenergic agonists.
The activation induced by these substances was competetively inhibited by
β-blocking agents, indicating that the receptor sites mediating the stimulatory effects of catecholamines are of the β-adrenergic type. The order of
potency (isoproterenol > adrenaline = noradrenaline > β_2-adrenergic agonists)
supports the contention that the β-adrenergic receptors coupled to the human
fat cell adenylate cyclase are of the β_1-subtype.*

*Whilst the major emphasis of the study of a new β-blocking drug is on the
cardiovascular system, it is important to determine its action on the metabolic responses in man. Even slight changes in lipid and carbohydrate metabolism have implications for long-term β-blocking therapy in the treatment
of hypertensive patients who are already prone to ischemic heart disease
because of their hypertension. It is well known that catecholamines have
many effects in vivo which tend to complicate the estimation of the antilipolytic potency of β-blocking agents. There is, therefore, a need for
new tests which will relate efficacy to selectivity of action.*

*The adenylate cyclase is the physiological relevant target of β-adrener-
gic catecholamines. The relative effects of various beta-blocking agents on
the isoproterenol-activated human fat cell adenylate cyclase are in good
agreement with their effects in intact cell preparations[26-28]. These findings, therefore, raise the possibility of using the human fat cell adenylate cyclase for estimating the effects of new β-adrenergic substances on
the mtabolism of human adipose tissue.*

*As opposed to rat adipose tissue human fat cells have been shown to con-
tain alpha- as well as β-adrenergic receptor sites mediating antagonistic
catecholamine effects[3,29]. Our data confirm and extend the findings of
Burns and Langley[30] that both types of adrenergic receptors are coupled
to the adenylate cyclase system in human fat cells. The observed stimulatory action of the naturally occuring catecholamines, adrenaline and noradrenaline, is the balance between opposing alpha- and β-adrenergic effects*

198

with the ß-component as the predominant one. Metabolic studies suggest
that the relation of alpha-/beta-adrenergic responsiveness is different
in different body regions[31,32]. The reduced responsiveness of the gluteal
adenylate cyclase towards the stimulatory action of adrenaline might reflect these regional differeneces in the relation of alpha-/beta-adrener-
gic responsiveness. Such a relationship, however, remains to be established
in future studies. Nevertheless our finddings about the reduced responsiveness of the gluteal enzyme towards the stimulatory effect of adrenaline
demonstrate that human adipose tissue cannot be regarded as uniform in all
areas.

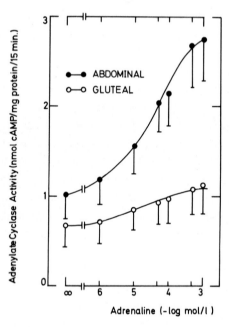

Fig. 5. Log-Dose Response Curve for Adrenaline in Membrane Preparations
from the Abdomen and the Buttock of the same Subjects.

Values are mean ± SEM of six experiments carried out in triplicate.
(from Kather et al., Europ. J. Clin. Invest. 7, 595-597, 1977)

Prostaglandins have been reported to stimulate lipolysis under certain
conditions[22,33]. However, their main effect appears to be an ihibitory one
on the mobilization of free fatty acids and glycerol from adipose tissue
of various species[22,34]. This inhibitory effect is associated with a decrease of intracellular cAMP[22,34,35]. Since prostaglandins are synthesized
in response to catcholamines in rat adipocytes[36,37] it has been proposed

that these C-20 fatty acids might act as feed back inhibitors of hormone-
stimulated lipolysis at the level of enzymes involved in the formation of
cAMP[38]. We have shown that the human fat cell adenylate cyclase reflects
the hormone-responsiveness of the intact tissue in many aspects. It is,
therefore, unlikely that stimulation of the human fat cell adenylate cyclase
is a non physiological artefact. Our findings thus support the view that
that prostaglandins may play an important role in human fat cell function
but cast doubt on the validity of the negative feed back concept for human
adipose tissue.

Mainly based on the negative feed back concept of prostaglandin action
Curtis-Prior[39] previously suggested that metabolic obesity is caused by
overproduction of prostaglandins. He concluded that aspirin, which inhibits
prostaglandin synthesis, might protect against hypertensive heart disease
and myocardial infarction by lowering the incidence of overweight. However,
in a joint clinical study with doses of aspirin at least five times higher
than those required for complete inhibition of prostaglandin synthesis in
human platelets we have observed no weight loss over two years[41].
Our biochemical and clinical data, therefore, suggest that more needs to
be found out about the physiological effects of prostaglandins on human
fat cell function before prostaglandin antagonists or sythetase inhibitors
are tried in the obese.

CONCLUSIONS

The human fat cell adenylate cyclase reflects the hormone-responsiveness
of the intact tissue in many aspects, suggesting that this membrane-bound
effector system of hormone action might be useful in gaining further insight in the hormonal regulation of human fat cell function. The adenylate
cyclase assay requires considerably less material than metabolic studies.
This system, therefore, should be most suitable in performing systematic
studies on problems related to the effects of age and diet or concerning
the pathogenesis of metabolic disorders such as diabetes or obesity. The
investigation of these problems should be essential not only in understanding the pathogenesis, but also in the search of drugs useful in the therapy
pertaining to such disorders.

The physiological meaning of the stimulatory effects of prostaglandins
is difficult to assess at this time. The effects of these C-20 fatty acids
on intact fat cells are suggestive for an operating feed back inhibition
of the adenylate cyclase. Further studies are necessary on the possible existence of other members of the prostaglandin family inducing an inhibition
instead of stimulating the human fat cell adenylate cyclase.

ACKNOWLEDGEMENTS

*This work was supported by grants of the Deutsche Forchungsgemeinschaft,
Bonn-Bad Godesberg, F.R.G. The authors wish to thank Mrs. I. Ring for
excellent technical assistence.*

REFERENCES

1. *Birnbaumer, L. (1973) Biochim. Biophys. Acta, 300, 129-158.*

2. *Steinberg, D., Meyer, S.E.,Khoo,J.C., Miller, E.A., Fredholm, B., Eichner,R.
   (1975) Adv. Cyclic Nucleotide Res.,5, 549-568.*

3. *Burns,T.W., Langley, P.E. and Robison, G.H. (1972) Adv. Cyclic Nucleotide
   Res.,1, 63-85.*

4. *Manganiello, V. and Vaughan, M. (1972) J. Lipid Res.,13, 12-16.*

5. *Cooper, B., Weinblatt, F. and Gregerman, R.I. (1977) J. Clin. Invest.,59,
   467-474.*

6. *Kather, H. and Geiger, M. (1977) Europ. J. Clin. Invest.7, 363-371.*

7. *Kather, H. and Simon, B. (1977) J. Clin. Invest.,59, 730-733.*

8. *Rodbell, M. (1972) in Methods in Cyclic Nucleotide Research, Chasin, M. ed.,
   Marcel Dekker, New York, pp. 101-124.*

9. *Salomon, Y., Londos, C. and Rodbell, M. (1974) Anal. Biochem.,58, 541-548.*

10. *Lowry, O.H., Rosebrough, N.J., Farr, A.L. and Randall, R.J. (1951)
    J. Biol. Chem.,193, 265-275.*

11. *Rodbell, M. (1975) J. Biol. Chem.,250, 5826-5834.*

12. *Kather, H., Zöllig, K. and Simon, B. (1978) Horm. Metab. Res.,10, 46-49.*

13. *Kather, H. and Simon, B. (1976) Clin. Chim. Acta,73, 497-504.*

14. *Cooper, B., Partilla, J.S. and Gregerman, R.I. (1975) J. Clin. Invest.,
    56, 1350-1353.*

15. *Cooper, B., Partilla, J.S. and Gregerman, R.I. (1976) Biochim. Biophys.
    Acta,445, 246-258.*

16. *Poupon, R. (1975) Biomedicine (Paris),23, 438-442.*

17. *Kather, H., Vogt, B. and Simon, B. (1977) Klin. Wschr.,55, 625-628.*

18. *Kather, H. and Simon, B. (1977) Metabolism,26, 1179-1185.*

19. *Kather, H., Zöllig, K., Simon, B. and Schlierf, G. (1977) Europ. J. Clin.
    Invest., 7, 595-597.*

20. *Kather, H., Vogt, B. and Simon, B. (1977) Experientia, 33, 541-542.*

21. *Kather, H. and Simon, B. (1977) Res. Comm. Chem. Pathol. Pharmacol., 18,
    11-18.*

22. *Carlson, L.A. (1965) Ann. N.Y. Acad. Sci., 131, 119-142.*

23. *Kather, H. and Simon, B. (1977) J. Cyclic Nucleotide Res., 3, 199-206.*

24. *Sinha, T., Thajchayapong, P., Queener,S.F., Allen, D.O. and Bell, N.H. (1976)
    Metabolism, 25, 251-260.*

25. *Lands, A.M., Arnold, A., Mc Anliff, J.P., Induena, F.P. and Brown, T.G.
    (1967) Nature, 214, 597-598.*

26. Harms, H.H. and Van der Meer, J. (1975) Br. J. Clin. Pharmacol.,2, 311-315.

27. Frisk-Holmberg, M. and Östman, J. (1977) J. Pharmacol. Exptl. Therap., 200, 598-605.

28. Wenkeova, J., Kuhn, E. and Wenke, M. (1976) Europ. J. Pharmacol.,37, 91-95.

29. Rosenquist, U. (1972) Acta Med. Scand., 192, 361-369

30. Burns, T.W. and Langley, P.E. (1975) J. Cyclic Nucleotide Res., 1, 321-328.

31. Kissebah, A.H., Vydelingum, N., Adams, P.W. and Wynn, V. (1978) Fifth Interntl. Congress of Endocinology, Diabetes and Obesity, Marseille, Abstract.

32. Arner, P., Engfeldt, P., Nowak,J. and Östman, J. (1978) Fifth Interntl. Congress of Endocrinology, Diabetes and Obesity, Abstract.

33. Butcher, R.W. and Baird, C.E. (1968) J. Biol. Chem., 243, 1713-1717.

34. Rosenquist, U. and Efendic, S. (1971) Acta Med. Scand., 190, 341-345.

35. Gilbert, C.H. and Galton, D.J. (1974) Horm. Metab. Res., 6, 229-233.

36. Dalton, C. and Hope, W.C. (1974) Prostaglandins, 6, 227-242.

37. Shaw, J.E. and Ramwell, P.W. (1968) J. Biol. Chem., 243, 1498-1503.

38. Bergström, S. (1967) Science, 157, 382-391.

39. Curtis-Prior, P.B. (1975) Lancet, I, 897-899.

40. Kather, H., Walter, E. and Simon, B. (1978) Lancet, II, 111.

Lipoprotein Metabolism and Endocrine Regulation
L.W. Hessel and H.M.J. Krans editors
© ECSC, EEC, EAEC, Brussels-Luxembourg, 1979
Published by Elsevier/North-Holland Biomedical Press-Amsterdam

HORMONE-STIMULATED PHOSPHATIDYLINOSITOL BREAKDOWN AND ITS RELATIONSHIP TO
HORMONE-STIMULATED CALCIUM MOBILISATION.

R.H. MICHELL

Department of Biochemistry, University of Birmingham, P.O. Box 363, Birmingham
B15 2TT (UK)

SUMMARY

It appears likely that there is a substantial family of hormone receptors
whose main intracellular message is a rise in the Ca^{2+} ion concentration in the
cytosol of target cells. These receptors also activate phosphatidylinositol
breakdown, but in a Ca^{2+}-independent manner, and this reaction may be involved
in some general unitary mechanism by which many different receptors bring about
mobilisation of Ca^{2+} in target cells. Amongst these receptors are the α-adrenergic, vasopressin and angiotensin receptors of liver, and probably the α-adrenergic receptors of adipose tissue. The role of phosphatidylinositol metabolism in
cellular responses to insulin is much less clear. The idea that inositol lipids
are implicated in endocrine control of lipid and lipoprotein metabolism is
strongly supported by the imbalance of these processes which characterises
inositol-deficient animals.

INTRODUCTION

The idea that cAMP is an intracellular second messenger which transmits to
the cell interior a wide variety of hormonal messages that are detected by hormone receptors at the cell surface has grown from the clear starting point provided by Sutherland's discovery that this nucleotide was synthesised in adrena-
line-treated dog liver and that it could cause activation of glycogen phosphorylase. Subsequently, almost every known hormonal effect has been investigated to
see whether it might be mediated through the production of cAMP as a second
messenger[1]. As a result of these studies there is evidence that quite a large
number of hormones exert at least some of their effects on cells by the activation of adenylate cyclase, but it has also become clear that many cell surface
receptors must provoke cellular responses in other ways. Indeed, this was
always to be expected since many hormones produce effects quite different from,
and sometimes opposite to, the effects evoked in the same cells by hormones
which employ cAMP as their second messenger.

The search for other second messengers which, together with cAMP, form the
intracellular language by which hormone receptors at cell surfaces communicate

with intracellular enzymes has proceeded at a much less decisive pace, maybe because it could not follow the same pattern of divergence away from a clear point of departure. For a time it appeared that the control of cellular cGMP levels would provide such a point of departure, with the elevation of cGMP levels in heart by stimulation of muscarinic cholinergic receptors as one of the crucial early observations. This was not to be, since little evidence has since been found in support of the idea that levels of intracellular cGMP have profound effects on cellular function[2].

Ca^{2+} AS AN INTRACELLULAR MESSENGER

The other candidate as an intracellular messenger which has recently received substantial support is the Ca^{2+} ion. Here the evidence is far better, even though the mechanisms by which activation of a variety of cell surface receptors can bring about a rise in the Ca^{2+} ion concentration ($[Ca^{2+}]$) in the cytosol compartment of cells is still a matter of considerable dispute. Table 1 includes a number of receptors which appear, on the basis of current evidence, to bring about many of their effects in cells as a result of a rise in cytosol $[Ca^{2+}]$. It will be apparent that here we have another family of receptors that share an intracellular effector and that comprise a group at least as large as the family for which cAMP is the second messenger. Also in Table 1 are certain other receptors which are known to stimulate phosphatidylinositol metabolism in target cells, but whose effects on Ca^{2+} mobilisation are not clear. The reason for their inclusion will become clear later.

So far as I am aware, there is no cell known in which the Ca^{2+} concentration in the cytosol compartment is in equilibrium with the external environment. Indeed, even in unicellular organisms any rise in cytosol $[Ca^{2+}]$ from the micromolar or submicromolar range towards levels which approach those outside the cell's causes gross disorganisation of cell activity. It therefore, seems reasonable to conclude that the maintenance of a low cytosol $[Ca^{2+}]$ by outward pumping - and hence the potential control of cells through elevation of cytosol $[Ca^{2+}]$ by leakage into the cytosol compartment from the exterior or from sequestered pools within the cell (e.g. in mitochondria) - may be a universal and essential attribute of all cells, or at least of all eukaryote cells. By contrast, the fact that certain strains of cells in culture can survive quite well without adenylate cyclase and hence with minimal cellular levels of cAMP indicates that this may be part of a less universally essential control system.

Why then has it taken so long for attention to focus on Ca^{2+} as a general intracellular control ligand, even though its central importance in particular

TABLE 1

RECEPTORS WHOSE EFFECTS ON APPROPRIATE TARGET CELLS ARE MEDIATED BY Ca^{2+} AND/OR
WHICH STIMULATE PHOSPHATIDYLINOSITOL (PI) METABOLISM

Unless otherwise indicated, original references can be found in references 3-5

Stimulus	Responses involve Ca^{2+}	Stimulation of PI metabolism
Muscarinic cholinergic	Yes	Yes
α-adrenergic	Yes	Yes
5-hydroxytryptamine	Yes	Yes
Histamine (H_1-receptors)	Yes	Yes
Pancreozymin	Yes	Yes
Bombesin	Yes	Yes
Substance P	Yes	Yes
Angiotensin	Yes	Yes
Vasopressin	Yes(some)	Yes
Antigens and other secretogogues (mast cells)	Yes	Yes
fmet-leu-phe	Yes	Yes
Thyrotropin	Yes? (some)	Yes
Parathyrin	Yes? (some)	Yes
ADP, thrombin, collagen	Yes	Yes
Membrane depolarisation	Yes	Yes
Glucose or mannose (pancreatic islets)	Yes	Yes
Ocytocin	Yes	?
Bradykinin	Yes	?
$PGF_{2α}$	Yes	?
Thyroliberin	Yes[8]	?
Luliberin	Yes[9]	?
Receptors controlling protozoan ciliary activity	Yes	?
Nerve growth factor	?	Yes[6,7]
Various other cellular proliferative situations	Yes?	Yes

tissues such as skeletal muscle and heart has long been appreciated. The answer
probably lies in two areas. First, it is extremely difficult to accurately
measure $[Ca^{2+}]$ within the cytosol compartment of cells and to unequivocally
identify the source of the Ca^{2+} which is mobilised during hormonally-induced

rises in cytosol $[Ca^{2+}]$. Methods for the former measurement include Ca^{2+}-sensitive dyes (e.g. arsenazo III), photoproteins (aequorin or obelin) or electrodes, which cannot yet be reliably admitted to most cells. Measurement of fluxes of ^{45}Ca, the method by which the latter unknown is usually assessed, have almost as many interpretations as there are experimenters collecting the data. Thus, decisions about the importance or otherwise of Ca^{2+} in initiating particular cell responses usually have to be taken on the basis of a quite finely balanced judgement (or, as far as sceptics are concerned, a guess) as to the overall meaning of a variety of experimental observations which, taken individually, would be inconclusive. Many pharmacologists and physiologists have operated successfully, if unhappily, within these experimental limitations, but this is not the sort of situation in which most biochemists like to become involved. The second major obstacle to the clear understanding of the intracellular control function of Ca^{2+} has lain in the diversity of directions from which relevant information has come. Most scientists confine themselves to a single discipline (often the study of a single tissue, metabolic pathway or hormone). But key data on the role of Ca^{2+} as a mediator of receptor-controlled effects have come from studies of the control of processes as diverse as contraction of smooth muscle[10-12], secretion of neurotransmitters and proteins[13-15], enhanced cellular permeability to K^+ ions[14-17] and hepatic glycogenolysis[18-20].

However, a very healthy aspect of any discipline which finally becomes coherent as a result of the convergence of many different threads of evidence, as appears now to be happening to the Ca^{2+} field, is that the final resolution of major problems, if there is to be one, can draw upon thinking which has happened quite independently in many different contexts: this cannot so easily happen in a closely focussed and divergently evolving world such as that inhabited by cyclic nucleotide workers. Inevitably, though, such initial diversity of approach leads to a substantial difficulty in the synthesis of unifying ideas, simply because of the complexity and variety of the information which needs to be reconciled.

PHOSPHATIDYLINOSITOL METABOLISM IS STIMULATED BY RECEPTORS WHICH CONTROL CELLULAR Ca^{2+} MOBILISATION

We were lucky to enter this field along a route quite different from that followed by most experimenters. We were analysing, in several tissues with several stimuli, an effect which was widespread and which appeared likely to have a single explanation wherever it was observed. This was the 'phospholipid effect' or 'phosphatidylinositol effect', a response first found in secretory tissues in the 1950s and later detected in a wide variety of cells stimulated by many, but not all, ligands which control cells through interactions with receptors at the cell surface[3-5,21,29]. This response appears to be initiated by hormonally stimulated breakdown of phosphatidylinositol (PI) followed by a compensatory resynthesis of this lipid which, in ^{32}P-labelled tissue, causes an increase in labelling of PI with [32]P (Fig. 1).

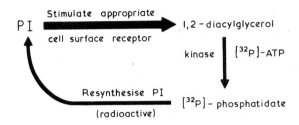

Fig. 1 Probable events in receptor-controlled PI breakdown and resynthesis.

It was only after we had realised that this is usually a response to receptors which do not control adenylate cyclase (i.e. to receptors for which the second messenger(s) appeared to be unknown)[3,21] that we noticed that the many effective receptors share two very interesting features: they usually bring about an increase in cellular cGMP levels and their actions appear to involve Ca^{2+} ions in some essential way (see ref 22 and Table 1). At about the same time, evidence was emerging which indicated that a rise in cellular cGMP levels is often little more than an indicator of a rise in cytoplasmic $[Ca^{2+}]$, (i.e. that this change is only one amongst the many responses to activation of these receptors which are mediated by a rise in cytosol $[Ca^{2+}]$). We were therefore very surprised when we found that the 'PI response' was not a consequence of a rise in intracellular Ca^{2+} concentration (see 4,5). This observation that the PI responses evoked by receptors whose main physiological effect appears to be the elevation of cytosol $[Ca^{2+}]$ concentration are Ca^{2+}-independent was the main factor which provoked us to suggest that PI breakdown might be a key event in bringing about the Ca^{2+} mobilisation that can be triggered by activation of any receptor in the Ca^{2+}-mobilising family.

Implicit in this suggestion was an unitary inference which had not been so clearly expressed until that time, namely that all members of this substantial family of Ca^{2+}-mobilising receptors might employ a fundamentally similar mechanism for bringing about a rise in cytosol $[Ca^{2+}]$. Although this type of unity had previously been considered as a possibility when more than one Ca^{2+}-mobilising receptor was found to operate in a single tissue (e.g. in controlling smooth muscle contraction), it is apparently not an idea which has until recently had much appeal across a broad spectrum of hormones and tissues (e.g. see 15).

Fortunately, however, this idea was eminently falsifiable. For example, if PI breakdown is really a reaction essential to the mechanisms of action of all Ca^{2+}-mobilising cell-surface receptors then it must accompany the operation of all of these receptors in all of the tissues in which they operate. So far, about four years of work aimed at testing this far-reaching prediction have failed to dissociate the activity of Ca^{2+}-mobilising receptors from stimulation of PI metabolism. In addition, they have strengthened the evidence that this response, unlike other more 'physiological' responses, is itself not a consequence of a rise in cytosol Ca^{2+}-concentration. The current situation is therefore that we have an unbroken correlation between Ca^{2+} mobilisation by receptors and Ca^{2+}-independent stimulation of PI breakdown by the same receptors (Table 1). Thus PI breakdown remains most easily explained as an event which has some essential role in the mechanisms of action of all of the receptors in a large family which uses Ca^{2+} as its intracellular messenger, but without any clear indication as to how PI breakdown contributes to this process (for reviews see refs. 3-5, 21, 29).

In addition to identifying a reaction which may be mechanistically important in the function of Ca^{2+}-mobilising receptors, this set of observations also has a second important consequence. It suggests, on the basis of numerous experiments which have been undertaken with the direct aim of either breaking or extending an existing correlation, that there is indeed a unity in at least one of the cellular responses to stimulation of all members of a family of diverse receptors. This may be the strongest argument yet available in support of the view that in looking for the modes of action of all of these Ca^{2+}-mobilising receptors we may indeed be looking for a single unitary mechanism. If correct, this conclusion would be of fundamental importance to studies of the cellular role of Ca^{2+} (in much the same way that the earlier conclusion that all members of another receptor family probably control adenylate cyclase by a single type of mechanism brought unity to that field).

MOBILISATION OF Ca^{2+} BY RECEPTORS: WHERE FROM AND HOW?

Detailed studies of calcium mobilisation by receptors, usually by using ^{45}Ca, have been done with a wide variety of cells. It is fortunate for a discussion of lipoprotein metabolism that some of the best studies have recently been with rat hepatocytes, but the bad news is that the situation even in this cell is still confused. A point upon which none of the major groups working on the

control of carbohydrate metabolism in this tissue appear to disagree is that
when the hepatocyte is stimulated with α-adrenergic agonists, with vasopressin
or with angiotensin there is a rapid activation of glycogen phosphorylase which
is brought about as a result of a rise in cytosol $[Ca^{2+}]$[18-20]. These hormones
also stimulate gluconeogenesis, stimulate PI breakdown and provoke a rapid incorporation of ^{32}P into PI[22-24]. Here, however, agreement ends. The simplest way
in which to assess the origin of the Ca^{2+} which activates phosphorylase is to
remove extracellular Ca^{2+} and see if the glycogenolytic response disappears. In
several studies this has been the observed result[18-20]. This suggests, as a
obvious explanation, that activation of these receptors causes an increase in
plasma membrane permeability to Ca^{2+} and that this ion then flows into the cell
down its substantial electrochemical gradient. In support of this view, there
have also been studies in which an influx of external ^{45}Ca into hepatocytes has
been seen very soon after stimulation by any of these hormones[19,20]. However,
if this was the only effect of stimulation, the net effect upon the stimulated
cell would inevitably be to cause an increase in its total calcium content.
This was the result in one study in which cells were stimulated with adrenaline
for an hour[25], but in two other studies in which calcium movements were followed
within the first few minutes (activation of phosphorylase occurs within a minute
or two) there was an early fall in cellular calcium content as a result of
stimulation[24,27]. This must mean that these stimulated cells rapidly released
to the exterior some of the calcium which they contained before stimulation,
and it seems quite likely that one of the intracellular origins of this calcium
was from mitochondria[26,27]. One of these studies also included a demonstration
that hepatocytes which had been only briefly depleted of Ca^{2+} could still
respond with glycogenolysis to any of these three hormones[26]. [It has also
been shown that α-adrenergic stimuli and angiotensin (vasopressin was not
tested) can trigger efflux of hepatocyte K^+, a cellular response that is
normally brought about by a rise in cytosol $[Ca^{2+}]$, even in a Ca^{2+}-free medium[17].
It is particulary interesting that in this study there appeared to be an easily
depleted cellular Ca^{2+} pool that was available to the two receptors in that a
second wave of K^+ efflux could not be evoked by repeated stimulation[17].]

The characteristics just described for the hepatocyte have many parallels in
other tissues which exhibit responses controlled by Ca^{2+}-mobilising receptors.
In most cases cells can show rapid responses to stimuli even when not supplied
with external Ca^{2+}, but only continue to respond to stimulation for prolonged
periods if external Ca^{2+} is made available continuously[10,14,16,17,28,29]. In
all such situations PI metabolism is stimulated, but only after further studies will
we understand: (a) the relative contributions to these cellular responses of

changes in cell surface permeability to Ca^{2+} and of Ca^{2+} liberation from intracellular pools; (b) the way in which activation of a receptor at the cell
surface provokes release of Ca^{2+} from an as yet unidentified intracellular site;
and (c) the role of Ca^{2+}-independent PI breakdown in this pattern of events.

PI METABOLISM AND CELL RESPONSES TO INSULIN

The mechanism of action of the insulin receptor is still an enigma: it does
not appear to belong to either of the receptor families discussed so far, i.e.
the cAMP and Ca^{2+} families. In the liver, in particular, this view is supported
by the clear difference between the actions of insulin, of either glucagon or
β-adrenergic stimuli, and of the three Ca^{2+}-mobilising receptors. Many years ago,
however, there was a report which suggested that insulin might cause a specific
stimulation of PI turnover, at least in adipocytes[30]. This phenomenon was later
analysed in much greater detail by Stein, who concluded that the changes in
lipid labelling caused by insulin were probably unspecific effects caused by
changes in the general pattern of phosphate utilisation in insulin-stimulated
adipocytes[31]: the original observation of enhanced PI labelling therefore
appeared trivial.

Recently, though, there has been an unexpected and provocative new twist to
the insulin story. As a tailpiece to a recent review[32] and in an abstract[33],
Czech has reported that insulin does indeed have specific effects upon PI
metabolism, but in a way quite different from other hormones. What is reported
in an increase in the rate of turnover of the fatty acids of PI which occurs
only in the PI of the plasma membrane. Moreover, he also reports that PI added
externally to adipocytes has a stimulatory effect on glucose entry into the
cells which resembles the effect of insulin.

Though fascinating, there are no details yet available of the experiments
upon which these conclusions have been based and so judgement upon their significance must be reserved.

INOSITOL AS A LIPOTROPIC FACTOR

When considering specific ideas about the possible role of inositol phospholipids in membrane function it is easy to forget that inositol first attracted
attention as a lipotropic growth factor[34]. In particular, animals deficient in
this trace nutrient develop a severe fatty liver which can be alleviated simply
by administration of inositol[35,36]. In the gerbil, there is also evidence that
inositol deficiency can cause an intestinal lipodystrophy[37,38]. However, much
of the early work designed to illuminate the aetiology of these conditions used
rather extreme dietary regimens in which factors other than inositol deficiency

may have contributed to the observed phenomena: for, example, the diet used by Hanaler[35] and by Yagi & Kotaki[36] was high in carbohydrate, low in protein and lacked B vitamins.

Recently, however, Tomita and his colleagues have developed a much quicker and more controllable dietary method for producing an inositol-responsive fatty liver in rats whose growth rate, at least in the short term, is unchanged[39]. This consists of feeding a reasonably balanced sucrose-rich diet which contains vitamins and also substantial quantities of protein (casein) and fat (hydrogenated cottonseed oil). To this is added 0.5% of phthalylsulphathiazole, in order to suppress the growth of intestinal microorganisms which synthesise inositol. The triacylglycerol contents of the livers of normal animals transferred to this diet rose 2.6-fold within a week and 5.3-fold in two weeks, and dietary inositol both prevented this lipid accumulation and corrected it within a week.

It seems likely that there are at least two processes which contribute to the accumulation of lipid in the livers of inositol-deficient animals, namely a decreased ability of the liver to secrete lipoproteins and an increase in mobilization of fatty acids from adipose tissue to liver. Evidence for the former comes from studies such as those of Yagi & Kotaki[36], who showed that endogenously synthesised cholesterol was retained for longer in the livers of inositol-deficient rats than of healthy animals. However, it is also well-known that inositol deficiency can perturb lipid metabolism severely in yeast, which does not secrete the synthesised lipid. It therefore seemed likely to Tomita that factors other than those which control lipoprotein secretion might be involved in the lipid loading of inositol-deficient liver, and he has now shown that one such factor may be a substantial increase in the rate at which fatty acids are released from adipose triacylglycerol into the bloodstream of inositol-deficient animals. This was directly demonstrated by experiments in which the fat pads of anaesthetised animals were surgically externalised, incubated with labelled palmitate and then returned to the abdomen. During the following 24 h more than twice as much labelled fatty acid was transferred to the liver in the inositol-deficient animals as in the controls[40]. This effect was abolished by bupranolol, indicating that a major cause of this increased fatty acid mobilisation is activation of the β-adrenergic receptors of the adipose tissue[41]. Enhanced fatty acid mobilisation in the inositol-deficient rats was not prevented by adrenalectomy, but was alleviated by hexamethonium and reserpine, suggesting that the increased adrenergic input to the adipose tissue was through the sympathetic nervous system rather than through a rise in circulating catecholamine levels[40,41]. This, of course, simply moves the ultimate cause of inositol-deficient fatty liver one stage further away from the liver, presumably to a functional impairment of some central nervous mechanism that is involved in regulating the activity of the sympathetic nervous input to adipose tissue: whether other tissues are sympathetically hyperstimulated during inositol deficiency appears to be unknown. Whatever the cause of this change in nervous activity, it could help us understand the role of inositol in the nervous system (maybe in the neurotransmitter receptors of the nervous system?). In addition, inositol deficiency could well prove a valuable tool for the experimental manipulation of lipoprotein metabolism. It is unlikely, however, that the inositol status of an animal will often contribute appreciably to the normal control of lipoprotein metabolism, simply because inositol deficiency does not occur as an accidental deficiency disease.

REFERENCES

1. Robison, G.A., Butcher, R.W. & Sutherland, E.W. (1971) Cyclic AMP, Academic Press

2. Goldberg, N.D. & Haddox, M.C. (1977) Ann. Rev. Biochem. 46, 823-896

3. Michell, R.H. (1975) Biochim. Biophys. Acta, 415, 81-147.

4. Michell, R.H., Jafferji, S.S. & Jones, L.M. (1977) in Metabolism and Function of Lipids (Bazan, N.G., Brenner, R.R. & Giusto, N.M., eds.) pp 447-464, Plenum Press.

5. Michell, R.H. (1978) Trends in Biochemical Science, in press.

6. Lakshmanan, J. (1978) Biochem. Biophys. Res. Commun. 82, 767-775.

7. Lakshmanan, J. (1978) FEBS Letters, 92, 159-162.

8. Tashjian, A.H., Lomedico, M.E. & Maina, D. (1978) Biochem. Biophys. Res Commun. 81, 798-806

9. Hopkins, C.R. & Walker, A.M. (1978) J. Cell Biol. in press

10. Triggle, D.J. (1971) Neurotransmitter-Receptor Interactions, Academic Press

11. Hurwitz, L. & Suria, A. (1971) Ann. Rev. Pharmacol. 11, 303-326

12. Bolton, T.B. (1979) Physiol. Rev. in press.

13. Douglas, W.W. (1976) in Stimulus-Secretion Coupling in the Gastrointestinal Tract (Case, R.M. & Goebbell, H., eds.) pp 17-29, MTP Press, Lancaster

14. Berridge, M.J. (1975) Adv. Cyclic Nucleotide Res. 6, 1-98.

15. Rasmussen, H. & Goodman, D.A.P. (1977) Physiol. Rev. 57, 421-509.

16. Putney, J.W. (1977) J. Physiol. (London) 268, 139-149.

17. Putney, J.W., personal communication

18. Hems, D.A., Rodrigues, L.M. & Whitton, P.D. (1978) Biochem. J. 172, 311-317.

19. Keppens, S., Vandenheede, J. & De Wulf, H. (1977) Biochim. Biophys. Acta 496, 448-457.

20. Assimacopoulos-Jeannet, F., Blackmore, P.E. & Exton, J.H. (1977) J. Biol. Chem. 252, 2662-2669.

21. Lapetina, E.G. & Michell, R.H. (1973) FEBS Letters, 31, 1-10.

22. Kirk, C.J., Verrinder, T. & Hems, D.A. (1977) FEBS Letters 83, 267-271.

23. Kirk, C.J., Verrinder, T. & Hems, D.A. (1978) Biochem. Soc. Trans., in press

24. Billah, M.M. & Michell, R.H. (1978) Biochem. Soc. Trans., in press

25. Foden, S. & Randle, P.J. (1978) Biochem. J. 170, 615-625.

26. Blackmore, P.F., Bromley, F.T., Marks, J.L. & Exton, J.H. (1978) J. Biol. Chem. in press.

27. Chen, J.-L., Babcock, D.F. & Lardy, H.A. (1978) Proc. Natl. Acad. Sci. USA 75, 2234-2238.

28. Michell, R.H. (1979) in Companion to Biochemistry (Bull, A.T. et al., eds) in press, Longman, London

29. Jones, L.M. & Michell, R.H. (1978) Biochem. Soc. Trans., 6, 673-688

30 De Torrentegui, G. & Berthet, G. (1966) Biochim. Biophys. Acta 116, 477-482

31. Stein, J.M. & Hales, C.N. (1974) Biochim. Biophys. Acta 337, 41-49

32. Czech, M.P. (1977) Ann. Rev. Biochem. 46, 359-384.

33. Czech, M.P. & Waters, B.K. (1977) Diabetes 26, 367.

34. Gavin, G. & McHenry, E.W. (1941) J. Biol. Chem. 139, 485

35. Handler, P. (1946) J. Biol. Chem. 162, 77-85

36. Yagi, Y. & Kotaki, A. (1968) Ann. N.Y. Acad. Sci. 165, 710-725.

37. Hegsted, D.M., Hayes, K.C., Gallagher, A. & Hanford, H. (1973) J. Nutr. 103, 302-307.

38. Knoes, J.F., Hegsted, D.M. & Hayes, K.C. (1973) J. Nutr. 103, 1448-1453.

39. Hayashi, E., Maeda, T. & Tomita, T. (1975) Biochim. Biophys. Acta, 360, 134-145

40. Hayashi, E., Maeda, T. & Tomita, T. (1974) Biochim. Biophys. Acta 360, 146-155

41. Hayashi, E. Maeda, T., Hasegawa, R. & Tomita, T. (1978) Biochim. Biophys. Acta in press.

Lipoprotein Metabolism and Endocrine Regulation
L.W. Hessel and H.M.J. Krans editors
© ECSC, EEC, EAEC, Brussels-Luxembourg, 1979
Published by Elsevier/North-Holland Biomedical Press-Amsterdam

RECEPTORS OF INSULIN, GLUCAGON, GROWTH HORMONE AND PROLACTIN IN THE ISOLATED
LIVER CELLS OF THE OBESE ZUCKER RAT[1] THEIR IMPLICATIONS IN THE OVERPRODUCTION
OF LIPOPROTEINS.

Y. BROER, M. FOUCHEREAU-PERON, M. LABURTHE, and G. ROSSELIN
Unité de Recherche de Diabétologie et d'Etudes Radio-Immunologiques des Hormones
Protéiques, U.55 (Institut National de la Santé et de la Recherche Médicale),
E.R.A. n° 494 (Centre National de la Recherche Scientifique), Hôpital Saint-
Antoine, 184 Rue du Faubourg Saint-Antoine, Paris 12°, France.

ABSTRACT
    Plasma levels of insulin, glucagon, growth hormone and prolactin were related
to their specific receptor sites in hepatocytes of the genetically obese Zucker
rat in the fed state.
    The number of receptors for each hormone were similar in obese and in lean
littermate, despite a dramatic increase of insulin and a decrease of growth
hormone levels in plasma observed in the fatty rat. In addition glucagon induced
cyclic AMP levels were more greatly increased in the obese than in the lean;
this indicates a higher sensitivity of liver to the glucagon action. Thus, it
was suggested that the overproduction of lipoproteins by the liver of the obese
Zucker rat is facilited in the feeding period by the effectiveness of hormones
on liver: increase of the availability of substrats which in liver cells are
precursors for apoproteins and triglycerides synthesis; and prevalent stimulation of lipogenesis pathway by insulin.

    The Zucker fatty rat represents a form of extrem obesity which is transmitted
by a recessive mutant gene "fa"[2]. This obesity which is noticeable at 3-4 weeks
of age, is later associated with spectacular hyperlipemia[3], hyperinsulinemia[4,5],
but slightly elevated blood glucose levels[4]. The unlarged adipose depots of the
adult fatty rat result of both hypertrophy[6] and hyperplasia[7,8] of fat cells.
Adipose tissue exhibits a highly elevated lipogenesis[9], and liver an overproduction of lipoproteins in blood[10] with an increase of lipogenetic enzyme activity
[11-13]. The hyperlipemia is characterized by an elevation of all serum lipids[14].
Very low density lipoproteins are increased several fold and 75% of their mass
are triglycerides compared with 60% in littermate rats[14]. Low and high density
lipoproteins are increased two fold and have similar lipid composition than

those of the controls. Apoproteins are also elevated and the increase of lipoprotein lipase activity in the obese can be related to a greater amount of subunit apoprotein peptide (ApoC)[14], as in man. Overproduction of lipoprotein by the liver is related to high levels of protein synthesis[15] and RNA polymerase activity[16] and to high triglyceride synthesis derived from carbohydrates[17].

Hyperinsulinemia is favoured by elevated concentration in pancreas[17,18] and enhanced insulin release[19]. Although hyperinsulinemia is the most characteristic abnormality of the endocrine changes observed in the genetically obese Zucker rat, neuroendocrine disturbance involving the hypothalamus pituitary axis have been described and are associated with: hyperphagia[20,21], polyuria[22], sterility[2], delayed oestrus[23], hypothyroidism[24], impaired control of TSH secretion[25], disturbance of body fluids regulation[22], low plasma growth hormone concentration[26], reduced noradrenalin content in the hypothalamus paraventricular nucleus and increased noradrenalin in the median eminence[27], reduced levels of arginine-vasopressin in the pituitary gland[28].

EXPERIMENTAL ANIMALS (Fed rats)

	Body (g)	Liver (g)	Pancreas (g)	Pituitary (mg)
	WEIGHTS			
LEAN Mean ± SE	(25) 194 ± 4	(16) 5.7 ± 0.7	(10) 1.24 ± 0.05	(9) 10.4 ± 0.5
OBESE Mèan ± SE	(21) 380 ± 9	(9) 11.2 ± 0.2	(10) 0.96 ± 0.02	(10) 11.1 ± 0.7
P.values	< 0.001	< 0.001	NS	NS

Table 1-a: The P values (impaired t test) refer to statistical comparison between parameter of the lean and of the obese; NS means no significant. Number of rats are given in parenthesis.

An extensive study of the hormonal control of lipogenesis in the fatty rat is not our purpose. Rather our purpose was to determine a system which makes it possible to directly measure the interaction of hormones with liver in that genetic model of hyperlipemia. By this way it is possible to know to what extend the first step of hormone action on liver is involved in the metabolic defect of

HORMONE CONTENTS in the PLASMA and in the GLANDS (FED RATS)

	IRI		GLI		GROWTH HORMONE		PROLACTIN	
	Plasma (μU/ml)	Pancreas (U/g)	Plasma (ng/ml)	Pancreas (μg/g)	Plasma (μU/ml)	Pituitary (μg/mg)	Plasma (ng/ml)	Pituitary (μg/mg)
LEAN Mean ± SE	(15) 113 ± 14	(11) 1.39 ± 0.02	(11) 0.32 ± 0.18	(11) 6.95 ± 0.38	(15) 13.4 ± 1.8	(16) 16 ± 2	(7) 74.8 ± 19.3	(9) 2 ± 0.4
OBESE Mean ± SE	(15) 691 ± 132	(12) 3.90 ± 0.09	(12) 0.38 ± 0.12	(12) 7.95 ± 0.15	(8) 7.3 ± 1.2	(9) 15.4 ± 2.2	(10) 113.8 ± 12.6	(10) 1.4 ± 0.1
P Values	< 0.001	< 0.001	NS	NS	< 0.01	NS	NS	NS

Table 1-b: The P values (impaired t test) refer to statistical comparison between parameter of the lean and of the obese; NS means no significant. Number of rats are given in parenthesis.

obese rat. Furthermore, it will indicate if the modification of hormonal concentration in blood, which is observed in fatty rat, results in any change in the number of corresponding receptors in liver. Indeed, it has been shown that in some conditions, the cell can reduce the number of receptors depending on the amount of hormone to which it is exposed. This "down regulation" phenomenom has been involved for explaining the insulin resistance of ob/ob mouse and of some human obesities[29]. Such a phenomenom has been investigated in the fatty rat for insulin and growth hormone; glucagon and prolactin receptors have also been studied.

Twelve week-old females were chosen because at that time, the syndrome is fully present with the maximum level of insulin in blood[30]. Plasma levels of insulin[31], glucagon[32], GH and PRL[33] were determined by radioimmunoassay. Binding sites characteristics of insulin, glucagon, GH and PRL were studied on enzymatically isolated liver cells of fatty rat and compared to its lean littermate as described previously[1]. Cyclic AMP accumulation was determined by radioimmunoassay[34,35]. The characteristics of these animals are indicated in tables 1-a and 1-b. Body and liver *weights* of the obese were about twice than those of the lean, pancreas and pituitary weights were similar. *Plasma* insulin levels were significantly higher and plasma GH levels were significantly lower in the obese compared to the lean. Plasma glucagon and PRL levels were similar. In *pancreas*, IRI

NUMBER OF MOLECULES OF INSULIN AND GLUCAGON BOUND PER LIVER CELL

HORMONE	FASTED RATS		FED RAT	
	LEAN	OBESE	LEAN	OBESE
Insulin (nM)	(13)	(14)	(16)	(15)
0.03	1,113 ± 134 ‡	699 ± 75	1,009 ± 103	864 ± 96
16	(9)	(9)	(13)	(13)
	122,600 ± 13,000	124,000 ± 12,000	119,400 ± 9,000	132,500 ± 17,000
Glucagon (nM)	(9)	(9)	(13)	(13)
0.03	609 ± 47 †	560 ± 113	1,181 ± 122	924 ± 142
28	(9)	(9)	(13)	(13)
	114,800 ± 25,000 *	116,000 ± 27,000	214,000 ± 25,000	167,000 ± 24,000

Table 2: Incubations were performed at 30 C, during 60 min in KRP-BSA 3% pH 7.5, with liver cells 1 x 10^6 ml. NS : binding in presence of 100 µg/ml insulin or glucagon. When the number of hormone molecules bound in fasted rats (both lean and obese) was different from those of the corresponding fed animals, significance is given by: * p < 0.02, † p < 0.001. When the number of hormone molecules bound in lean rats (both fasted and fed) was different from those of the corresponding obese animals, significance is given by ‡ p < 0.02. Number of experiments is given in parentheses.

levels were significantly higher in the obese compared to the lean, GLI levels were similar. In *pituitary glands*, concentration of GH and PRL were similar, indicating a deficiency of GH secretion in the obese rat.

Quantitative analysis of the specific receptors of insulin, glucagon (Table 2) and measure of the glucagon induced cyclic AMP accumulation (figure) in isolated hepatocytes, as shown in previous study[1], give the following results. First: *insulin binding* of the liver cell receptor is decreased in the obese Zucker rat when compared to the lean, but only in the 24 hr fasted state and at low insulin concentration; insulin binding is increased in the fasted lean but not in the fasted obese at least after a 24 hr fast. Secondly: *glucagon binding* is similar in the obese and in the lean, glucagon binding is decreased in the fasted rats, both obese and lean. Thirdly: glucagon stimulated *cyclic AMP accumulation* is higher in the fed obese than in the other situations. Several comments can be made. The nutritional state does alter the glucagon binding: fasting results in a reduced number of glucagon receptor sites[36]. Glucagon binding is not the unique factor involved in the increase of cyclic AMP accumulation, since similar degrees of site occupancy in all the groups cause a higher accumulation only in the fed obese. These results with insulin binding somewhat differ from those reported in the obese hyperglycemic mouse. In the ob/ob mouse, the receptor defect is apparent over a wide range of insulin concentration[37]. Further, fasting causes a dramatic improvement of insulin binding in the ob/ob mouse[38].

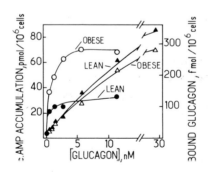

Relationship between glucagon-stimulated cAMP accumulation ●— o and glucagon specifically bound ▲— △ to isolated liver cells from fed rat. Incubations were performed as in Table 2 in presence of 1 mM theophylline for cAMP experiments[1].

Growth hormone and prolactin in liver have similar metabolic action and show, at least in part, a common receptor site. The amount of human GH and ovine PRL specifically (and not specifically) bound to hepatocytes was similar in lean and obese rats, however the specific binding of labeled hGH was about three-fold that of oPRL (Table 3). Effective doses for 50% displacement (ED 50) of labeled hGH and oPRL by native hGH, oPRL and bGH (Table 4) were not significantly different between lean and obese, except for ^{125}I-hGH displaced by hGH: ED 50 is lower in obese than in lean (14.4 versus 20.8 ng/ml) indicating a higher GH affinity in obese than in lean. Thus in the obese Zucker rat, GH levels in plasma is low, but the presence in hepatocytes of growth hormone binding sites of higher affinity than in lean suggests that the metabolic effect of the hormone on liver is fully retained.

HORMONES BOUND per 10^6 CELLS (% of TOTAL RADIOACTIVITY ADDED)

Labeled Hormones (ng/ml)	Binding		Lean		Obese
hGH (1.6)	Specific	(7)	19.94 ± 2.80	(7)	18.09 ± 3.2
	Non specific		1.87 ± 0.53		1.60 ± 0.63
oPRL (1.7)	Specific	(5)	6.38 ± 1.38	(5)	4.14 ± 0.37
	Non specific		1.09 ± 0.31		0.81 ± 0.13

Table 3: Incubations were performed at 22C during 4 h in similar conditions than in table 2. Liver cells at .5 x 106/ml. NS binding was determined in presence of 10 µg/ml hGH or oPRL. Each value in the mean ± SEM of n experiments (given in parenthesis).

One of the main features of liver cells in the fatty rat is the maintenance of the same pattern of *insulin* receptor-site: in such a model of hyperinsulinemia it was shown that in the fed state, the specific binding of labeled insulin to isolated hepatocytes was similar in obese and lean rats, and slightly decreased in the obese compared to the lean in the fasted state. Those findings were partly supported by results obtained with liver plasma membranes[48]. However, the number of insulin receptors in liver plasma membranes of the fatty rat is much lower than those observed by using liver cells, indicating that the type of preparation used might influence the number of receptors found. In the fasted state, insulin binding with fatty liver cells exhibits a modest decrease almost similar to that observed with peripheral mononuclear cells in obese patients after an overnight fast[39].

Thus contrarily to other models of hyperinsulinemia where high insulin levels result in a down regulation of insulin[29], the number of insulin receptor sites in hepatocytes from fed or fasted obese is sufficient for a maximal effect of the hormone.

Several arguments suggest that insulin is effective in stimulating lipogenesis in liver: insulin stimulates the incorporation of ^{14}C glucose into lipids released by the liver[40]. Direct effect of insulin in stimulating acetyl-CoA carboxylase and free-fatty synthetase was described[41], and is well related to the increase of those enzymes in fatty rat liver[11-13]. The effect of insulin on liver lipogenesis was further suggested by the fact that lowering insulin by streptozotocin results in a decrease in lipid synthesis in fatty rat[42].

		ED 50 (ng/ml)		
TRACER		hGH	oPRL	bGH
^{125}I-hGH	LEAN	(7) 20.8 + 2.2	(5) 17.7 + 8.8	(2) 800 + 200★
	OBESE	(6) 14.4 + 1.4	(6) 41.3 + 9.2	(2) 2,000 + 500
	P	< 0.05	NS	NS
^{125}I-oPRL	LEAN	(3) 14.4 + 2.4	(5) 33.6 + 3	(2) 4,140 + 340
	OBESE	(4) 14.8 + 2.8	(5) 30.1 + 1.9	(2) 7,500 + 3,500
	P	NS	NS	NS

Table 4: Effective dose for 50% displacement (ED 50) for ^{125}I-iodo hGH and oPRL binding to hepatocytes from lean and obese female Zucker rat. Experimental conditions as in Table 3. NS binding for bGH was determined in presence of 20 µg/ml hormone. Data are expressed as means + SEM. p < 0.05 refers to statistical comparison between lean and obese. ★ p < 0.02 refers to statistical comparison between displacement of labeled hGH and oPRL by cold bGH in lean rats. NS means no significant. Number of experiments given in parentheses.

The number of *glucagon* receptors in liver fatty rat is submitted to the same regulation as in normal rat; it is higher in fed than in fasted state[36]. The most striking observation is the higher level of glucagon-induced cyclic AMP accumulation in the fed obese than in the fed lean rat despite a similar number of glucagon binding sites. This fact is not due to an increase biological potency of glucagon[18] or to a decrease in the degradation of this hormone by liver cells in fatty rat[1]. Rather it suggests a lower cyclic nucleotide phosphodiesterase activity in obese than in lean rat. Those findings are well correlated to the following facts: 1) in fatty rat liver glycogen content is lower than in the lean control[17]. 2) Some aminoacids catabolizing enzymes has been found increased in fatty[11]. 3) Enzymes associated with gluconeogenesis, which are normally considered to be depressed in hyperinsulinemia, are also increased[13].

On the contrary, a possible role of glucagon deficiency in the evolution or maintenance of lipemic status has been suggested[43]. This hypothesis was proposed because: 1) glucagon have hypolipemic action in mammals[44], either by reduction of hepatic triglycerids secretion and decreased of fatty acids[56] or apoprotein synthesis; 2) low glucagon levels has been found in hyperlipemia such as carbohydrate induced hyperglycemia[45]; 3) glucagon deficiency or glucagon resistance have also been suggested in fatty rat, because low glucagon levels have been found in those animals[46]. However, it appears that low glucagon levels are observed mainly in the fasted state or after hypoglycemia. In fed fatty rat, glucagon is normal[18,47] or only slightly decreased[46]. Furthermore, long term administration of pharmacological doses of glucagon causes hypolipemia in fatty rat as in control, through to a less extent in fatty than in lean animals[48]. These data, together with the high sensitivity of liver cyclic AMP system to the glucagon stimulation in the fatty rat, indicate that deficiency of glucagon, or glucagon resistance is not responsible for the overproduction of lipids in fatty rats. At the opposite, it could be supposed that optimal effect of glucagon in fed state could favour glycogenolysis, aminoacid input, gluconeogenesis and enhance available substrates for apoprotein synthesis.

Despite decreased blood *growth hormone* levels in fatty[26], specific receptor sites are not different in liver of lean and obese rats. However the effective dose for 50% displacement of labeled GH bound to hepatocyte by native GH is lower in obese than in lean, indicating a higher affinity of GH to the cells of obese than those of its lean littermate. Thus, full biological activities of GH and PRL present in the blood can be expected on the liver of fatty rat. Growth hormone, and to a less extent, prolactin have been demonstrated to increase intracellular accumulation of aminoacids[49], ornithine decarboxylase[50] and

ARN polymerase activities[51], somatomedine production[52]. The reduced lipogenesis due to GH in liver of normal rat[53] is probably overcome in fatty rat by the predominant effect of insulin. Indeed, it has been shown that GH, as the other pituitary hormones is not responsible for the fatty obesity, since complete hypophysectomy blocks the continued development of obesity but does not eliminate the adiposity established prior the hypophysectomy [53]. The maintenance of growth hormone activity on liver cells may explain the development of the liver which reaches in fatty rat twice the size observed in lean control.

In conclusion, hyperproduction of lipid in fatty rat is associated to: 1) hyperinsulinemia without dramatic loss of insulin receptors; 2) hypersensitivity of glucagon cyclic AMP system in the liver without decrease of glucagon level in the fed state; 3) maintenance of growth hormone receptors.

It may be suggested that the hepatic production of lipoproteins in fatty rat is facilitated by the effectiveness of hormones on liver occuring at two different steps during the feeding period: 1) increase of the availability of substrates which in liver cells are precursors for apoproteins and triglycerides synthesis; 2) prevalent stimulation of lipogenic pathway by insulin. This system is fully effective in presence of an excess of fuels due to the hyperplagia of these animals[2,20]. When fatty rats are fasted, overproduction of lipids by liver persists[54] for a long time. This is likely due to the persistence of high insulin level[30] and the decrease in the fasting induced glucagon [55]. In these fasting conditions, the hyperlipemic effect of insulin remains prominent.

This work was supported by INSERM (contrat n° 78 5 030 4).

REFERENCES
1. Broer, Y. et al. (1977) Endocrin. 101, 236-249
2. Zucker, L.M., Zucker, T.F. (1961) J. Hered. 52, 275-278
3. Zucker, L.M. (1965) Ann. N.Y. Acad. Sci. 131, 447-458
4. Zucker, L.M., Antoniades, H.N. (1970) Fed. Proc. 29, 379
5. York, D.A. et al. (1972) 21, 277-284
6. Bray, G.A. (1969) Proc. Soc. Exp. Biol. Med. 131, 1111-1114
7. Johnson, P.R. et al. (1971) J. Lipid Res. 12, 706-714
8. Lemonnier, D., Alexiu, A. (1974) in the Regulation of the Adipose Tissue Mass. Amsterdam, Excerpta Medica Foundation, pp. 158-173
9. York, D.A., Bray, G.A. (1973) Horm. Metab. Res. 5, 355-360
10.Schonfeld, G.C.Pfleger, B. (1971) Am. J. Physiol. 220, 1178-1181
11.Martin, J. (1974) Life Sci. 14, 1447-1453
12.Taketomi, S. et al. (1975) Horm. Metab. Res. 7, 242-246
13.Spydevold, S.O., Greenbaum, A.L. (1978) Eur. J. Biochem. 89, 329-339
14.Schonfeld, G. et al. (1974) J. Lipid Res. 15, 457-464
15.Fillios, L.C., Saito, S. (1965) Metabolism 14, 734-745

16.Fillios, L.C., Yokono, 0. (1966) Metabolism 15, 279-285
17.Lemonnier, D. et al. (1974) Diabetologia 10, 1-5
18.Laburthe, M. et al. (1975) Diabetologia 11, 517-526
19.Stern, J.S. et al. (1975) Am. J. Physiol. 228, 543-548
20.Zucker, T.F., Zucker, L.M. (1962) Proc. Soc. Exp. Biol. Med. 110, 165-171
21.Bray, G.A., York, D.A. (1972) Am. J. Physiol. 223, 176-179
22.York, D.A., Bray, G.A. (1971) Proc. Soc. Exp. Biol. Med. 136, 798-801
23.Saiduddin, S. et al. (1973) Endocrin. 93, 1251-1256
24.Bray, G.A., York, D.A. (1971) Endocrin. 88, 1095-1099
25.York, D.A. et al. (1972) Endocrin. 90, 67-72
26.Martin, R.J. et al. (1978) Horm. Metab. Res. 10, 187-192
27.Cruce, J.A. et al. (1976) Brain Res. 101,165-170
28.Crowley, W.R. et al. (1978) J. Endocr. 77, 417-418
29.Kahn, C.R., Roth, J. (1969) Am. J. Clin. Path. 5, 358-359
30.Zucker, L.M., Antoniades, H.N. (1972) Endocrn. 90, 1320-1330
31.Rosselin, G., Dolais, J. (1967) Sté Fse Biol. Clin. "Les Isotopes - Applica-
   tions biocliniques" Expansion Sci. Ed. 1, 189-217
32.Unger, R.H. et al. (1961) J. Clin. Invest. 40, 1280-1289
33.Utiger, R.D. et al. (1962) J. Clin. Invest. 41, 254
34.Steiner, A.J. et al. (1970) in Greengard, P. and Costa, E. (eds) Advances
   in Biochemical Psychopharmacology, Raven Press, New York 3, 89
35.Broer, Y. et al. (1972) C.R. Acad. Sci. Paris 275, 619-622
36.Fouchereau-Péron, M. et al. (1976) Endocrin. 98, 755-760
37.Kahn, C.R. et al. (1973) J. Biol. Chem. 248, 244-250
38.Le Marchand, Y. et al. (1977) Diabetes 26, 582-590
39.Archer, J.A. et al. (1975) J. Clin. Invest. 55, 166-174
40.Letarte, J., Fraser, T.R. (1969) Diabetologia 5, 358-359
41.Lakshmanan, M.R. et al. (1975) Arch. Biochem. Biophys. 169, 737-745
42.Godbole, V., York, D.A. (1978) Diabetologia 14, 191-197
43.Eaton, R.P. et al. (1974) Lancet 2, 1545-1547
44.Aubry, F. et al. (1974) J. Metabolism 23, 225
45.Eaton, R.P., Kipnis, D.S. (1969) Am. J. Physiol. 217, 1153
46.Eaton, R.P. et al. (1976) Am. J. Physiol. 230, 1336-1341
47.Bryce, G.F. et al. (1977) Horm. Metab. Res. 9, 366-370
48.Mahmood, H.A. et al. (1978) Diabetologia 14, 405-412
49.Jefferson, L.S. et al. (1975) J. Biol. Chem. 250, 197-204
50.Richards, J.F. (1975) Biochem. Biophys. Res. Commun. 63, 292-299
51.Chen, H.W. et al. (1972) Biochim. Biophys. Acta 287, 90-97
52.Williams, J.P.G., Hugues, S. (1974) J. Endocr. 63, 585-586
53.Raben, M.S. (1973) in Methods in Investigative and Diagnostic Endocrinology,
   Berson, S.A. and Yalow, R.S. (eds) Am. Elsevier Publishing Company, 261-267
54.Bloxham, D.P. et al. (1977) Horm. Metab. Res. 9, 304-309
55.Unger, R.H. et al. (1962) J. Clin. Invest. 41, 682-689
56.Meikle, A.W. et al. (1973), Proc. Soc. Exp. Biol. Med. 143, 379-387

Lipoprotein Metabolism and Endocrine Regulation
L.W. Hessel and H.M.J. Krans editors
© ECSC, EEC, EAEC, Brussels-Luxembourg, 1979
Published by Elsevier/North-Holland Biomedical Press-Amsterdam

DISCUSSION ON CHANGES IN RECEPTORS AND RESPONSIVENESS.

Paraphrased and annotated by H.M.J. Krans, Dept. Endocrinology and Metabolic
Diseases, University Hospital, Rijnsburgerweg 10, 2333 AA Leiden, The Netherlands.

Galton : Dr. Gliemann, and perhaps Dr. Krans, how much of the insulin bound to
the fat cell is internalized and which fraction of the internalized insulin is
actively involved in the cell?

Gliemann : About 95% of the material extracted from the cells was active insulin
which could stimulate transport of 3-O-methylglucose (3-OMG). But the situation
is complicated. Insulin is actively turned over on the receptor. Insulin comes
from the membrane into the medium and it is degraded. I do not know how much is
internalized. Kahn and Baird (J.B.C., 253, 4900 (1978)) have just reported that
35% of the label associated with fat cells at $37^{\circ}C$ is not insulin anymore. This
means it is converted to something else which is now within the cell. What is
collected in the cell is activity which is not insulin. This is at variance
with our results, where we could extract a much higher amount of the label. In
liver cells the situation is different. The radio-activity is collected some
micrometers within the the plasma membrane, (e.g. P. Gorden et al, Science,
200, 782 (1978) Ed.) but we do not know if this is insulin.

Krans : Carpentier said in the recent meeting of the E.A.S.D. in Zagreb that it
takes about 45 till 60 minutes before labeled "insulin" can be demonstrated
some micrometers from the mebrane. The activity stays there and does not come
into the nucleus. Remember that Goldfine is advocating an active role of insulin in the nucleus (e.g. I.D. Goldfine, PNAS 74, 1368 (1977) Ed.).

Galton : Is the activity in the cell an important fraction for action?

Gliemann : We do not know, it is not the same type of action as you will see
for the LDL-receptor, where during the steady state only 20% is outside the
cell and most is inside the cell. If you block the internalization of the
complex you can increase the binding a lot. This is not seen with insulin.
Another difference is that buffers like amoniumchloride blocked the degradation
of the epidermal growth factor and may be of LDL. This does not happen to insulin.

Tomasi : The slow dissociation rate is more or less a general phenomenon of
peptide hormones and may point to an internalization of the hormone. Do you
have data on membranes or ghosts? Is there the dissociation rate higher? A

second question: do you think that the greater discharge rate induced by higher concentrations of unlabeled hormone is sufficient justification to talk about negative co-operativity?

Gliemann : The dissociation is non-linear. This means it is not a simple binding system. The label comes from different pools. However, the fact that the vanishing of hormone is not mono-exponential does not justify a conclusion that something has gone into the membrane or into the cell. In many studies you will see that after full dissociation of the hormone still 60% of the binding remains and never decreases further. This is an artifact. In a good experimental system everything comes off with a halftime of 8 till 10 minutes. Only 6% is left after 60 minutes. In a profile of 60%, label other than insulin must be taken up. The small acceleration of the dissociation by addition of a high amount of cold insulin is insufficient proof of negative co-operativity.

Krans : 1. To account for some differences of the studies reported by us and other authors both Gliemann and we measured the very early effects of insulin on glucose transport. Others like Freychet measured a late effect of insulin on enzyme activity. 2. I did not expand on the uptake of insulin into the membrane. In the fluid bilayer of the membrane, the receptor is not just sitting there, but it is exposed, can be dislocated and pass into the membrane, but this proces takes some time. The movement of the receptor may be one of the mecha- nisms by which insulin intrudes into the membrane and insulin is transported through the membrane. Studies with isolated membranes do not give much informa- tion if you cannot clearly discriminate between the inside and the outside of the membranes. Keeping these factors in mind it is very complicated to build a model which can account for the internalization of the hormone. You have to keep the options open.

Gliemann : The effect of high concentrations of insulin on glucose transport is fully expressed in 40 seconds.

Krans : And the equilibrium of the binding of insulin is much slower.

Kempen : Dr. Krans, why did you use phospholipase in your studies?

Krans : Phospholipase may transform the structure of phospholipids and affect the fluidity of the membranes. Are the changes induced by phospholipases comparable to what is seen in diabetes? To extract the phospholipids quantati- vely from purified fat cell membranes is very difficult. Besides this the hydrophobic part of the triglycerides in the fat cell may be connected with and influenced by the structure of the phospholipids involved. It may be that insulin changes the physical state of the membrane.

Wieringa : Insulin has hydrophylic and hydrophobic parts. It could have some
interaction with phospholipids and in this way partly penetrate the membrane.
This may have to do with the remaining 6% of insulin bound discussed by Gliemann.
Michell : How is the 3 dimensional structure of insulin related to the binding
to the receptor and action on the surface?
Gliemann : The structure of insulin is complicated. In binding a large number
of the aminoacids in the centre as well as in the periphery, are involved,
which you cannot modify without changing the affinity. You cannot change very
much in the insulin molecule before the tertiary structure collapses completely.
The B 22-26 and the carboxy terminal part in the A-chain come together with the
amino terminal part of the A-chain. They constitute together the binding part.
What happens after the binding is difficult to say. In some circumstances it is
cleaved off. Binding induces degradation. Degradation and binding are going
together. Lowering of the temperature lowers the degradation, but the transport
systems as such are also changed. Otherwise the degradation is very constant.
Chicken or hagfish insulin, which have a very different structure, show the
same amount of degradation, and changes in pH have little influence.
Brindley : Dr. Krans 1. Does the K_m of insulin binding change if you alter the
temperature? 2. Did you try surfactant agents which do not destruct the membrane? Do they affect glucose transport? 3. Did you prepare adipocytes from
animals fed on polyunsaturated fat?
Krans : 1. We measured the effect of change in temperature on transport. The
correlation with the effect of change in temperature on binding is in progress.
Answer to other questions 2 and 3 is no, except that we used phospholipase.
Gliemann : The effect of lowering the temperature is to cut down the degradation of bound insulin. The steady state of binding increases and the apparent
affinity increases. With the change in binding the response changes too. This
makes things very complicated.

Tomasi : Dr. Kather, how can you imagine one adenylate cyclase located in a
membrane to work with four receptors; it seems difficult to be sure that you
are not working with different populations of cells with different receptors.
Kather : In the mobile receptor model it is clear that adenylate cyclase can be
coupled to several receptors. Recent work by Levitzky strongly supports this
model.
Johnston : Growth hormone has been shown to be lipolytic in vivo; how does it
work in this system?
Kather : Growth hormone has a long term effect. We were looking for short term

effects.

Brunzell : What is the effect of the various calcium concentrations and PTH on hormone-sensitive lipase?

Kather : Calcium has an inhibitory effect on all hormones involved. PTH works without added extra calcium. I did not study the effect of insulin on PTH or epinephrin-stimulated lipolysis.

Ebert : We found an inhibition of adenylate cyclase by insulin.

Kather : Nobody who studies adenylate cyclase likes to work with insulin. There was a recent report in Febs letters, (c.f. Z.Kiss, Febs Letters, 92, 29 (1978) Ed.) that the inhibitory effect of insulin is mediated by adenosin.

Krans : But adenosin is an inhibitor of adenylate cyclase by itself.

Galton : Dr. Michell, is stimulation of endocytosis in leucocytes also associated with PI breakdown?

Michell : We have observed that uptake of opsonized particles by poly-morpho-nuclear leucocytes induces the PI effect, but it is difficult to decide whether the effect is related to the binding, the surrounding or the internalization step. However, recent work has shown that the peptide formyl-methionyl-leucyl-phenylalanine, a strong chemotactic agent in PMN leucocytes, also induces the PI effect. It is significant that Ca is involved in the chemotactic response.

Tomasi : Why should PI specifically been involved, and not another phospholipid?

Michell : Not known. First the whole set of events must be studied in broken cell systems.

Tomasi : Is there any new information on cyclic inositol phosphate?

Michell : The importance of this substance oscillates month by month. The idea of its being a possible intracellular messenger was put forward by us some five years ago, before the physiological evidence on this family of receptors was going to lead us to the hypothesis that calcium was the messenger of these receptors. Now the position of cyclic inositol phosphate is redundant. However, there are situations in which hormones act in the absence of extracellular calcium, drawing upon an intracellular reserve, and in these cases cyclic inositol monophosphate may perhaps play a role as a messenger from the hormone receptor on the plasma membrane, to the internal calcium store. At the moment, however, there are no firm data supporting this idea.

Kempen : The first step in PI-breakdown is the production of diglyceride by phospholipase C. Is there any inhibitor known for this enzyme?

Michell : No, but if it exists, it must be a broad spectrum antagonist for this whole family of receptors and a marvellous poison.

Hülsmann : What does lanthanum do to the PI-effect?

Michell : There is only one report, dealing with the effect of acetylcholine on the parotid gland; lanthanum ions inhibited the PI-response in that case.

Wieringa : How is PI distributed among both lipid leaflets of the plasma membrane?

Michell : There is only information available for the case of the red blood cell. Most of the PI seems to be at the inside of the plasme membrane as appears from the availability of PI for phosphorylation by intracellular ATP, and from phospholipase C (PI-specific) treatments.

Gliemann : What is the evidence for the increase in Ca^{2+}-concentration in the hepatocyte after exposure to vasopressin?

Michell : First, the absence of a vasopressin effect in Ca-free media; secondly, the occurrence of a rapid Ca-influx after vasopressin treatment.

Gliemann : What do you think at the moment about the involvement of PI in the action of insulin on the fat cell?

Michell : This hormone has been on and off the list alternatingly during the last years. At the moment, there is some evidence that insulin stimulates the turnover of fatty acids of PI in the plasma membrane of adipocytes, and that PI addition to intact fat cells produces an enhanced glucose uptake. However, there is no firm reason to maintain insulin on the list, since its action on the hepatocyte is very different from that of vasopressin, angiotensin II and alpha-adrenergic compounds, which act via the Ca-message, and stimulate PI-turnover.

Tomasi : What do you think of the following kind of reasoning: hormonal stimulation of adenylate cyclase is PI-dependent; insulin promotes PI-breakdown; ergo, insulin can inhibit adenylate cyclase.

Michell : The experimental support for the involvement of PI in the receptor-modulation of adenylate cyclase is weak: Dr. Levey's experiments have not been confirmed. (e.g. G.S. Levey, Glucagon receptor and adenylate cyclase, Metabolism, 24, 301 (1975) Ed.). I rather believe that stimulation of PI-breakdown can inhibit the cyclase by increasing the intracellular calcium concentration.

Mannaerts : Dr. Broer would you conclude that although the insulin effects in liver are normal, adipose tissue is insulin-resistant? Despite high insulin levels the FFA levels are high, or is the FFA removal decreased in these animals?

Broer : Lipolysis is increased. More is not known.

Gliemann : Did Cushman and Salans not find in Zucker rats a decreased binding of insulin, a decreased arabinose uptake and a decreased sensitivity for insulin with increased lipolysis? It is difficult to correlate increased lipolysis with insulin receptors.

Broer : In ob/ob rats we found decreased receptors for insulin.

Kather : Regarding the increased FFA levels Vaughan (e.g. V.C. Manganiello, F. Murad and M. Vaughan, J. Biol. Chem., 246, 2195 (1971) Ed.) described that insulin can be lipolytic. Does anybody know if there is evidence in vivo about the lipolytic effect of insulin? It is an interesting possibility that properties of hormones change.

Galton : In maturity onset diabetics you find high insulin levels with increased lipolysis but an elevated lipolytic hormone is missing. This may suggest that insulin in high doses is lipolytic. The only evidence is, however, in vitro not in vivo.

Brunzell : The measurement of FFA levels in presence of high triglyceride levels is difficult. Even at $-50^{\circ}C$ spontaneous hydrolysis occurs. If you hydrolyse 1% of the triglycerides you triple FFA level. It can be stopped by adding a compound called paraoxon (diethyl-paranitrophenyl-phosphate). It is an anticholinesterase. You can partly circumvent the problem by measuring glycerol.

Broer : We did not add anything like that.

Mannaerts : Glucagon increases the cAMP response. Does glucagon inhibit the glycolysis and may be the lipogenesis at the acetylcarboxylase step too?

Broer : Glucagon acts on the liver. Glycogen is lower in the obese than in the lean litter mate, lactate is preferential used over glucose. The glycogenolytic enzymes are increased. Glucagon may primarily act on glycogenolysis.

Brindley : Glucocorticoids have also a permissive effect. They may interact through insulin. They may affect the gluconeogenesis.

Broer : We did not study glucocorticoids.

Johnston : Cortisol potentiates some actions of glucagon and it potentiates the inhibition of lipolysis by other hormones.

Krans : We found that the effects of fasting on insulin binding was much better expressed after 3 days of fasting than after 1 day. Do you know what happens to binding and insulin effect if you extend the fasting period?

Broer : We did not try.

Gliemann : Fasting normalises (increases) the number of receptors in ob/ ob mice.

Broer : Insulin receptors were slightly increased in the fasted state. The insulin concentrations fell.

Brunzell : Cleary and Greenwood found in obese and lean litter mates of Zucker

rats retrospectively that the adipose tissue LPL per cell was higher in the
obese animals. It is fascinating that they found the same thing as we found in
humans: if one takes a rat which is supposed to be obese (and one has to do
that in retrospect) and pair-feeds him with a lean litter-mate his LPL increases
to much higher levels and stays higher until one allows him to eat and gain
weight. Only then his LPL comes down. So LPL may be a determinant for fat cell
size (M.P. Cleary et al, Fed. Proc., 37, 675 (1978) Ed.).

Birkenhäger : Glucagon binding increased in the fed state. Is this normal? I
would have expected that it was lowered. Glucagon levels fall during feeding.

Tomasi : Glucagon was more effective in adenylate cyclase stimulation but
binding was similar. This is uncommon. Can you account herefore by difference
in glucagon inactivation.

Broer : The degradation of glucagon was similar in obese and normal animals.

(Editors comment: Extensive investigations on lipid metabolism of the Zucker
rat including cholesterol turnover studies, LCAT activities and effect of
fasting on circulating lipid and insulin levels have been published recently by
H. de Waard, "Effects on lipid and glucose metabolism of diets with different
types of fat and sugar in male fatty Zucker rats", Thesis Agricultural University,
Wageningen, The Netherlands, 1978).

PATHWAYS OF LIPID METABOLISM IN CELLS AND ORGANS

Lipoprotein Metabolism and Endocrine Regulation
L.W. Hessel and H.M.J. Krans editors
© ECSC, EEC, EAEC, Brussels-Luxembourg, 1979
Published by Elsevier/North-Holland Biomedical Press-Amsterdam

MICROTUBULES AND ACTIN MICROFILAMENTS IN LIPOPROTEIN SECRETION BY ISOLATED
RAT HEPATOCYTES*

M. Prentki, G. Gabbiani, C. Chaponnier, and B. Jeanrenaud**
Laboratoires de Recherches Médicales and the Département de Pathologie,
64 Avenue de la Roseraie, 1205 Geneva, Switzerland

ABSTRACT

The effects of phalloidin and cytochalasin D (drugs which, respectively,
stabilize and destabilize actin microfilaments) as well as those of colchicine
(a drug which interferes with the function of microtubules) have been tested on
isolated rat hepatocytes. The release of triglycerides, an index of very low
density lipoprotein secretion, was inhibited by phalloidin or cytochalasin D,
and accompanied by an increase in cellular triglycerides. At the electron mi-
croscopic examination, triglyceride accumulation was represented by fat droplets
and vesicle-enclosed very low density lipoprotein-like particles. Similar effects were obtained by the addition of colchicine. When used at maximal concentrations, phalloidin plus colchicine or cytochalasin plus colchicine had additive effects, suggesting different sites of action for these drugs. Total protein
or albumin secretion was only very slightly inhibited by phalloidin or cytochalasin, while colchicine had a marked inhibitory effect upon these secretory
processes. Using various phalloidin analogs, a correlation was observed between
their respective ability to stabilize F-actin in vitro, and their effects on
triglyceride secretion. In conclusion, phalloidin and cytochalasin D inhibit
lipoprotein secretion, an effect that possibly results from a modification of
actin microfilament function; colchicine inhibits lipoprotein and protein secretion, an effect that probably results from an interference with the microtubular
system. The additive effect of phalloidin (or cytochalasin D) and colchicine suggests that microfilaments and microtubules may possibly have complementary functions in the release of lipoproteins. Finally, the observation that phalloidin or

---

*As the present studies are not published yet, no data are given in the tables
but only trends of changes.
**Guest speaker, Head of Laboratoires de recherches médicales.

cytochalasin D inhibits triglyceride but not protein secretion while colchicine inhibits both processes suggests that the intracellular routes are, at least in part, different for the two types of secretory products and therefore differently regulated.

INTRODUCTION

In the liver, as in many other tissues, the microtubular system appears to be implicated in secretory processes[1-7].

It has been claimed that microtubules and a precursor pool of free tubulin exist in a dynamic equilibrium. To substantiate such a concept, we have previously used a method that allows for the measurement, in the intact liver, of these two states of the microtubular system, i.e. the structured microtubular one and that of unstructured free tubulin[8]. We came to the conclusion that the liver contains a colchicine-binding protein which, considering its intracellular distribution, its specificity for colchicine and its several similarities to purified brain tubulin, can be identified as being the hepatic microtubular protein, i.e. tubulin[8]. In addition, a good agreement between the dose-dependent binding kinetics of colchicine of either liver high speed supernatant or purified liver tubulin, and the actual inhibitory effect of colchicine upon hepatic secretory processes was observed[1,4,8]. Furthermore, while the _total_ amount of tubulin remained essentially constant upon liver perfusion with colchicine, liver microtubules disappeared in a dose-dependent manner in the presence of the drug. From these experiments, we concluded that there exists, in the liver, an assembly-disassembly cycle of microtubules, and that colchicine interferes with this cycle through its binding to free tubulin thus preventing polymerization of tubulin into microtubules[9]. As colchicine is inhibitory to lipoprotein and protein secretion (without changes in their synthesis)[1], we further thought that this inhibitory effect of the drug might be related to its interrupting effect upon the assembly-disassembly cycle of microtubules[9,10]. According to this view, this cycle might be a key feature of the intracellular migration and eventual secretion of vesicles containing secretory products. One could for instance postulate (although it is difficult to prove it) that microtubules could grow in a given direction while depolymerizing at their tail end or vice versa, thereby "pushing" or "dragging" secretory vesicles to the vascular pole of the hepatocytes.

By analogy with the microtubular system, the existence of a polymerization-depolymerization cycle of actin could represent an additional system for controlling secretory processes of liver cells. Two families of drugs appear to interfere with actin microfilaments. Firstly, the cytochalasins, which destabilize the actin filament structure, although their precise mode of action is still unsettled[11]. While cytochalasin B inhibits transmembrane glucose transport in various cell types[12,13], cytochalasin D does not[12]. Furthermore, cytochalasin D is 8-10 times more potent in altering cell shape of cultured fibroblasts than the B analog[12]. Secondly, the cyclic peptide phalloidin from the genus amanita[14], which has been shown _in vitro_ to react stoechiometrically with actin, to enhance the rate of actin polymerization and to stabilize the F-actin structure[15-17].

The effects of phalloidin and cytochalasin D on the secretory processes of isolated rat hepatocytes were therefore investigated, alone, as well as in the combined presence of colchicine.

RESULTS

Effects of phalloidin, cytochalasin D and colchicine on hepatic secretory processes. Triglyceride output (an index of very low density lipoprotein (VLDL) secretion) by isolated hepatocytes, was linear for 2 hours. In the presence of phalloidin (10^{-5}M) or cytochalasin D (3 μg/ml), the output of triglycerides into the medium was markedly curtailed from 30 min of incubation onwards (Table 1). The effects of phalloidin and cytochalasin D on triglyceride secretion were dose-dependent. Actually, phalloidin used at 10^{-4}M and cytochalasin D at 20 μg/ml decreased triglyceride output to the same extent than phalloidin 10^{-5}M and cytochalasin D, 3 μg/ml. Due to this, subsequent experiments were all carried out with 10^{-5}M phalloidin or 3 μg/ml cytochalasin D. Of further interest was the observation (Table 1) that the decrease in triglyceride output brought about by phalloidin or cytochalasin was accompanied by an accumulation of triglycerides within the hepatocytes, such that total triglycerides (i.e. cellular + medium triglycerides) was identical in control and phalloidin or cytochalasin-treated cells. Similar results were obtained with colchicine, i.e. the presence of the drug resulted in a decrease in triglyceride output by hepatocytes, an effect that could be accounted for by an increase in cellular triglycerides. Moreover, the combined addition of colchicine + phalloidin (or colchicine + cytochalasin D) used at maximal concentrations had additive effect, as depicted by Table 1. At the electron microscope, such an accumulation of triglycerides in the phalloidin-treated cells, corresponded to the presence (never seen to that extent in control cells) of both lipid droplets and vesicles containing VLDL-like particles, although lipid droplets were conspicuously more numerous than vesicles containing VLDL. Analogous ultrastructural changes have been previously noted in colchicine-treated livers[1-3].

As shown in Table 2, phalloidin not only decreased labelled protein secretion but also total protein synthesis (by about 25%), while cytochalasin D barely changed protein secretion or synthesis. In marked contrast, colchicine brought about a marked decrease in labelled protein secretion without altering overall protein synthesis (Table 2). Similar data with either one of the three drugs were obtained when albumin output was measured. To decide whether the inhibitory effect of phalloidin upon triglyceride secretion previously noted was secondary to such decrease in protein synthesis (since VLDL synthesis and release require apoprotein formation), it was necessary to dissociate protein synthesis from protein and triglyceride secretion. To do this, the release, in the presence of cycloheximide, of hepatic triglycerides and proteins previously labelled during a preincubation of hepatocytes with labelled precursors was investigated. Using this technique, it was found that phalloidin reduced only slightly the release of prelabelled proteins into the medium, while that of prelabelled triglycerides was again markedly curtailed[18].

TABLE 1

SCHEMATIC REPRESENTATION OF THE EFFECT OF PHALLOIDIN, CYTOCHALASIN D AND COLCHICINE ON TRIGLYCERIDE (TG) SECRETION BY ISOLATED RAT HEPATOCYTES

Addition	TG secreted into the medium (A)	Cellular TG (B)	Total TG (A+B)
Phalloidin	decreased	increased	unchanged
Cytochalasin D	decreased	increased	unchanged
Colchicine	decreased	increased	unchanged
Colchicine + phalloidin	markedly decreased	markedly increased	unchanged

Isolated hepatocytes incubated in the presence of 1 mM oleate-albumin for 2h. The changes noted are those compared to control, untreated cells. Phalloidin, colchicine: 10^{-5}M; cytochalasin D: 3μg/ml (From ref. 18,19).

TABLE 2

SCHEMATIC REPRESENTATION OF THE EFFECT OF PHALLOIDIN, CYTOCHALASIN D AND
COLCHICINE ON LABELLED AMINO ACID INCORPORATION INTO PROTEINS OF ISOLATED
RAT HEPATOCYTES

Addition	Labelled proteins secreted into the medium (A)	Labelled cellular proteins (B)	Total labelled proteins (A+B)*
Phalloidin	decreased	decreased	decreased
Cytochalasin D	slightly decreased	slightly decreased	slightly decreased
Colchicine	decreased	increased	unchanged

Isolated hepatocytes incubated with ^{14}C-amino acid mixture. The changes noted
are those compared to control, untreated cells. Phalloidin, colchicine :
10^{-5}M; cytochalasin D: 3µg/ml (From ref. 18,19).
* index of overall protein synthesis.

Specificity of phalloidin for microfilaments. As phalloidin has been
well documented to interact and bind to muscle actin in vitro[15], the following
experiments were carried out, to suggest similar specificity in the liver. It
was observed (Table 3) that the monocyclic secophalloidin that does not react
with F-actin[15,16], and therefore does not protect it from heat denaturation,
had no effect either on triglyceride secretion by isolated hepatocytes. For the
other phallopeptides including phalloidin, a reasonable fit between protective
effect from heat denaturation of F-actin and inhibitory effect upon triglyceride secretion was observed (Table 3).

SUMMARY

Although we have studied the effects of phalloidin upon hepatic secretory
processes in more detail than those of cytochalasin D, the most prominent finding of these studies was that either one of these drugs caused a marked, rapid
decrease in triglyceride (VLDL) secretion. Similar results were obtained with
colchicine. In phalloidin-, cytochalasin D-, or colchicine-treated cells, the
diminution of triglyceride secretion was accompanied by intracellular triglyceride accumulation, resulting in unimpairment of total triglyceride formation
(i.e. cell + medium). This accumulation of lipids was represented at the electron microscope by an accumulation (never seen to such an extent in control

240

cells) of vesicles containing VLDL-like particles as well as free lipid droplets. These data suggest that the intracellular migration of VLDL had been, at some ill-defined step(s), interfered with by either one of these drugs. Furthermore, the combined addition of phalloidin and colchicine (or of cytochalasin D and colchicine) used at maximal concentrations resulted in an inhibition of trigly- ceride output that was greater than that observed with one single drug, sugges- ting that their respective site of action was different. Cytochalasin D or phalloidin had only a very slight inhibitory effect upon protein secretion. This was in marked contrast with the results obtained with colchicine in which a marked inhibition of triglyceride as well as of proteins secretion was obser- ved in the presence of the drug[1,4,19].

TABLE 3

SCHEMATIC REPRESENTATION OF THE RELATIONSHIP BETWEEN STABILIZATION OF F-ACTIN BY VARIOUS PHALLOPEPTIDES AND THEIR RESPECTIVE EFFECT ON TRIGLYCERIDE SECRETION BY ISOLATED RAT HEPATOCYTES

Addition	Exp. A : Relative turbidity of F-actin solution	Exp. B : Triglyceride secretion
	(% of control)	
0	100	100
Secophalloidin	96	91
Phalloidin sulfoxid A	67	85
Phalloidin sulfoxid B	24	73
Phalloidin	12	40

Exp. A: Protective effect of phallopeptides (10^{-5}M) on F-actin (10^{-5}M) from denaturation by heating to 70°C for 3min in 0.1 M KCl, 1mM Tris, pH 7.4. Data from reference 20, used for comparison with exp. B with authors' authorization.
Exp. B: Hepatocytes from fed rats incubated for 2h in the presence of 1mM oleate-albumin. All drugs (5.10^{-5}M), except phalloidin (10^{-5}).

Taken together, these observations suggest that : 1) in isolated hepatocytes, a normal equilibrium between G- and F-actin may be necessary for the secretion of VLDL. When this equilibrium is presumably altered either by phalloidin (sta- bilizing F- actin) or cytochalasin D (destabilizing F- actin), a decrease in liver lipoprotein secretion results; 2) this is in keeping with the concept, previously reported[9,10], that a normal equilibrium between a polymerized and depolymerized state of the microtubular protein, tubulin, is needed for a normal hepatic secretion of VLDL to occur. Indeed, when such an equilibrium is altered by colchicine, a decrease in lipoprotein secretion also results; 3) it is conceivable that the microfilamentous system (as interfered with by phalloidin or cytochalasin D) and the microtubular one (as interfered with by colchicine) may have a complementary role in the secretory process of lipoproteins; 4) it appears that some of the intracellular migratory routes of proteins and lipoproteins probably differ as the secretion of proteins is inhibited by colchicine only, while that of lipoproteins is inhibited by colchicine, phalloidin as well as cytochalasin D.

ACKNOWLEDGEMENTS

We are greatly indebted to Miss M. Brunsmann, Miss C. Grillet and Miss M.-C. Clottu for their excellent technical assistance. This work has been supported by grants 3.2180.76, 3.1540.77 and 3.6920.76 of the Swiss National Research Foundation, Berne, Switzerland, and a grant-in-aid of Zyma, Nyon, Switzerland.

REFERENCES

1. Le Marchand, Y., Singh, A., Assimacopoulos-Jeannet, F., Orci, L., Rouiller, Ch. and Jeanrenaud, B. (1973) J. Biol. Chem., 248, 6862-6870.

2. Orci, L., Le Marchand, Y., Singh, A., Assimacopoulos-Jeannet, F., Rouiller, Ch. and Jeanrenaud, B. (1973) Nature, 244, 30-32.

3. Stein, O. and Stein, Y. (1973) Biochim. Biophys. Acta, 306, 142-147.

4. Le Marchand, Y., Patzelt, C., Assimacopoulos-Jeannet, F., Loten, E.G. and Jeanrenaud, B. (1974) J. Clin. Invest., 53, 1512-1517.

5. Stein, O., Sanger, L. and Stein, Y. (1974) J. Cell Biol., 62, 90-103.

6. Singh, A., Le Marchand, Y., Orci, L. and Jeanrenaud, B. (1975) Europ. J. Clin. Invest., 5, 495-505.

7. Redman, C.M., Banerjee, D., Howell, K. and Palade, G.E. (1975) J. Cell Biol., 66, 42-59.

8. Patzelt, C., Singh, A., Le Marchand, Y., Orci, L. and Jeanrenaud, B. (1975) J. Cell Biol., 66, 609-620.

9. Patzelt, C., Singh, A., Le Marchand, Y. and Jeanrenaud, B. (1975) in Microtubules and Microtubule Inhibitors, Borgers, M. and De Brabander, M. eds., North-Holland Publishing Company, Amsterdam, pp. 165-176.

10. Patzelt, C., Le Marchand Y., and Jeanrenaud B. (1976) in The Liver. Quantitative aspects of structure and function, Preisig, R., Bircher, J., Paumgartner, G. eds., Editio Cantor-Aulendorf, pp. 17-31.

11. Tannenbaum, J., Tannenbaum, S.W. and Godman, G.C. (1977) J. Cell. Physiol., 91, 225-238.

12. Atlas, S.J., and Lin, S. (1978) J. Cell Biol., 76, 360-370.

13. Loten, E.G., and Jeanrenaud, B. (1974) Biochem. J., 140, 185-192.

14. Wieland, T. (1968) Science, 159, 946-952.

15. Wieland, T. (1977) in Advances in enzyme regulation, Weber, G. ed., 15, pp. 285-300.

16. Löw, I. and Wieland, T. (1974) FEBS (Fed. Eur. Biochem. Soc.) Lett., 44, 340-343.

17. Gabbiani, G., Montesano, R., Tuchweber, B., Salas, M. and Orci, L. (1975) Lab. Invest., 33, 562-569.

18. Prentki, M., Chaponnier, Ch., Jeanrenaud, B. and Gabbiani, G. submitted for publication.

19. Prentki, M. and Jeanrenaud, B. in preparation.

20. De Vries, J.X., Schäfer, A.J., Faulstich, H. and Wieland, Th. (1976) Hoppe-Seyler's Z. Physiol. Chem., 357, 1139-1143.

Lipoprotein Metabolism and Endocrine Regulation
L.W. Hessel and H.M.J. Krans editors
© ECSC, EEC, EAEC, Brussels-Luxembourg, 1979
Published by Elsevier/North-Holland Biomedical Press-Amsterdam

REGULATION OF HEPATIC TRIACYLGLYCEROL SYNTHESIS AND LIPOPROTEIN SECRETION BY DIET AND HORMONES

DAVID N. BRINDLEY, HELEN P. GLENNY, P. HAYDN PRITCHARD, JUNE COOLING, SUSAN L. BURDITT AND SYLVA PAWSON

Department of Biochemistry, University of Nottingham Medical School, Queen's Medical Centre, Nottingham NG7 2UH (U.K.)

ABSTRACT

The effects of diet on the synthesis of hepatic glycerolipids and the secretion of lipoproteins are discussed in relation to changes in the concentrations of insulin, glucagon, thyroxine and glucocorticoids in the blood. A low ratio of insulin/glucagon ensures that the flux of fatty acids in the liver is diverted to β-oxidation and phospholipid synthesis when the supply of fatty acids is low. However, if the supply of fatty acids increases then the excess is sequestered as triacylglycerol. Thyroxine promotes the synthesis of triacylglycerols, but this probably reflects a general increase in metabolic turnover rather than a net stimulation in triacylglycerol synthesis. Cortisol administration increases the activity of phosphatidate phosphohydrolase in the liver, the net synthesis of triacylglycerol and the secretion of very low density lipoproteins. The synthesis of triacylglycerols and their accumulation in the liver can be increased in starvation, diabetes, stress, liver damage, and after feeding diets rich in saturated fat, ethanol, sucrose, fructose, sorbitol and glycerol. It is proposed that these effects can be partly explained by the cortisol-mediated control of phosphatidate phosphohydrolase activity. The implications of these observations are discussed in relation to atherosclerosis and premature ischaemic heart disease.

INTRODUCTION

The TG* that are synthesized in the liver may be temporarily stored there before subsequent metabolism of the FA by the enzymes of β-oxidation. Alternatively, the TG may be secreted by the liver in VLDL and transported to other organs. If the rate of TG synthesis exceeds the rate at which they are

---

*Abbreviations: DG = diacylglycerol; FA = fatty acid; GP = glycerol phosphate; HDL = high density lipoprotein; LDL = low density lipoprotein; PA = phosphatidate; PC = phosphatidylcholine; PE = phosphatidylethanolamine; PL = phospholipid; TG = triacylglycerol; VLDL = very low density lipoprotein. Enzyme abbreviations are shown in Fig. 1.

244

used for β-oxidation and lipoprotein synthesis, then a fatty liver occurs. The secretion of TG also involves the secretion of cholesterol since this is a component of VLDL. TG is subsequently removed from VLDL by lipoprotein lipase and the cholesterol is left in the circulation in LDL. Thus an enhanced rate of VLDL production leads to an increased appearance of LDL. An increased concentration of LDL in the blood is considered to be a risk-factor in atherosclerotic disease[1]. In addition, an increased synthesis of TG and VLDL by the liver could contribute to obesity.

PC is produced by the same metabolic pathway as TG and it shares the same precursor, namely DG (Fig. 1). PC is secreted by the liver in VLDL and in HDL of which it is a major component. It is also used for membrane synthesis within the liver and for the production of bile. High circulating concentrations of HDL are associated with a low incidence of ischaemic heart disease[1],

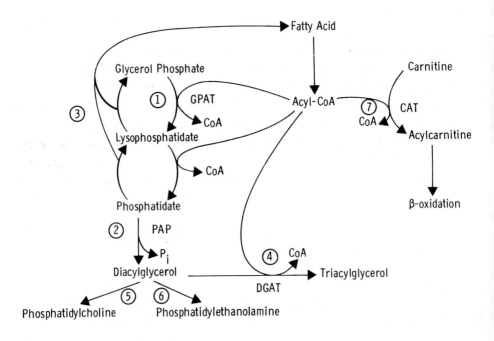

Fig. 1. Pathways of glycerolipid synthesis and β-oxidation. Enzyme activities are indicated by: (1) Glycerol phosphate acyltransferase (EC 2.3.1.15); (2) Phosphatidate phosphohydrolase (EC 3.1.3.4); (3) Phospholipase A type activities; (4) Diacylglycerol acyltransferase (EC 2.3.1.20); (5) Choline phosphotransferase (EC 2.7.8.2); (6) Ethanolamine phosphotransferase (EC 2.7.8.1); and (7) Carnitine acyltransferase (EC 2.3.1.21).

and there appears to be a reciprocal relationship between the concentrations of TG and HDL in the blood[2]. Little is known about the mechanisms for controlling the secretion of VLDL and HDL, although the factors that influence VLDL secretion have been reviewed[3].

One facet of this problem is the regulation of FA metabolism in the liver. It is important to know what factors control the partitioning of FA a) into β-oxidation rather than into glycerolipid synthesis and b) into the synthesis of PL rather than into TG. In particular, it is necessary to understand the effects of changing our dietary and hormonal status on these events. Our knowledge of the control of glycerolipid synthesis is not as advanced as that in many other areas of biochemistry because of the inherent difficulties of working with lipids and the enzymes that metabolize lipids. However, patterns of control are beginning to emerge and these will be the subject of this article. The discussion will concentrate on the effects of insulin, glucagon, thyroxine and glucocorticoids, since it is possible to postulate how these hormones might alter the activity of enzymes involved in hepatic glycerolipid synthesis.

RESULTS AND DISCUSSION

The role of insulin and glucagon in regulating the balance between β-oxidation and the synthesis of TG, PC and PE

It is well known that the fate of FA entering the liver is dramatically affected by the ratio of insulin/glucagon in the circulation. When this ratio is high the esterification of FA to TG is favoured, whereas the rate of β-oxidation is decreased. Conversely, at low ratios of insulin/glucagon there is often an increased ketogenesis combined with a decreased rate of TG synthesis[3,4]. The synthesis of PC and PE is far less sensitive to the effects of starvation than that of TG[4,5]. These observations indicate two possible sites for the control of FA metabolism by insulin and glucagon: a) the branch-point for the metabolism of acyl-CoA esters by GPAT and CAT and b) the branch-point for the metabolism of DG by DGAT, choline phosphotransferase and ethanolamine phosphotransferase (Fig. 1).

Starvation decreases the activity of both the mitochondrial and the microsomal GPAT in the liver, although these results have not always been obtained[6]. In this condition the activity of CAT is increased, and these changes would, in themselves, favour the diversion of FA into the pathway of β-oxidation[7]. However, the activity of the microsomal GPAT is not significantly altered in diabetes[8,9], whereas that in the mitochondrial fraction is decreased[9].

Conversely, perfusing livers with insulin specifically increases the activity of the mitochondrial enzyme[10]. These results, and the different sensitivities of the GPAT in the two fractions to N-ethylmaleimide, indicate that these activities are catalysed by different proteins[10]. This may be particularly significant since it is at the mitochondrial outer membrane that one would expect the competition for acyl-CoA esters between the pathways of β-oxidation and esterification to take place. Moreover, it is the mitochondrial enzyme that is sensitive to changes in the glucagon/insulin ratio. However, the major site for the synthesis of TG is normally thought to be in the endoplasmic reticulum. It is interesting to consider that there might be a further level of control that regulates the flux of FA between mitochondria and the endo-plasmic reticulum. Possibly FA binding proteins might participate in this[11].

The mechanisms that produce the decreased activity of GPAT in diabetes and starvation are not known for certain. The changes in the microsomal GPAT may be controlled by Ca^{2+} accumulation, since this is correlated with a decreased rate of PA synthesis from glycerol phosphate[12]. The synthesis of PA was decreased in microsomal fractions obtained from livers perfused with dibutyryl-cyclic-AMP[12]. Also the uptake of Ca^{2+} was higher in male rats than in females, whereas the synthesis of TG and the secretion of TG from the livers in females exceeded that in the males[12,13]. It may also be relevant that PAP activity is inhibited by Ca^{2+}[14].

The GPAT activity in adipose tissue can be inactivated by a phosphorylation reaction[15]. This is achieved by incubation with ATP, Mg^{2+} and a cyclic AMP-dependent protein kinase. GPAT activity can be regenerated by incubating with alkaline phosphatase[15], but it is not yet certain whether this mechanism operates in liver.

The insulin/glucagon ratio could also be responsible for an acute regulation of CAT activity. When this ratio is high acetyl-CoA carboxylase activity is increased, and the concentration of malonyl-CoA in the cells rises[16]. This inhibits CAT and the oxidation of FA. Conversely, when this ratio falls, acetyl-CoA carboxylase activity declines and the decrease in malonyl-CoA concentration relieves the inhibition on CAT, thus facilitating β-oxidation[16].

An additional mechanism for controlling the balance between glycerolipid synthesis and β-oxidation could occur at the point of PA breakdown. PAP activity in the liver changes rapidly and dramatically in the same direction as the potential of the liver to synthesize TG[6,17]. The liver also has the ability to deacylate PA back to GP (Fig. 1). The rates of the latter reactions in the microsomal plus supernatant fractions of livers of rats fed glucose or saline are similar to that of DG synthesis[18]. Thus, if the phospholipase A type activities compete for PA with PAP, then the balance between these activites could be involved in controlling the overall rate of TG synthesis. This also means that some of the FA that are incorporated into PA could be cycled back to the unesterified FA pool, and could therefore have a further chance of being oxidized [17].

Nothing is known about the hormonal control of the enzymes that deacylate PA. It is known that insulin does not maintain the hepatic activity of PAP since this activity is increased in experimental diabetes[8]. Furthermore, feeding rats with glucose did not increase PAP activity[18], even though we now know that the serum insulin concentrations in these rats was increased by about 2-fold. It is also interesting to note that the addition of insulin to cultures of hepatocytes does not alter the rate at which FA are incorporated into TG, PC and PE[19]. However, glucagon does give a marked decrease in the rate of TG synthesis, whereas it has little effect on the synthesis of PC and PE[19]. Thus it preferentially channels DG into PL synthesis. The mechanism of this control is not certain, but a major factor in regulating PC and PE synthesis is the availability of CDP-choline and CDP-ethanolamine[20,21].

One of the major factors that regulates the balance between β-oxidation and the synthesis of different glycerolipids is the supply of FA to the liver. Low insulin/glucagon ratio ensures that FA are diverted into the more essential pathways of energy production[3] and PL synthesis[19] when the supply of FA is low. However, if the supply of FA in these conditions exceeds the capacity for β-oxidation and the ability to synthesize PC and PE, then the excess FA are converted to TG. It appears that the capacity of the liver to synthesize TG in starvation is not diminished[22], and the rate of TG production and VLDL secretion is often increased in diabetes[23].

Effects of thyroid hormones on the synthesis of TG

Thyroid hormones stimulate the rate of TG synthesis in liver and heart, but they have the opposite effect in adipose tissue[24]. Homogenates obtained from the livers of rats treated with L-thyroxine (0.5 mg/Kg of body weight for 5 days) showed the same rate of incorporation of GP into glycerolipid, but a greater proportion of the products were isolated as DG and TG. These results indicate that the activity of PAP or DGAT is increased (Fig. 1). Direct measurement of PAP activity in the soluble fraction demonstrated that it was increased by thyroxine when expressed per mg of protein, but that it was not increased significantly in terms of its content in the liver[25]. The rate of hepatic glycerolipid synthesis *in vivo* was also measured in this study, and a relative increase in the incorporation of [^{3}H]glycerol into TG was observed. There also appeared to be relatively less [^{14}C]palmitate and [^{3}H]glycerol accumulating in PA, but the results were not statistically significant[25]. An increased activity of hepatic PAP has been reported in experiments where 1 mg of L-thyroxine/Kg of body weight was administered to rats for seven days, but there was no significant increase when the duration of the treatment was decreased to 4 h (Communicated by Lehtonen, Savolainen and Hassinen at the 8th Linderstrøm-Lang Conference, 1978). It is therefore likely that the activity of PAP can be increased in the liver by injecting thyroid hormones, but that the increase occurs relatively slowly and is less dramatic than that described in the following section.

The hepatic activity of DGAT increases in rats treated with triiodo-thyronine[26]. This result is compatible with measurements made on the rate of glycerolipid synthesis in rat liver *in vivo*[25]. In these experiments the relative proportion of injected [^{14}C]palmitate and [^{3}H]glycerol isolated in DG was decreased, whereas that in TG was increased.

These increases in TG synthesis may contribute to the increased concentration of circulating VLDL that has been reported in hyperthyroid states[27]. However, a large proportion of the TG that is synthesized in the liver in these conditions is preferentially oxidized within the liver, and the secretion of VLDL can be decreased[28,29]. This is in agreement with the hypo-triglyceridaemia that has been observed in thyrotoxic patients[30]. The increased degradation of hepatic TG is probably catalysed by an acid lipase that increases in activity after thyroxine treatment[31]. The increased turnover of TG is a further example of substrate cycling leading to a thermogenic effect that is often observed with thyroxine. It is also known that this hormone stimulates simultaneously the synthesis and β-oxidation of FA in the liver[28].

Effects of glucocorticoids on the synthesis of hepatic TG and the secretion of VLDL

The activity of PAP in the liver changes more rapidly and dramatically than other enzymes of glycerolipid metabolism in response to stimuli that affect the synthesis of hepatic TG[6,17,32]. These changes parallel the capacity of the liver to synthesize TG, although this capacity, as in starvation, may not always be expressed.

The activity of hepatic PAP is clearly not maintained by insulin since it is increased in diabetes[8,33] and in starvation[34,35]. A significant increase in this activity was seen in the livers of rats between 6 and 10 h after feeding was stopped (Fig. 2). The activity remained high (Fig. 2) and was still

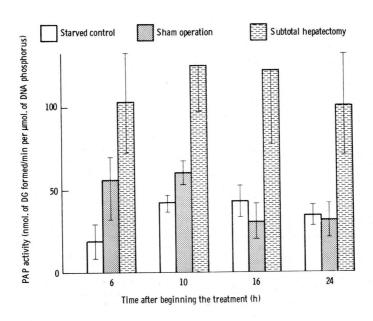

Fig. 2. Effect of starvation, sham operation and subtotal hepatectomy on the activity of hepatic PAP. The results are taken from Mangiapane et al.[35] and are reproduced by permission of the Biochem. J. The values are expressed as means ± S.D.

observed after 36-40 h[34]. The stress of removing 80% of the liver produced a PAP activity that was about 5.5-fold higher than that in the starved controls 6 h after the operation (Fig. 2). This increase in specific activity was maintained until 24 h after the operation. The sham-operated controls showed a smaller increase in PAP activity at 6-10 h after operation, and the activity declined to approach that in the starved rats after 16 h.

Starvation, diabetes and surgery produces metabolic stress that is characterized by an increased flux of FA from adipose tissue to the liver. The liver will preferentially oxidize these FA, but if the FA supply exceeds the capacity for β-oxidation, then the excess are converted to TG. The increased activity of PAP facilitates this protective mechanism that enables the liver to dispose of potentially toxic acyl-CoA esters and to regenerate CoA[17]. The increased synthesis of TG can contribute to the appearance of the fatty liver that can accompany starvation[36,37], diabetes[33], and partial (or subtotal) hepatectomy[35]. It also partly explains the hypertriglyceridaemia that often accompanies diabetes[23].

The hormones that are most likely to control the activity of PAP in these stress conditions are the glucocorticoids, and some evidence has been obtained

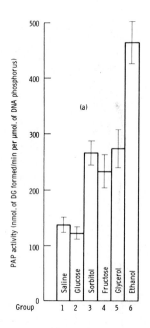
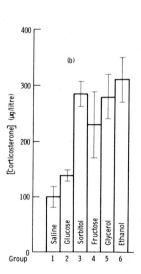

Fig. 3. Effect of feeding saline, glucose, sorbitol, fructose, glycerol and ethanol on the hepatic activities of PAP and on the concentration of serum corticosterone. Rats were fed with ethanol (5 g/kg body weight) or with iso-calaric glucose, sorbitol, fructose, glycerol or with the equivalent volume of 0.15 M-NaCl[18]. The results in Section (a) are taken from Sturton et al.[18] and show the activity of PAP in the microsomal and supernatant fractions 6 h later. These are reproduced by permission of the Biochem. J. Section (b) shows the serum concentrations of corticosterone at 90 min after feeding in similar group each composed of four rats. Results are given as means ± S.E.M.

to support this hypothesis. Injecting rats for 5 days with cortisol produced a 2.8-fold increase in the soluble PAP activity of the liver[25]. This change was accompanied by an increase in the relative rate at which TG was synthesized in the liver, and by an increased flux of PA to DG. Injecting corticotropin had similar, though not identical effects on the hepatic synthesis of glycero-lipids[25]. Cortisol and other glucocorticoids are known to produce fatty livers[38,39] and to increase the secretion of VLDL[40,41].

Increases in blood glucocorticoid concentrations are also probably responsible for the increased PAP activity observed after feeding with ethanol, sorbitol, glycerol and fructose. Evidence for this proposal is given in Fig. 3. Compared with the saline or glucose treated controls, rats fed with ethanol showed a 3.4-3.8 fold increase in the combined microsomal and soluble PAP activities in their livers after 6 h[18]. The equivalent increases obtained with sorbitol, fructose, and glycerol were about 2-fold. All of these changes were preceded at 90 min after feeding by similar patterns of increase in the concentration of corticosterone in the serum (Fig. 3b). Other measurements show that the increase for ethanol persisted for longer than that observed after feeding fructose, glycerol and sorbitol, and this could explain the greater increase in PAP activity.

Evidence has also been presented that the increased PAP activity is one of the factors that predisposes the liver to synthesize increased quantities of TG after ethanol ingestion[42-44]. These findings are compatible with earlier observations that an intact pituitary-adrenal axis is necessary for the development of the ethanol-induced fatty liver[45,46]. Ethanol might provoke the increase in circulating glucocorticoids by stimulating the release of corticotropin and by damaging the liver, thus diminishing the degradation of glucocorticoids[47]. Prolonged feeding with sucrose (or fructose) has also been claimed to lead to hypercortisolism[48], and this type of chronic dietary modification is known to maintain high activities of PAP in the liver[49]. The increased synthesis of TG that is caused by consuming diets rich in ethanol[50,51], fructose[48,52], glycerol[53,54], and sorbitol[55] is manifested by the accumulation of TG in the liver and by hypertriglyceridaemia.

Rats that were pretreated with benfluorex prior to ethanol administration showed much smaller increases in PAP activity[44], in TG synthesis and in TG accumulation in their livers[43]. This drug is also known to have hypotriglyceridaemic effects[43]. It is possible to inhibit TG synthesis in liver slices by adding benfluorex or related compounds to the incubations[56]. These drugs interact with PA and in the presence of Mg^{2+} inhibit PAP activity[57]. However, the decreased activity of PAP that was isolated from the livers of rats treated with benfluorex prior to ethanol could not be explained by this mechanism[44]. Preliminary experiments in our laboratory have indicated that the ethanol-induced increase in plasma corticosterone concentrations is less marked in the benfluorex-treated rats. These experiments provide further evidence that glucocorticoids are part of the mechanism that causes the changes in FA metabolism after ethanol ingestion.

It is widely believed that ethanol diverts FA into TG by changing the redox state of the liver[50,51]. This increases the availability of GP and decreases the hepatic oxidation of FA to CO_2[50]. The metabolism of glycerol and sorbitol has a similar effect in increasing the availability of NADH and GP[58]. Fructose is also readily converted to GP and dihydroxyacetone phosphate, but this need not involve changes in the redox state[58,59]. There is also evidence that alterations in GP concentration alone cannot account for the ethanol-induced stimulation of hepatic TG synthesis[60-62]. Furthermore, it is unlikely that benfluorex prevents the ethanol-induced effects on FA esterification by altering the hepatic redox state, since it does not significantly alter the rate of ethanol oxidation to CO_2[43].

Changes in the composition of dietary fat can also alter the rate of hepatic TG synthesis and the partitioning of FA between TG and PL. Feeding rats a diet enriched with corn oil favours the synthesis of PC rather than TG when compared with diets enriched with starch or lard[63]. This probably results partly from the increased activity of choline phosphotransferase and also the preferential incorporation of polyunsaturated DG into PC[63]. Feeding lard appears to increase the rate at which FA are incorporated into hepatic glycerolipids and this is accompanied by an increased PAP activity[63]. The introduction of rapeseed oil into the diet is known to produce an abnormally high stress response in rats resulting in increased concentrations of serum corticosterone and a fatty infiltration of tissues[64]. Feeding the long chain FA that are found in lard probably has a similar effect[64]. This again implicates glucocorticoids in increasing PAP activity[63], in the production of fatty livers[65,66], in the increased synthesis of VLDL[67], and in the hypertriglyceridaemia[65,67-69] that accompanies the feeding of diets rich in saturated and monounsaturated FA.

High plasma concentrations of cortisol are associated with conditions of excessive fat accumulation such as in Cushing's disease and obesity[70,71]. Cortisol appears to be involved in increasing the rate of FA synthesis in the liver in obesity, although its effects may be mediated through insulin[72-74]. The increased synthesis of TG in the livers and adipose tissue of obese animals is probably facilitated by an increased activity of PAP in these organs[32].

It is known that adrenalectomized animals fail to develop fatty livers in response to the hepatotoxic effects of phosphorus, ethionine, and colchicine, or in starvation, diabetes, partial hepatectomy and in other forms of metabolic stress. There is evidence that adrenalectomy has direct effects on the liver that cannot be entirely accounted for by defective mobilization of FA from adipose tissue[70,75]. The preceding discussion has shown that one of the effects of glucocorticoids is probably to increase the activity of PAP in the liver and thereby stimulate TG synthesis.

The mechanism by which PAP activity is increased is not known. However, it seems likely that corticosteroids stimulate the synthesis of PAP in the liver, since the increased activity that is produced by subtotal hepatectomy is blocked when the rats are pretreated with actinomycin D[35]. The rapid decline in PAP activity between 10 and 16 h after sham-operation (Fig. 2) also suggests that PAP may be rapidly degraded. These changes could account for a long-term metabolic control, but it is also likely that short-term control exists. A stimulating factor which has a molecular weight of between 8,000-16,000 has been described[76], and it is also suggested that polyamines control PAP activity[77]. It is not known whether PAP activity is controlled by covalent modification.

CONCLUDING REMARKS

In the foregoing discussion an attempt has been made to summarize the effects of insulin, glucagon, thyroxine and glucocorticoids on the synthesis of TG and the secretion of VLDL. The information that is available concerning the effects of other hormones is less complete, and their specific effects on individual enzymes of glycerolipid synthesis are not well understood. Of particular interest are the sex hormones which are known to exert profound effects on lipid metabolism. Such differences may contribute to the different rates of coronary thrombosis in men and premenopausal women.

The hormonal status of animals is largely influenced by diet and the inter-action between this and the response to hormonal change has been emphasized. Particular attention has been placed on the effects of diet on the circulating concentrations of glucocorticoids which increase TG synthesis and the secretion of VLDL. Evidence has been presented that the consumption of diets rich in sucrose, fat and alcohol is accompanied by increased plasma concentrations of glucocorticoids. This in turn increases the activity of PAP in the liver and stimulates the synthesis and secretion of TG. Eating excessive quantities of saturated fat and of sucrose has been widely implicated in producing adverse changes in the concentration of circulating lipoproteins and in the development of atherosclerosis. Glucocorticoids may be involved in producing these changes. They are also prominent in regulating metabolism in diabetes and in stress. These conditions also constitute risk factors for atherosclerosis and coronary thrombosis, and they are characterized by increased PAP activities and increased TG synthesis in the liver. Furthermore, it is likely that the increases in TG synthesis that are produced by saturated fat and sucrose are amplified in a stressed person.

A greater understanding of these effects must be part of the basis for formulating future policies on dietary recommendations with respect to dimin-ishing the risk of premature atherosclerosis and ischaemic heart disease.

254

ACKNOWLEDGEMENTS

We thank the Medical and Science Research Councils of Great Britain for financial support.

REFERENCES

1. Glueck, C.J., Mattson, F. and Bierman, E.L. (1978) New Eng. J. Med., 298, 1471-1474.

2. Shaefer, E.J., Anderson, B.W., Brewer, H.B., Levy, R.I., Danner, R.N. and Blackwelder, W.C. (1978) Lancet, 2, 391-393.

3. Mayes, P.A. in International Encyclopedia of Pharmacology and Therapeutics, Peters, G. ed., Section 24, Pergamon Press, Oxford, pp.125-174.

4. Groener, J.E.M. and van Golde, L.M.G. (1977) Biochim. Biophys. Acta, 487, 105-114.

5. Iritani, N., Yamashita, S. and Numa, S. (1976) J. Biochem. (Tokyo), 80, 217-222.

6. Brindley, D.N. (1978) in Regulation of Fatty Acid and Glycerolipid Metabolism, Dils, R. and Knudsen, J. eds., Pergamon Press, Oxford and New York, pp.31-40.

7. Aas, M. and Daae, L.N.W. (1971) Biochim. Biophys. Acta, 239, 208-216.

8. Whiting, P.H., Bowley, M., Sturton, R.G., Pritchard, P.H., Brindley, D.N. and Hawthorne, J.N. (1977) Biochem. J. 168, 147-153.

9. Bates, E.J. and Saggerson, D. (1977) FEBS Lett. 84, 229-232.

10. Bates, E.J., Topping, D.L., Soorana, S.P., Saggerson, D. and Mayes, P.A. (1977) FEBS Lett. 84, 225-228.

11. Wu-Rideout, M.Y.C., Elson, C. and Shrago, E. (1976) Biochem. Biophys. Res. Commun. 71, 809-816.

12. Soler-Argilaga, C., Russel, R.L. and Heimberg, M. (1977) Biochem. Biophys. Res. Commun. 78, 1053-1059.

13. Soler-Argilaga, C. and Heimberg, M. (1976) J. Lipid Res. 17, 605-615.

14. Brindley, D.N., Bowley, M., Sturton, R.G., Pritchard, P.H., Cooling, J. and Burditt, S.L. in Enzymes of Lipid Metabolism, Gatt, S., Freysz, L. and Mandel, P. eds., Plenum Publishing Corp., New York, pp.227-234.

15. Nimmo, H.G. and Houston, B. (1978) Biochem. J., 176, in the press.

16. McGarry, J.D., Mannaerts, G.P. and Foster, D.W. (1977) J. Clin. Invest., 60, 265-270.

17. Brindley, D.N. (1978) Int. J. Obesity, 2, 7-16.

18. Sturton, R.G., Pritchard, H.P., Han, L-Y. and Brindley, D.N. (1978) Biochem. J., 174, 667-670.

19. Geelen, M.J.H., Groener, J.E.M., De Haas, C.G.M., Wisserhof, T.A. and van Golde, L.M.G. (1978) FEBS Lett. 90, 57-60.

20. Infante, J.P. (1977) Biochem. J., 167, 847-849.

21. Åkesson, B. and Sundler, R. (1977) Biochem. Soc. Trans., 5, 43-48.

22. McGarry, J.D., Meier, J.M. and Foster, D.W. (1973) J. Biol. Chem. 248, 270-278.

255

23. Nikkilä, E.A. (1974) Proc. R. Soc. Med., 67, 662-665.

24. Roncari, D.A.K. and Murthy, V.K. (1975) J. Biol. Chem., 250, 4134-4138.

25. Glenny, H.P. and Brindley, D.N. (1978) Biochem. J., 176, in the press.

26. Young, D.L. and Lynen, F. (1969) J. Biol. Chem. 244, 377-383.

27. Nikkilä, E.A. and Kekki, M. (1972) J. Clin. Invest. 51, 2103-2114.

28. Diamant, S., Gorin, E. and Shafrir, E. (1972) Eur. J. Biochem. 26, 553-559.

29. Keyes, W.G. and Heimberg, M. (1978) Fed. Proc. Fed. Am. Soc. Exp. Biol., 37, 258A.

30. Tulloch, B.R., Lewis, B. and Fraser, T.R. (1973) Lancet, 1, 391-394.

31. Coates, P.M., Brown, S.A., Lau, H., Krulich, L. and Koldovsky, O. (1978) FEBS Lett. 86, 45-48.

32. Fallon, H.J., Lamb, R.G. and Jamdar, S.C. (1977) Biochem. Soc. Trans., 5, 37-40.

33. Murthy, V.K. and Shipp, J.C. (1976) Diabetes, 25, 378.

34. Vavrečka, M., Mitchell, M.P. and Hübscher, G. (1969) Biochem. J., 115, 139-145.

35. Mangiapane, E.H., Lloyd-Davies, K.A. and Brindley, D.N. (1973) Biochem. J., 134, 103-112.

36. Mayes, P.A. (1962) Metabolism, 11, 781-799.

37. Gillman, J., Gillman, C. and Savage, N. (1962) Metabolism, 11, 800-813.

38. Hill, R.B. and Droke, W.A. (1963) Proc. Soc. Exp. Biol. Med., 114, 766-769.

39. Ožegović, B., Rode, B. and Milković, S. (1975) Endokrinologie, 66, 128-134.

40. Klausner, H. and Heimberg, M. (1967) Am. J. Physiol., 212, 1236-1246.

41. Reaven, E.P., Kolterman, O.G. and Reaven, G.M. (1974) J. Lipid Res., 15, 74-83.

42. Savolainen, M.J. (1977) Biochem. Biophys. Res. Commun. 75, 511-518.

43. Pritchard, P.H. and Brindley, D.N. (1977) J. Pharm. Pharmacol., 29, 343-349.

44. Pritchard, P.H., Bowley, M., Burditt, S.L., Cooling, J., Glenny, H.P., Lawson, N., Sturton, R.G. and Brindley, D.N. (1977) Biochem. J., 166, 639-642.

45. Brodie, B.B. and Maickel, R.P. (1963) Ann. N.Y. Acad. Sci., 104, 1049-1058.

46. Maickel, R.P. and Brodie, B.B. (1963) Ann. N.Y. Acad. Sci., 104, 1059-1064.

47. Mendelson, J.H. (1971) in The Biology of Alcoholism, Kissin, B. and Beglester, H. eds., vol. 1, Plenum Press, New York, pp.513-544.

48. Yudkin, J. (1978) Lipids, 13, 370-372.

49. Lamb, R.G. and Fallon, H.J. (1974) Biochim. Biophys. Acta 348, 179-188.

50. Lieber, C.S. (1974) Lipids, 9, 103-116.

51. Hawkins, R.D. and Kalant, H. (1972) Pharmacol. Rev., 24, 67-156.

52. Waddell, M. and Fallon, H.J. (1973) J. Clin. Invest., 52, 2725-2731.

53. Nikkilä, E.A. and Ojala, K. (1964) Life Science, 3, 1021-1023.

256

54. Narayan, K.A. and McMullen, J.J. (1978) Fed. Proc. Fed. Am. Soc. Exp. Biol., 37, 258.

55. Lederer, J., Masri, H. and Niethals, E.W. (1978) Ann. Endocrinol., 39, 157-158.

56. Brindley, D.N. and Bowley, M. (1975) Biochem. J., 148, 461-469.

57. Bowley, M., Cooling, J., Burditt, S.L. and Brindley, D.N. (1977) Biochem. J., 165, 447-454.

58. Rawat, A.K. and Menahan, L.A. (1975) Diabetes, 24, 926-932.

59. Pereira, J.N. and Jangaard, N.O. (1971) Metabolism, 20, 392-400.

60. Kalant, H., Kanna, J.M. and Bustos, G.O. (1972) Biochem. Pharmacol., 21, 811-819.

61. Estler, C.J. (1974) Res. Exp. Med., 163, 95-100.

62. Abrams, M.A. and Cooper, C. (1976) Biochem. J., 156, 33-46.

63. Glenny, H.P., Bowley, M., Burditt, S.L., Cooling, J., Pritchard, H.P., Sturton, R.G. and Brindley, D.N. (1978) Biochem. J., 174, 535-541.

64. Hülsmann, W.C. and Stam, H. (1979) in Lipoprotein Metabolism and Endocrine Regulation, Hessel, L.W. and Krans, H.J.M. eds., Elsevier/North-Holland Biomedical Press, Amsterdam, pp. 287-295.

65. Bruckdorfer, K.R., Kari-Kari, B.P.B., Khan, I.H. and Yudkin, J. (1972) Nutr. Metab., 14, 228-237.

66. Laitinen, M., Hietanen, E., Vaino, H. and Hänninen, O. (1975) Lipids, 10, 461-466.

67. Chait, A., Onitir, A., Nicoll, A., Rabaya, E., Davies, J. and Lewis, B. (1974) Atherosclerosis, 20, 347-364.

68. MacDonald, I. (1971) Proc. Nutr. Soc. 30, 72A-73A.

69. Waterman, R.A., Romsos, D.R., Tsai, A.C., Miller, E.R. and Leveille, G.A. (1975) Proc. Soc. Exp. Biol. Med. 150, 347-351.

70. Rudman, D. and Di Girolamo, M. (1971) in The Human Adrenal Cortex, Cristy, N.P. ed., Harper and Row, New York, pp.241-255.

71. Herberg, L. and Coleman, D.L. (1977) Metabolism, 26, 59-99.

72. Salmon, D.M.W. and Hems, D.A. (1973) Biochem. J., 136, 551-563.

73. Diamant, S. and Shafrir, E. (1975) Eur. J. Biochem., 53, 541-546.

74. Kirk, C.J., Verrinder, T.R. and Hems, D.A. (1976) Biochem. J., 156, 593-602.

75. Ramey, E.R. and Goldstein, M.S. (1957) Physiol. Rev., 37, 155-195.

76. Roncari, D.A.K. and Mack, Y.W. (1975) Biochem. Biophys. Res. Commun. 67, 790-796.

77. Lamb, R.G. and Blank, W.L. (1977) Pharmacologist, 19, 182.

Lipoprotein Metabolism and Endocrine Regulation
L.W. Hessel and H.M.J. Krans editors
© ECSC, EEC, EAEC, Brussels-Luxembourg, 1979
Published by Elsevier/North-Holland Biomedical Press-Amsterdam

SYNTHESIS AND SECRETION OF LIPOPROTEIN LIPIDS BY ISOLATED RAT HEPATOCYTES

HERMAN JAN KEMPEN

Gaubius Institute, Health Research Organization TNO, Herenstraat 5d, Leiden
(The Netherlands)

SUMMARY

It is shown in this report that it is feasible to study the release of lipoprotein lipids by isolated hepatocytes during short (60') incubations. The
results indicate that the release of unlabeled or radiolabeled lipids from hepatocytes of fed rats is generally similar to that from the perfused rat liver.
The molar proportion of triacylglycerol to phospholipid is smaller than one in
the hepatocytes but about two in the medium; likewise the proportion of esterified to free cholesterol is higher in the medium than in the cells. Calculation
of specific activities of labeled lipids in cells and medium shows that equili-
bration of newly synthesized lipids with the pool of "secretory" lipids is most
rapid for triacylglycerol, and slowest for free cholesterol.

The majority of radiolabeled triacylglycerol and free and esterified sterols
in the medium are precipitated by addition of phosphotungstate and $MgCl_2$, in
the presence of "carrier" rat serum. This suggests that these lipids are released as VLDL particles. About half of the labeled phospholipids in the medium do
not precipitate by this treatment, indicating their presence in HDL. The
release, but not the synthesis, of labeled triacylglycerol is strongly inhibited
by colchicine. Release of labeled phospholipid is much less affected.

Addition of oleic acid to the incubation medium elevates the cellular level
of triacylglycerols, but does not result in enhanced release of this lipid into
the medium, in contradistinction to published findings in the perfused liver.
This points to a defect in the assembly and/or export of triacylglycerol-
containing lipoprotein. However, addition of rat serum causes both an increase
in the cellular level and an elevation of the release of triacylglycerols, as
has been observed earlier with the perfused liver.

Glucagon is found to depress *de novo* synthesis of fatty acids, but not that
of sterols. The hormone has no effect on the percent release of labeled lipids
in the medium.

INTRODUCTION

The liver and intestinal mucosa are responsible for the production of the
very low density lipoprotein (VLDL) and high density lipoprotein (HDL) occurring

258

in the plasma. The role of the liver has been studied in the past by means of liver slices and of the isolated perfused organ, which preparations have been shown to synthesize and secrete both VLDL[1-14] and HDL[1-4,6,10,11,13,14]. The production of VLDL is increased by addition of fatty acid to the perfusate[4,7], and is also modified by hormones[15-19]. About the regulation of the HDL production no information has yet appeared.

The newly synthesized lipids are secreted as complexes with apoproteins. VLDL, containing triacylglycerol, phospholipid and cholesterol as lipids, possesses apo-B, apo-C and apo-E, while HDL has apo-A, apo-C and apo-E proteins, in complex with phospholipid and cholesterol[20]. There is only scant information on the mechanisms which are involved in the assembly of the lipo-protein particles from lipid and apo-proteins[8,9,12], and none at all on the distribution of newly synthesized lipids among VLDL and HDL. It is the purpose of our study to obtain a more thorough understanding of these processes, and the ways in which they are regulated. This regulation may occur by way of variations in the flow of lipoprotein precursors towards the liver, as well as by hormonal or neural influences, alone or in conjunction with altered sub-strate flow. Obviously, knowledge of the nature of the substrate regulation is required before hormonal actions can be fully understood.

Since isolated hepatocytes have been shown during recent years to be a good model for the study of many functional and metabolic aspects of the intact liver, we have decided to explore the usefulness of this preparation for our aims. Our first results, presented here, confirm and extend the finding of others using isolated rat hepatocytes in suspension[21-23], and provide new data on the secretion of sterols and sterol esters.

MATERIALS AND METHODS

Animals. Male Wistar rats, obtained from the Centraal Proefdierenbedrijf TNO, Zeist, The Netherlands, were used in this study. They were housed in an airconditioned room (20°C), with a daily period of darkness from 18.00 p.m. to 8.00 a.m. From their arrival they were fed a regular chow containing 60% (by weight) carbohydrate, 22% protein and 4% fat; at least one week before sacrifice they were fasted one night, and thereafter fed _ad libitum_ a diet containing 67% carbohydrate, 22% protein and no added fat (less than 0.1%). Water was given in bottles. Animals with a body weight between 200 and 300 g were used for hepatocyte preparation.

Isolation and incubation of hepatocytes. The method of hepatocyte isolation was essentially that of Seglen[24]. Experiments were started between 10.00 and 11.00 a.m. After induction of ether anaesthesia the abdomen was opened and the portal vein cannulated. A non-recirculating perfusion was done with 250 ml Ca-free Krebs-Henseleit medium buffered with 20 mM Hepes and 25 mM bicarbonate (KHHB). Thereafter the liver was perfused in the circulatory mode with KHHB containing 1.2 mM $CaCl_2$, 50 mg% collagenase and 1% fatty acid-free bovine serum albumin during 15'. The liver capsula surrounding the lobes was then cut, and the hepatocytes were freed by shaking the lobes in about 100 ml KHHB with Ca. The suspension was filtered through a 80 m pore screen, and the cells were washed 4 times by centrifugation and resuspension in KHHB. All media were kept at 37°C and gassed with 95% oxygen and 5% carbon dioxide. The cells were final-ly resuspended to a volume of about 25 ml, and used for incubation without further delay. One ml cell suspension was put on a tared watch glass and dried at 95°C, in order to determine the cell concentration in terms of dry weight.

Incubations were carried out in 30 x 106 mm glass tubes fitted with screw caps. The tubes were filled with 1.0 ml suspension (30-50 mg dry weight) and further additions to a final volume of 2.5 ml. The media contained either 2% fatty acid-free albumin (complexed in some experiments with oleic acid), or 40% (v/v) dialysed rat serum as protein. As radioactive tracers were added 625 µCi ^3H_2O, 0.5 µCi $[1-^{14}C]$-acetate, 0.5 µCi $[2-^{14}C]$-mevalonate or 0.75 µCi $[1-^{14}C]$-oleate per incubation. The tubes were gassed with the 95% oxygen - 5% carbon dioxide mixture before closing, and then incubated in a Dubnoff meta-bolic shaker kept at 37°C with 100 strokes per minute. After 60' the tubes were centrifuged for 15' at 3,000 x g, and the supernatant (medium) carefully aspirated with a Pasteur pipet.

Lipid extractions and analyses. The cell pellets were resuspended in 3.0 ml water, and lipids were extracted according to Bligh and Dyer[25] by the consecutive admixture of 12 ml chloroform:methanol (1:2), 4 ml chloroform and 4 ml water. After separation of the phases by centrifugation, the lower layer was quantitatively aspirated and blown dry under nitrogen. The lipid residue was subjected to the same cycle of solvent additions and treatments, and the final residue dissolved in a small volume of chloroform. Part (1.2 ml) of the incubation medium was extracted in the same way. When incubation media contain-ing ^3H_2O and 40% rat serum were incubated in the absence of hepatocytes and then extracted according to this procedure, the lipid extract contained no radioactivity.

An aliquot of the lipid extract was mixed with 10 ml scintillation fluid and counted. Another part was applied as a streak on a thin layer plate of silica, and developed in chloroform:methanol (98:2), and then for a greater distance in hexane:chloroform (60:25). This results in the clear separation of phospho-

lipids, monoacylglycerols, free fatty acids, sterols, diacylglycerols, triacylglycerols, sterolesters and hydrocarbons (in order of increasing R_f). The
lipids were stained by iodine vapour, identified with the help of reference
lipids spotted on the same plate, scraped off with a spatula, mixed with 10 ml
scintillation fluid in a counting vial (the phospholipid-containing silica was
first soaked with 1 ml methanol), and counted. Recovery of radioactivity from
the thin layer was usually better than 90%.

Chemical determinations of lipid levels in cells and media were done as
follows: triacylglycerol by the method of Giegel et al.[26] with triolein as
standard; free and esterified cholesterol in the media by an enzymatic
method[27]; free cholesterol in the cell extract by dissolving an aliquot of
the lipid extract in isopropanol, and mixing this with the same enzymatic
reagent mixture; cholesterolesters in the cells as free cholesterol after
isolation of the esters by thin layer chromatography, elution from the silica
with chloroform, saponification of the esters in alcoholic KOH, extraction of
the liberated free cholesterol with hexane, and dissolving the dried residue in
isopropanol; phospholipid as phosphorus after destruction according to Böttcher
et al.[28], using egg lecithin as standard.

In some experiments the VLDL and LDL in the incubation medium were separated
from the other (lipo-)proteins in the medium by precipitation according to the
method of Burstein[29]. The media that contained no serum were mixed with rat
serum to a final concentration of 40% (v/v) serum, offering "carrier" lipoprotein for the precipitation of the labeled VLDL. To 1 ml of the serum containing
medium 100 μl 4% (w/v) sodium phosphotungstate and 25 μl 2 M $MgCl_2$ were
added, and after the tubes had stood for 30' at room temperature they were
centrifuged for 5' at 3,000 x g. The supernatant was carefully aspirated, and
lipids were extracted from pellet and supernatant as described above.

Other analytical techniques. Lipoprotein electrophoresis was done on polyacrylamide gels with the "Quick Disc" lipoprotein kit from Canalco (Rockville,
Md, USA). Adenine nucleotide levels were determined by standard methods[30,31],
after quenching of hepatocyte incubations with $HClO_4$ and neutralization with
K_2CO_3. Sodium and potassium were measured with a flame photometer.

Materials. Pure porcine glucagon was a generous gift of Eli Lilly Co.
(Indianapolis, In, USA). Radioactive tracers were purchased from the Radio-
chemical Centre, Amersham, England, with the following specific activities:
^3H_2O as 45 mCi/mole; $[1-^{14}C]$-acetate as 58 mCi/mmole; $[2-^{14}C]$-mevalo-
nate as 25.5 mCi/mmole; $[1-^{14}C]$-oleate as 56 mCi/mmole. Scintillation counting was done in Insta-fluor[R] (Packard) in a Packard 2425 spectrometer. Collagenase was Type II from Worthington; fatty-acid-free bovine serum albumin was

from Sigma.

Rat serum was prepared freshly for each experiment from the blood of 3 rats
fed the regular chow. The blood was punctured from the aorta, allowed to clot
for 1 h at room temperature and 1 h at 4°C, and then centrifuged for 20' at
3,000 x g. The serum was collected and dialysed against 3 changes of 1 liter
150 mM NaCl, 10 mM Hepes, pH 7. 4. Preparation of albumin-oleate complexes was
done according to Spector and Hoak[32], yielding solutions of 5% (w/v) albumin
in KHHB with 3-4 mM oleate.

RESULTS AND DISCUSSION

Characterization of the hepatocyte preparation. The structural and metabolic integrity of the isolated hepatocytes has been verified in various
manners. Uptake of trypan blue is never observed by more than 15% of the freshly isolated cells. After 10' incubation of hepatocytes with ^3H_2O or ^3H-
inuline and centrifugation for 30 secs in a Beckman microfuge B, the inuline
(i.e. extracellular) space in the pellet is only 36 ± 3% of the water space. At
this moment the cells have intracellular sodium and potassium concentrations of
46 ± 5 and 161 ± 3 mEq/liter intracellular water, respectively (means ± SEM of
3 preparations), calculated from measured cation concentrations in the cell
pellet, and the proportions of intra- and extracellular water therein. Levels
of adenine nucleotides after 30' incubation in KHHB are 8.2 ± 0.5, 2.0 ± 0.4 and
0.9 ± 0.4 μmol/g dry weight for ATP, ADP and AMP respectively (mean ± SEM of 5
preparations). The initial glycogen content of the hepatocytes of rats fed the
normal chow is between 800 and 1200 μmoles glycogen-glucose/g dry weight.
During incubation in KHHB at 37°C this level decreases (and glucose appears) at
a rate of 100-200 μmole/g dry weight/h. The basal rate of glucose production
can be increased by glucagon; we consistently find stimulations of about 25% by
as little as 10^{-14} M glucagon (Kempen, to be published). When rats are fasted
overnight, before the day of cell isolation, their hepatocytes contain less
than 1 μmole glycogen-glucose/g dry weight. These fasted cells are able to synthesize glucose from 10 mM lactate and 1 mM pyruvate at rates of 100-150 μmoles
glucose/g dry weight/h.

Lipid content and release in media without serum. The amount of various
lipoprotein lipids in isolated rat hepatocytes and in their incubation medium
after 60' incubation in KHHB are given in Table 1. It can be seen that the
proportion of the various lipids in the medium is very different from that
within the cells. Triacylglycerols constitute the majority of the medium
lipids, but not of the cell lipids, indicating the secretory destination of

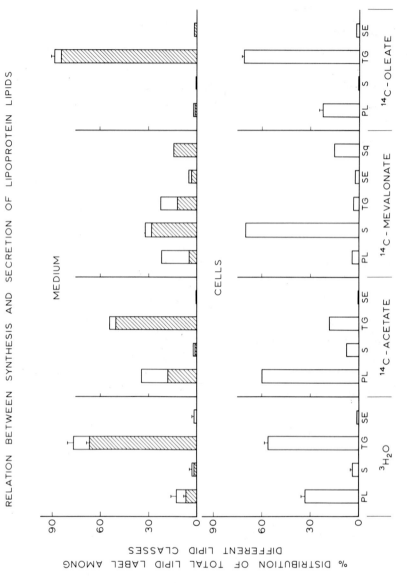

Fig. 1. Distribution of radioactivity among various lipid classes in cells (lower part) or medium (upper part) after 60' incubation of hepatocytes in KHHB. Data are given as percent of total lipid radioactivities, having the following values (in dpm/mg dry weight in cell- or medium-lipids respectively): with ^3H_2O: 262 ± 66, 32 ± 7; with ^{14}C-acetate: 1731, 172; with ^{14}C-mevalonate: 1506, 40; with ^{14}C-oleate: 13235 ± 1769, 3718 ± 1320.

at least a part of this lipid class in the cells.

TABLE 1

Lipid content of isolated rat hepatocytes and their medium after 60' incubation in KHHB containing 2% fatty acid-poor albumin. Data are means ± SEM of 4
experiments.

	Phospholipid	Triacylglycerol	Cholesterol	Cholesterolester
	(nanomoles per mg dry weight)			
In cells	106 ± 18	36.6 ± 12.2	14.0 ± 0.8	1.3 ± 0.1
In medium	3.4 ± 0.5	4.4 ± 0.9	1.0 ± 0.2	0.7 ± 0.3
(% in medium	2.9 ± 0.1	9.1 ± 1.7	7.0 ± 1.0	30.4 ± 6.6)

The data for the medium lipids are consistent with published results on
lipid release from the isolated perfused rat liver[5,14], although we find a
rather high phospholipid level in the medium. The latter is possibly caused
by the release of bile phospholipid in the incubation medium in our experiments.

In order to study the relation between lipid synthesis and secretion,
incubations were carried out in the presence of radioactive compounds, known
to label the lipoprotein lipids. Figure 1 shows the incorporation of radioactivity in the lipids of cells and medium, found after 60' incubation. In
Table 2 the amount of radio-activity in each lipid class in the medium is
given as percent of the total radioactivity in that lipid in cells plus
medium.

TABLE 2

Appearance of labeled lipids in the medium, expressed as percent of total
radioactivity in each lipid. Data are means ± SEM of the indicated number of
experiments.

Label-donor		Phospholipids	Triacylglycerol	Sterols	Sterolesters
^3H_2O	(n=4)	4.4 ± 1.0	14.1 ± 1.8	8.9 ± 2.9	21.1 ± 1.9
^{14}C-acetate*	(n=1)	4.4	19.9	2.2	13.1
^{14}C-mevalonate*	(n=3)			1.0 ± 0.3	4.7 ± 1.3
^{14}C-oleate*	(n=4)	2.3 ± 0.5	24.4 ± 3.9		17.7 ± 1.5

*added in tracer amounts.

The results give rise to the following comments.

1) The proportion of radioactivity in triacylglycerol to that in phospholipid is greater in the medium than in the cells. This is observed with ^3H_2O and ^{14}C-acetate (tracing the fate of newly synthesized fatty acid and of glyceride glycerol), as well as with ^{14}C-oleate (tracing the fate of exogenous fatty acid entering the liver from the blood). These findings confirm those of others, working with the isolated perfused rat liver[5,33] or with isolated rat liver cells[21]. Clearly, newly synthesized triacylglycerols remain in the cell for a shorter period than newly synthesized phospholipids or sterols.

2) With ^{14}C-mevalonate label is found predominantly in sterols and squalene. Radioactivity in phospholipid and triacylglycerol probably represents esterified farnesoic acid[34].

3) The percent labeled sterols in the medium is always lower than that of labeled sterolesters. At present it cannot be decided whether this is due to the higher rate of release of sterolesters than of free sterols from the cells (after esterification within the liver cells), or to the esterification of secreted free sterols by LCAT in the medium.

The question arises whether the lipids released in the medium represent lipoprotein lipids as they would have been secreted by the intact liver, or whether they normally are part of intracellular liver lipids, now released in the medium by cell desintegration. In the upper side of figure 1 the hatched part of the bars represents labeled lipid that is precipitated after addition of carrier serum, sodium phosphotungstate and $MgCl_2$. Treatment of human serum with phosphotungstate and $MgCl_2$ is known to result in the precipitation of apo-B containing lipoproteins (i.e. VLDL and LDL)[29]. As shown in figure 2 the same holds true for rat serum: the supernatant of the phosphotungstate-$MgCl_2$ treatment does not contain any visible VLDL and LDL on polyacrylamide gel electrophoresis (the stain at the interface of sample gel and stacking gel represents an excess of unused Sudan black). Figure 1 shows that the major parts of labeled triacylglycerol, sterols and sterolester are found in the precipitated fraction, suggesting their presence in VLDL or LDL particles. However, the possibility that these labeled lipids originally are not secreted as VLDL, but are absorbed on the (V)LDL of the carrier serum after the incubation, cannot be excluded. About half of the labeled phospholipid in the medium does not precipitate with phosphotungstate-$MgCl_2$; this part may represent HDL or bile phospholipid.

The probability that the labeled triacylglycerol is released in the medium by a secretory process (and not by cell desintegration) is further increased by the observation that its appearance in the medium is strongly inhibited by 20 μM colchicine (Table 3), a known inhibitor of microtubule-mediated processes. This

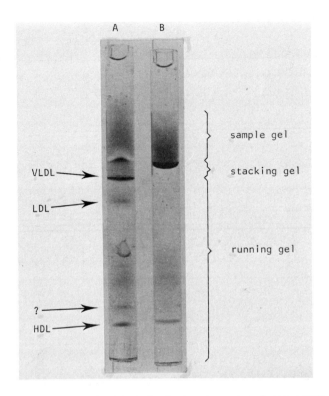

Fig. 2. Polyacrylamide gel electrophoresis of rat serum, before (A) or after (B) treatment with phosphotungstate and $MgCl_2$, as described in Materials and Methods.

finding has been reported earlier by others[21,23,35]. Colchicine has a smaller effect on the release of labeled phospholipid or sterolester (Table 3); the significance of this difference is as yet unclear.

TABLE 3

Effect of colchicine on incorporation of ^{14}C-oleate in lipids and their release into the medium. Hepatocytes (36.5 mg dry weight) are incubated in Krebs-Henseleit medium with 2% albumin and 5 µM ^{14}C-oleate ($1.6 \cdot 10^6$ dpm per incubation and with or without 20 µM colchicine.

	Phospholipids		Triacylglycerols		Sterolesters	
	Total dpm	% in medium	Total dpm	% in medium	Total dpm	% in medium
Control	151181	3.6	611424	34.0	10911	18.4
Colchicine	163062	3.1	615936	12.8	7088	13.0

The divergent fates of the different newly synthesized lipids may be visualized perhaps more clearly from the specific radioactivities of the lipids in cells or medium, as calculated from the data in Table 1 and Figure 1. In Table 4 the ratio is given between the specific activity in the medium and that in the cells for each lipid, as found with ^{14}C-mevalonate or ^{14}C-oleate.

TABLE 4

Specific activity in the medium, relative to the specific activity in the cells, for the various lipid classes after 60' incubation in KHHB.

	Phospholipids	Triacylglycerols	Sterols*	Sterolesters*
[14]C-mevalonate(2):	-	-	0.25 ± 0.12	0.40 ± 0.20
[14]C-oleate(3):	0.80 ± 0.34	4.2 ± 0.5	-	1.21 ± 0.37

*"specific activity" in these lipid classes is calculated as dpm in sterols or sterolesters per nanomol cholesterol or cholesterolester.

It may be concluded from the ^{14}C-mevalonate incorporation that the newly synthesized labeled cholesterol mixes slower with the pool of unlabeled cholesterol having a secretory destination, than with other intracellular cholesterol pools. After esterification with ^{14}C-oleate, the labeled phospholipids apparently can equilibrate to a greater extent with preexisting pools of phospholipid than the labeled triacylglycerols can do with preexisting triacylglycerol. The latter is consistent with the higher turnover of the "secretory" triacylglycerols than of those stored in the "lipid droplets", as described before[33].

Effects of addition of free fatty acid and of rat serum. Addition of oleate, complexed with albumin, in 0.5 to 1.0 mM concentration at the start of the incubation gives an increase in the triacylglycerol level in the cells, but not in the medium, after 60' incubation (Table 5). On the other hand, both the cellular level and the net release into the medium of triacylglycerol are elevated by addition of 40% (v/v) rat serum (Table 5). Addition of oleate lowers the percent release of radio-labeled triacylglycerol whereas with added rat serum an increase of this parameter is observed (Table 5; right column).

TABLE 5

Effect of oleate or rat serum on level and release of triacylglycerols in rat hepatocytes after 60' incubation.

	Level in cells	Net release in medium	% release of ^{3}H-TG (^{3}H$_2$O as label-donor)
			(in % of control)
Oleate (n=4)	126 ± 12*	92 ± 3*	63 ± 13*
Rat serum (n=5)	116 ± 5*	175 ± 38*	142 ± 18*

*significantly different from 100% (p < 0.05).

The lack of a stimulatory effect of added oleate on the release of unlabeled or tritiated triacylglycerol is surprising in view of the published data on fatty acid addition in the perfused rat liver[4,7,36]. Goh and Heimberg[36] find a highly significant increase in the output of triacylglycerol and cholesterol, and also an increased cholesterol synthesis, as compared to when oleate is not infused. They suggest that the latter effect is the result of the obligatory requirement of cholesterol for the secretion of triacylglycerols[36]. We have not observed an elevated ^{3}H-incorporation in sterols after incubation with oleate.

A lack of stimulation of lipid output by fatty acid has also been reported by others working with freshly isolated liver cells[21], although the effect seems to reappear when the hepatocytes are kept for 24 h in maintenance culture[37]. At present we have no explanation for the deviating behaviour of the isolated cells.

The increase in total triacylglycerol in cells and medium, found upon serum addition, is probably due to the fatty acids in the serum. The stimulated output of unlabeled or tritiated triacylglycerols in the presence of serum has earlier been noticed with the perfused rat liver[3,6]. The serum component responsible for this effect is not identified, but apparently resists dialysis. Possibly, the cholesterol and phospholipid, present in the serum and found to be taken up by the hepatocytes (results not shown), furnish the material for the packaging and export of the newly made triacylglycerols.

Effect of glucagon. The effect of 10^{-10} M glucagon on the synthesis and release of ^{3}H-labeled lipids during incubation with ^{3}H$_2$O is shown in Table 6. The incorporation of ^{3}H in phospholipids and triacylglycerols, but not in sterols, is significantly inhibited by the hormone; after saponification and extraction of the liberated fatty acids, the hormone effect is seen only in the fatty acid and not in the glyceride-glycerol moiety of these lipids. This indicates that glucagon inhibits the *de novo* synthesis of fatty acids, but not that of sterols, from endogenous precursors (mainly glycogen), in agreement wit published findings[38].

TABLE 6

Effect of glucagon (10^{-10} M) on synthesis and release of tritiated lipids during 60' incubation of rat hepatocytes in the presence of $^{3}H_{2}O$ (n=3).

	Phospholipids	Triacylglycerols	Sterols
		(in % of control)	
Incorporation of ^{3}H	84 ± 8*	83 ± 4*	111 ± 16
% release in medium	108 ± 14	92 ± 8	98 ± 10

*significantly lower than 100% ($p < 0.05$).

Glucagon (10^{-10} M) has no significant effects on the percent release of tritiated (Table 6) or unlabeled lipoprotein lipids from the hepatocytes. This is in contrast to the inhibitory effect of the hormone on the triacylglycerol output by the isolated rat liver perfused with added fatty acid[39]; however, free fatty acid was not added in our experiments with glucagon.

Further studies towards the combined effects of fatty acids, other serum components and hormones are in progress. Levels of apoproteins will be determined along with the lipids.

ACKNOWLEDGEMENTS

The author gratefully acknowledges the skilful technical assistance of Jan de Lange and Rens van Hevelingen, the helpful discussions with Louwrens Hessel, Jan Gevers Leuven and Louis Havekes, the technical advice of Coen van Gent, and the typing of the manuscript by Clara Horsting.

REFERENCES

1. Radding, C.M., Steinberg, D. (1960) J. Clin. Invest., 39, 1560-1569.
2. Haft, D.E., Roheim, P.S., White, A. and Eder, H.A. (1962) J. Clin.
    Invest., 41, 842-849.
3. Roheim, P.S., Miller, L. and Eder, H.A. (1965) J. Biol. Chem., 240, 2994-
    3001.
4. Heimberg, M., Weinstein, I., Dishmon, G. and Fried, M. (1965) Am. J.
    Physiol., 209, 1053-1060.
5. Windmüller, H.G. and Spaeth, A.E. (1966) J. Biol. Chem., 241, 2891-2899.
6. Windmüller, H.G. and Spaeth, A.E. (1967) Arch. Biochem. Biophys., 122,
    362-369.
7. Ruderman, N.B., Richards, K.C., Valles de Bourges, V. and Jones, A.L.
    (1968) J. Lipid Res., 9, 613-619.
8. Stein, O. and Stein, Y. (1967) J. Cell Biol., 33, 319-339.
9. Buckley, J.T., Delahuntey, T.J. and Rubinstein, D. (1968) Can. J.
    Biochem., 46, 341-349.
10. Marsh, J.B. (1971) in Plasma Lipoproteins, Smellie, R.M.S. ed.,
    Academic Press, New York, pp. 89-98.
11. Marsh, J.B. (1974) J. Lipid Res., 17, 85-90.
12. Glaumann, H., Bergstrand, A. and Ericsson, J.L.E. (1975) J. Cell Biol.,
    64, 356-377.
13. Nakaya, N., Chung, B.H. and Taunton, O.D. (1977) J. Biol. Chem.,
    252, 5258-5261.
14. Hamilton, R.L., Williams, M.C., Fielding, C.J. and Havel, R.J. (1976) J.
    Clin. Invest., 58, 667-680.
15. Mahley, R.W., Gray, M.E., Hamilton, R.L. and Lequire, V.S. (1968) J.
    Lab. Invest., 19, 358-369.
16. Wilcox, H.G., Woodside, W.F., Breen, K.J., Knapp, Jr. H.R. and
    Heimberg, M. (1974) Biochem. Biophys. Res. Commun., 58, 919-926.
17. Woodside, W.F. and Heimburg, M. (1976) J. Biol. Chem., 251, 13-23.
18. Chan, L., Jackson, R.L. and Means, A.R. (1977) Endocrinology, 100,
    1636-1643.
19. Tarlow, D., Watkins, P.A., Reed, R.E., Miller, R.S., Zwergel, E.E. and
    Lane, M.D. (1977) J. Cell Biol., 73, 332-353.
20. Eisenberg, S. (1975) Adv. Lipid Res., 13, 1-89.
21. Sundler, R., Åkesson, B. and Nilsson, Å. (1973) Biochem. Biophys. Res.
    Commun., 55, 961-968.

22. Jeejeebhoy, K.N., Ho, J., Breckenbridge, C., Bruce-Robertson, A., Steiner, G. and Jeejeebhoy, J. (1975) Biochem. Biophys. Res. Commun., 66, 1147-1153.

23. Gravela, E., Poli, G., Albano, E. and Dianzani, M.U. (1977) Exp. Molec. Pathol., 27, 339-352.

24. Seglen, P.O. (1976) Methods in Cellular Biol., 13, 29-83.

25. Bligh, E.G. and Dyer, W.J. (1959) Can. J. Biochem. Biophys., 37, 911-917

26. Giegel, J.L., Ham, A.B. and Clema, W. (1975) Clin. Chem., 21, 1575-1581.

27. Röschlau, R., Bernt, E. and Gruber, W. (1975) Z. Klin. Chim. Klin. Biochem., 12, 403-408.

28. Böttcher, C.J.F., Van Gent, C.M. and Pries, C. (1961) Anal. Chim. Acta, 24, 203-204.

29. Burstein, M. (1962) J. Physiol. (Paris), 54, 647-656.

30. Lamprecht, W. and Trautschold, I. (1970) in Methoden der enzymatische Analyse, Bergmeyer, H.U. ed., Chemie Verlag, Weinheim, pp. 2024-2033.

31. Jaworek, D., Gruber, W. and Bergmeyer, H.U. (1970) in Methoden der enzymatische Analyse, Bergmeyer, H.E. ed., Chemie Verlag, Weinheim, pp. 2051-2055.

32. Spector, A.A. and Hoak, J.C. (1969) Anal. Biochem., 32, 297-302.

33. Stein, Y. and Shapiro, B. (1959) Am. J. Physiol., 196, 1238-1241.

34. Christophe, J. and Popják, G. (1961) J. Lipid Res., 2, 244-257.

35. Le Marchand, Y., Singh, A., Assimacopoulos-Jeannet, F., Orci, L., Rouiller, C. and Jeanrenaud, B. (1973) J. Biol. Chem., 248, 6862-6870.

36. Goh, E.H. and Heimberg, M. (1973) Biochem. Biophys. Res. Commun., 55, 382-388.

37. Lamb, R.G., Wood, C.K., Landa, B.M., Guzelian, P.S. and Fallon, H.J. (1977) Biochim. Biophys. Acta, 489, 318-329.

38. Cook, G.A., Nielsen, R.C., Hawkins, R.A., Mehlman, M.A., Lakshmanan, M.R. and Veech, R.L. (1977) J. Biol. Chem., 252, 4421-4424.

39. Heimberg, M., Weinstein, J. and Kohout, M. (1969) J. Biol. Chem., 244, 5131-5139.

Lipoprotein Metabolism and Endocrine Regulation
L.W. Hessel and H.M.J. Krans editors
© ECSC, EEC, EAEC, Brussels-Luxembourg, 1979
Published by Elsevier/North-Holland Biomedical Press-Amsterdam

REGULATION OF HEPATIC FATTY ACID OXIDATION AND ESTERIFICATION

Guy P. MANNAERTS and Luc J. DEBEER

Laboratory of Pharmacology, School of Medicine, Katholieke Universiteit Leuven,

B-3000 Leuven, Belgium

I. *Hormonal regulation of free fatty acid partitioning between β-oxidation and triglyceride synthesis.*

Rates of hepatic fatty acid oxidation and esterification depend on two important factors : 1) fatty acid delivery to the liver and 2) the metabolic pattern of the liver itself. Both fatty acid delivery and the metabolic pattern of the liver are under nutritional and hormonal control.

Fatty acids are supplied to the liver via the plasma and their plasma levels are mainly determined by the rate of lipolysis in adipose tissue, which is increased in such conditions as starvation and uncontrolled diabetes. The main factor responsible for the increased lipolysis under these conditions appears to be insulin deficiency. Fatty acid uptake by the liver (and other organs) does not seem to be under hormonal control but depends on the plasma free fatty acid levels. Thus, in the intact organism, the starved and diabetic liver take up more fatty acids than the fed liver because of the elevated plasma levels. The fatty acids taken up by the liver are activated to their acyl-CoA esters and are used either for the synthesis of triglycerides, which will largely be reexported as part of very low density lipoprotein (VLDL) particles, or for the generation of energy during mitochondrial β-oxidation. The end product of mitochondrial β-oxidation, acetylCoA, is partly oxidized to CO_2 and H_2O in the Krebs cycle and partly converted to ketone bodies by the enzymes of the hydroxymethylglutarylCoA cycle. As the capacity of the Krebs cycle becomes rapidly saturated, the bulk of acetylCoA is converted to ketone bodies when rates of fatty acid oxidation are high. The pathways for triglyceride synthesis and β-oxidation are operative simultaneously, but the relative flux through each pathway is determined by the nutritional and hormonal state of the animal in such a way that there is a reciprocal relationship between rates of oxidation and esterification. Thus, for a given load of fatty acids the perfused liver of a fed animal will mainly esterify the incoming fatty acids and only a small portion will be oxidized. The converse is true for the perfused liver of a starved or a diabetic animal, which will preferentially oxidize the fatty acids[1]. The altered partitioning of the fatty acids between esterification and oxidation on transition from the fed to the starved state - and in diabetes as well - appears to be mediated primarily by excess of glucagon (see ref. 2 for review). The fact that only a small percentage of the incoming fatty acids is esterified by the starved or diabetic liver does not necessarily mean that the absolute amount is insignificant. *In vivo*, for example, the starved liver esterifies as much or even more than the fed liver, because the increased plasma free fatty acid levels are responsible for a highly increased fatty acid uptake[3]. Likewise, the increased rate of oxidation by the starved liver *in vivo* is the result of both the increased fatty acid supply and the preferential channeling of the fatty acids into the oxidation pathway.

Not only glucagon but also other hormones such as thyroid and sex hormones may influence fatty acid partitioning. Livers from hypothyroid rats display decreased rates of oxidation and increased rates of triglyceride synthesis, while livers from hyperthyroid rats show the opposite picture[4]. Livers from female rats oxidize less and esterify more than livers from male rats[5] and differences become even larger upon treatment of the female rats with ethynyl-estradiol[6]. Thus, as a rule, there exists a reciprocal relationship between esterification and oxidation. One notable exception is the liver from a clofibrate-treated rat. Despite a 3- to 4-fold increase in oxidation, this liver esterifies as much as the control liver[7].

II. Mechanisms that govern the partitioning of free fatty acids between β-oxidation and esterification.

Assuming that activation is not regulatory, partitioning between esterification and oxidation could theoretically be controlled at either the esterification arm, the oxidation arm or both. It has repeatedly been suggested that the main control point would lie at the esterification arm. Thus, the availability of α-glycerophosphate in the fed liver would drive esterification and thereby lower oxidation. However, McGarry and Foster could not find any negative correlation between oxidation rates and α-glycerophosphate levels, nor did they find lower α-glycerophosphate levels in starved than in fed livers[8]. It has also been proposed that the fate of the fatty acids might be determined mainly by adaptive changes in the amounts of glycerophosphate acyltransferase and carnitine palmitoyltransferase, the first enzymes specific for esterification and oxidation respectively. However, the hepatic capacity to synthetize triglycerides reflects the activity of phosphatidate phospho-hydrolase rather than that of glycerophosphate acyltransferase[9] and although an increase in the activity of carnitine palmitoyltransferase has been des-

cribed in homogenates from starved liver[10], we[3] and others[11] have been unable
to confirm these results. Mainly through the work of McGarry and Foster,
it has become increasingly clear that a major control point must lie at the
oxidation arm. These investigators provided strong evidence that on transition
from the fed to the starved state the activity - but not the amount - of the
carnitine palmitoyltransferase increases in the intact cell (but not in homogenates - see above) and that the increase in enzyme activity is responsible
for the observed increase in fatty acid oxidation (see ref. 2). In agreement
with this was the observation that livers from starved and diabetic rats had
elevated carnitine concentrations, which appear to drive the carnitine palmitoyltransferase I reaction[12]. More recently, malonylCoA, the first intermediate committed to fatty acid synthesis, was identified as another, and
likely the major determinant of the intracellular transferase activity. It
was found that malonylCoA potently suppresses fatty acid oxidation in homogenates through a specific inhibition of carnitine palmitoyltransferase
I[13,14]. The Ki of 1-2 μM is of the same order of magnitude as the intracellular malonylCoA levels. Subsequent work with isolated hepatocytes revealed a linear negative correlation between cellular malonylCoA content and
rates of fatty acid oxidation and showed that glucagon stimulates fatty acid
oxidation in hepatocytes from fed rats by lowering malonylCoA levels[15,16].
The hormone inhibits fatty acid synthesis most probably by interfering with
glycolysis at the level of pyruvate kinase and by interfering with fatty
acid synthesis itself at the level of acetylCoA carboxylase. Thus, it is
likely that in the fed state where fatty acid synthesis is brisk, malonyl-
CoA shuts off mitochondrial oxidation and thereby favors esterification.
In addition, the inhibitory levels of malonylCoA prevent the newly synthetized fatty acids from being oxidized. On transition from the fed to
the starved state glucagon excess likely causes a fall in malonylCoA levels
so that the inhibition of fatty acid oxidation is releaved. It is not known
yet whether the effects of the other hormones on fatty acid partitioning
are also mediated by changes in malonylCoA levels.

*III. Contribution of mitochondria and peroxisomes to overall fatty acid
oxidation in the liver.*

The mechanism described above for the reciprocal regulation of fatty acid
oxidation versus fatty acid synthesis and esterification was brought into
question by the discovery of Lazarow and de Duve[17] that not only mitochondria
but also liver peroxisomes are capable of oxidizing long chain acylCoA esters.
Like mitochondrial fatty acid oxidation, peroxisomal oxidation appears to

274

proceed via a mechanism of β-oxidation[18]. There are some interesting differences with mitochondria, however, such as the findings that the first
dehydrogenation step in peroxisomal oxidation involves the reduction of O_2
to H_2O_2, that peroxisomal oxidation is not inhibited by cyanide (since it
is not coupled to a phosphorylating system) and that peroxisomal fatty acid
oxidation may not be complete since only 5 acetylCoA equivalents were detected per equivalent palmitoylCoA oxidized[17,18]. It may also be mentioned
that the capacity of the peroxisomes to oxidize long chain fatty acids is
increased several-fold after treatment of rats with hypolipidemic compounds
such as clofibrate.

Mainly as a result of measurements of peroxisomal fatty acid oxidation
rates in purified subcellular fractions, it has been claimed that peroxisomal
oxidation may play an important role in overall hepatic fatty acid oxidation,
not only in the clofibrate-liver but in the normal liver as well, and the
role of the mitochondria has even been seriously questioned[18]. Obviously,
two important questions rose at this point. Firstly, what is the contribution
of each organelle to hepatic fatty acid oxidation and secondly, since in the
intact hepatocyte rates of fatty acid oxidation appear to correlate with
intracellular carnitine and especially malonylCoA levels, is peroxisomal
fatty acid oxidation also regulated by these compounds ? Recently, we made
an attempt to answer these questions for the normal and the clofibrate-liver.
Some of the experiments carried out with normal rat liver will be briefly
described below. A full account will be given elsewhere.

Using specific assay conditions we compared rates of mitochondrial and
peroxisomal fatty acid oxidation in whole liver homogenates. The specificity
of the assay conditions was established by comparing the subcellular distribution of fatty acid oxidation assayed under the appropriate conditions, with
the distribution patterns of mitochondrial and peroxisomal marker enzymes.
It was our purpose to keep the organelles as intact as possible. Consequent-
ly, gentle homogenizing procedures were used and fatty acid oxidation was
measured in isotonic media, in the absence of detergents and in the presence
of sufficient albumin to avoid detergent effects of the substrates.

In the intact cell free fatty acids and acylCoA esters are most likely
strongly bound to proteins and membranes so that their free concentrations
are kept low. Therefore, rates of mitochondrial and peroxisomal palmitoyl-
CoA oxidation were compared at low free substrate concentrations, obtained
by the addition of various amounts of albumin to the incubation mixtures
(Fig. 1). Mitochondrial oxidation rapidly increased with increasing substrate : albumin ratios and already reached a plateau at a ratio of 2.

At this substrate : albumin ratio a free palmitoylCoA concentration of .5 µM
was measured, indicating that mitochondrial oxidation was already saturated
at an extremely low free substrate concentration. Peroxisomal oxidation increased less rapidly and continued to rise at ratios where mitochondrial
oxidation was at its plateau, indicating that the affinity of the mitochondria for the substrate was markedly higher than the affinity of the peroxisomes. At all ratios tested peroxisomal oxidation was lower than mitochondrial except for the case where no albumin was present. Under these
conditions peroxisomal oxidation was maximal and roughly equal to mitochondrial oxidation at its plateau. Mitochondrial oxidation was severely
impaired in the absence of albumin, probably as a result of the detergent
effect of the substrate.

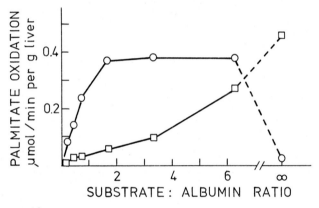

Fig. 1 : [1-^{14}C] palmitoylCoA oxidation in a whole liver homogenate versus
increasing substrate : albumin ratios. The palmitoylCoA concentration was
kept constant at 0.2 mM and various amounts of albumin were added to obtain
the ratios indicated. Oxidation rates represent the formation of acid soluble
labeled oxidation products and are expressed in terms of palmitate equivalents.
O-O : mitochondrial oxidation; □-□ : peroxisomal oxidation.

In a next series of experiments cofactor dependency was studied. Peroxisomal oxidation was Coenzyme A and NAD$^+$ dependent (in agreement with the
observations of Lazarow[17;18]), but was not stimulated by carnitine nor inhibited by inhibitors of carnitine palmitoyltransferase such as (+)-octanoyl-
carnitine or malonylCoA. These observations clearly established that a carnitine transfer step is not required for peroxisomal fatty acid oxidation.
As could be expected, mitochondrial oxidation was carnitine dependent and
strongly inhibited by (+)-octanoylcarnitine and malonylCoA.

Table 1 compares rates of peroxisomal palmitoylCoA oxidation in livers from fed rats and in livers from starved and diabetic animals which are characterized by increased rates of fatty acid oxidation. Starvation slightly increased peroxisomal fatty acid oxidation but the increase could be entirely accounted for by the shrinkage of the liver after 24 hours of starvation so that rates per total liver did not change. Alloxan-diabetic animals displayed slightly higher rates in the presence of albumin, but differences disappeared in the absence of albumin.

TABLE 1

PEROXISOMAL PALMITOYLCoA OXIDATION IN LIVER HOMOGENATES FROM FED, STARVED AND DIABETIC RATS

The substrate was 0.2 mM $[1-^{14}C]$ palmitoylCoA; oxidation rates represent the generation of acid soluble labeled oxidation products and are expressed as palmitate equivalents. Results are means $\pm$ S.E. of the number of experiments indicated in parentheses. $\bar{V}$ = palmitoylCoA : albumin ratio.

Animals	Peroxisomal oxidation $\bar{V} = 1.67$	Peroxisomal oxidation $\bar{V} = \infty$
	μmol per min per g liver	
Fed (12)	.090 $\pm$ .009	.644 $\pm$ .037
Starved (10)	.144 $\pm$ .008[*]	1.078 $\pm$ .039[*]
Alloxan-diabetic (6)	.138 $\pm$ .007[*]	.632 $\pm$ .051

[*]$P < .001$

Table 2 shows that 5 mM (+)-octanoylcarnitine, which selectively suppressed mitochondrial oxidation in homogenates, inhibited rates of oleate and palmitate oxidation in isolated intact hepatocytes by 87 % and 75 % respectively, suggesting that the bulk of fatty acid oxidation in the intact cell was carried out by the mitochondria. In line with these data was the observation that 2 mM KCN inhibited oleate and palmitate oxidation by approximately 80 %. The cyanide data must be interpreted with caution, however, since despite its cyanide-insensitivity peroxisomal oxidation might have been suppressed in an indirect way. One possibility would be that by lowering cellular ATP levels, cyanide might suppress fatty acid activation. The fact that esterification was not decreased by cyanide suggests, nevertheless, that glycolysis generated sufficient ATP to allow fatty acid activation. Since peroxisomal oxidation requires NAD^+, it might also be possible that cyanide would inhibit peroxisomal oxidation by reducing the cytosolic pyridine nucleotide pool.

This was apparently not the case since we found, quite unexpectedly, that lactate/pyruvate ratios were consistently higher in the absence of cyanide (24.5 + 6.1) than in its presence (12.6 + 2.2).

TABLE 2

EFFECT OF (+)-OCTANOYLCARNITINE AND CYANIDE ON FATTY ACID OXIDATION AND ESTERIFICATION IN HEPATOCYTES ISOLATED FROM FED RATS

The cells were preincubated for 15 min in Krebs-Henseleit bicarbonate buffer containing 2.3 % defatted albumin and incubated for another 15 min in the presence of 1 mM [1-^{14}C] oleate or 1 mM [1-^{14}C] palmitate. (+)-octanoyl-carnitine [(+)-OC] was present during the preincubation period; KCN was added together with the fatty acids. Results are expressed in terms of fatty acid equivalents (mean + S.E.). The term "Esterified Products" represents the sum of fatty acid equivalents incorporated in triglycerides plus phospholipids.

Additions	Acid soluble oxidation products		Esterified Products
	palmitate (n = 2)	oleate (n = 3)	oleate (n = 3)
	μmol fatty acid/10^8 cells per 15 min		
none	3.90	2.02 + .31	2.39 + .16
5 mM (+)-OC	.97	.27 + .06	-
2 mM KCN	.98	.39 + .09	2.89 + .09

Taken together our experiments strongly suggest that in the normal liver the bulk of fatty acid oxidation is mitochondrial. Our conclusion is based on the following lines of evidence. 1) On transition from the fed to the starved state the capacity of the liver to oxidize long chain fatty acids appears to be regulated by the cellular levels of carnitine and especially of malonylCoA. Neither carnitine nor malonylCoA affect peroxisomal oxidation. 2) The activity of the peroxisomal fatty acid oxidation pathway is unchanged in starvation and diabetes, although both conditions are characterized by an increased capacity of the liver to oxidize long chain fatty acids. 3) At low free substrate concentrations, a situation which most likely mimics that in the intact cell, mitochondrial oxidation is several-fold higher than peroxisomal oxidation. 4) The potent inhibition of fatty acid oxidation by cyanide and especially by (+)-octanoylcarnitine provides additional evidence that fatty acid oxidation is mainly mitochondrial.

The function of peroxisomal fatty acid oxidation remains unclear. Because of its lower substrate affinity peroxisomal oxidation might become important whenever - and for whatever reason - long chain fatty acylCoA would accumulate in the cell. Indeed, elevated concentrations of long chain acylCoA esters might suppress their own oxidation by the mitochondria either by inhibiting the adenine nucleotide translocator[19] or by inhibiting the carnitine palmitoyltransferase reaction[20].

REFERENCES

1. Mayes, P.A. and Felts, J.M. (1967) *Nature* (London), 215, 716-718.

2. McGarry, J.D. and Foster, D.W. (1976) *Am. J. Med.*, 61, 9-13.

3. Debeer, L.J., Thomas, J. and Mannaerts, G.P. Unpublished observations.

4. Heimberg, M. (1978) *Communication, 8th Linderstrøm-Lang Conference,* Tønsberg, Norway, June 28-30.

5. Soler-Argilaga, C. and Heimberg, M. (1976) *J. Lipid Res.*, 17, 605-615.

6. Weinstein, I., Soler-Argilaga, C. and Heimberg, M. (1977) *Biochem. Pharmacol.*, 26, 77-80.

7. Mannaerts, G.P., Thomas, J., Debeer, L.J., McGarry, J.D. and Foster, D.W. (1978) *Biochim. Biophys. Acta*, 259, 201-211.

8. McGarry, J.D. and Foster, D.W. (1971) *J. Biol. Chem.*, 246, 6247-6253.

9. Brindley, D.N. (1978) in *Regulation of Fatty Acid and Glycerolipid Metabolism*, Dils, R. and Knudsen, J. eds., Pergamon Press, Oxford, pp. 31-40.

10. Aas, M. and Daae, L.N.W. (1971) *Biochim. Biophys. Acta*, 239, 208-216.

11. DiMarco, J.P. and Hoppel, C. (1975) *J. Clin. Invest.*, 55, 1237-1244.

12. McGarry, J.D., Robles-Valdes, C. and Foster, D.W. (1975) *Proc. Natl. Acad. Sci. U.S.A.*, 72, 4385-4388.

13. McGarry, J.D., Mannaerts, G.P. and Foster, D.W. (1977) *J. Clin. Invest.*, 60, 265-270.

14. McGarry, J.D., Leatherman, G.F. and Foster, D.W. (1978) *J. Biol. Chem.*, 253, 4128-4136.

15. Cook, G.A., King, M.T. and Veech, R.L. (1978) *J. Biol. Chem.*, 253, 2529-2531.

16. McGarry, J.D. (1978) *Communication, 8th Linderstrøm-Lang Conference,* Tønsberg, Norway, June 28-30.

17. Lazarow, P.B. and de Duve, C. (1976) *Proc. Natl. Acad. Sci. U.S.A.*, 73, 2043-2046.

18. Lazarow, P.B. (1978) *J. Biol. Chem.*, 253, 1522-1528.

19. Shug, A., Lerner, E., Elson, C. and Shrago, E. (1971) *Biochem. Biophys. Res. Commun.*, 43, 557-563.

20. Bremer, J. and Norum, K.R. (1967) *J. Biol. Chem.*, 242, 1744-1748.

Lipoprotein Metabolism and Endocrine Regulation
L.W. Hessel and H.M.J. Krans editors
© ECSC, EEC, EAEC, Brussels-Luxembourg, 1979
Published by Elsevier/North-Holland Biomedical Press-Amsterdam

MECHANISM OF ACTION AND BIOLOGICAL SIGNIFICANCE OF PROSTAGLANDIN
E_2 AND PROSTACYCLIN IN THE LIVER

V.TOMASI, G.BARTOLINI, M.ORLANDI, C.MERINGOLO, O.BARNABEI

Laboratory of General Physiology, University of Bologna, 40126
Bologna (Italy)

INTRODUCTION

The surprisingly few studies dedicated to the role and mechanism
of action of prostaglandins in the liver, may be due to two reasons
a) on the basis of the pioneeristic studies of the Karolinska group
the liver,as well as the lung, were considered mainly as involved
in prostaglandin catabolism[1]; b) until recently,it has been difficult to demonstrate clear cut and reproducible effects of prostaglandins on liver function or metabolism.

In this article we summarize the available evidence indicating
that prostaglandin E_2 (PGE_2) and the newly discovered prostacyclin
(PGI_2), produced by distinct liver cell populations, play an important role in the control of liver functions.

BIOSYNTHESIS OF PGE_2 AND PGI_2 IN RAT LIVER

The first observation that the liver was capable of producing
prostaglandins is due to Dawson and Ramwell (see ref.2) who detected substantial amounts of prostaglandin E and F in liver perfusa-
tes. This observation has recently been confirmed by Carlson et al.
who also found that hypoxia was a potent stimulus for PGE formation
assayed by radioimmunoassay[3]. MacManus and Whitfield[4] reported the
production of PGE and $PGF_{2\alpha}$ in the whole organ and in liver homogenates incubated with arachidonate. Their data are in agreement
with those of Cohen and Jaffe[5] and Pace-Asciak and Rangaraj[6] who
detected PGE_2 produced in liver homogenates by mass spectrometry.

All of these data were obtained using the whole liver, which is
known to be an heterogeneous tissue composed by at least three
types of cells. PGE biosynthesis was investigated by using more
homogeneous cell populations: parenchymal cells (PC) and nonparenchymal cells (NPC) constituted by about 70% endothelial and 25%
Kupffer cells. These two populations were obtained by perfusing
rat liver with collagenase as described by Berry and Friend[7],
followed by density gradient centrifugation[8].

It was observed that both PC and NPC converted labeled arachidonate into PGE_2 and $PGF_{2\alpha}$; on a mg protein basis NPC were at
least 5-fold more active than PC. Quantitative analysis by radioimmunoassay, revealed that PC in presence of arachidonate produced
175 pg and NPC 1200 pg PGE / mg protein[9]. The higher amount of PGE
produced, the differences in the kinetic and in the effect of the
substrate concentration between PC and NPC, coupled with the

reports that endothelial cells of blood vessels produced a novel prostaglandin called prostacyclin[10], having PGE_1-like effects, prompted us to re-investigate the type of prostaglandins produced by the liver.

The best way to discriminate between PGE_2 and PGI_2 seems to use the platelet aggregation test, since PGE_2 is pro-aggregatory while PGI_2 is a potent inhibitor of aggregation[10]. We observed that while addition of a suspension of PC had little or no effect on arachidonate-induced aggregation, addition of as low as 13.5 μg of NPC suspension inhibited by 30% aggregation and 47.5 μg protein were completely inhibitory[11]. By using synthetic PGI_2 as standard we calculated that NPC produced 18.9 $\pm$ 4.6 ng per mg protein (mean $\pm$ s.e.m.,n=5), a figure which is in accordance with that reported by the Vane's group for blood vessels[12]. Thus, it appears that while PC produce mainly PGE_2 the major prostaglandin synthesized in NPC is PGI_2[11].

That rat liver endothelial cells do synthesize PGI_2, was confirmed by isolation of 6-keto-$PGF_{1\alpha}$ by thin layer chromatography of extracts of endothelial cells incubated with labeled arachidonic acid (Fig. 1). Although endothelial cells synthesize also PGE_2 and $PGF_{2\alpha}$, PGI_2 was found to be the major product of arachidonate metabolism. Tranylcypromine, an inhibitor of PGI_2 synthetase, reduced considerably the conversion of arachidonate into PGI_2[13]. Since endothelial cells constitute only 2.8% of the liver volume[6], it is not surprising that Pace-Asciak and Rangaraj[13] failed to detect the formation of 6-keto-$PGF_{1\alpha}$ in a total liver homogenate.

THE ROLE OF PROSTAGLANDINS IN THE LIVER

As stated in the introduction it has been difficult to demonstrate reproducible effects of PGE on liver metabolism. In 1972 Curnow and Nuttal[14], reported that PGE_1 administered intravenously to rats, decreased liver glycogen synthetase and increased phosphorylase activity, an action which is typical of hormones which act by increasing cyclic AMP levels. However, Exton et al.[15] were unable to observe a modification of cyclic AMP after a 30 min liver perfusion with PGE_1, a finding which was later confirmed by Levine[16].

On the other hand, in 1973 two groups reported that PGE_1 was capable of stimulating adenylate cyclase activity of particulate liver fractions[17,18], a finding which was confirmed using isolated rat liver plasma membranes[19]. In addition it was demonstrated that PGE_1 acted upon an adenylate cyclase-coupled receptor distinct from that for glucagon and epinephrine[19,20].Several lines of evidence indicated that PGE receptor was located on the outer side of liver cell plasma membrane and that PGE did not need to enter the cell in order to activate adenylate cyclase[20].

Zenzer et al.[21] observed that although PGE_1 stimulated adenylate cyclase of particulate fractions 4-fold, very high doses of PGE_1 (40 μg) administered to intact rats increased cyclic AMP only 2-fold,which compares with the 20-fold increase due to glucagon.

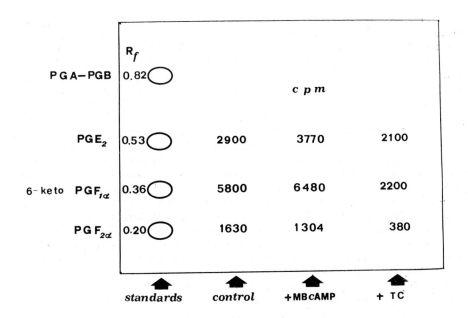

Fig. 1. Chromatographic identification of 6-Keto-PGF$_{1\alpha}$ in liver
endothelial cells. Aliquots (1.1-1.9 mg protein) of endothelial
cell homogenates in Krebs-Ringer containing 20 mM EDTA were incubated for 10 min at 37°C with 0.5-1.0 µCi ^{3}H-arachidonic acid (135Ci/m
mol) and 10 µg sodium arachidonate, in a final volume of 1 ml. At the
end of incubations the pH was adjusted to 3.5, samples were centrifuged at 2000 x g and the supernatants were extracted twice with 5
vol. of ethylacetate. The solvent was taken to dryness and the residue taken up with 0.2 ml CHCl$_3$-CH$_3$OH (1:1), 0.1 ml of a solution
containing 6-keto-PGF$_{1\alpha}$,PGF$_{2\alpha}$,PGE$_2$ and PGA$_2$ (20 µg each) was added and 0.15 ml was applied to silicic acid plates .Elution was car-
ried out first with ethylacetate-acetic acid-isoctane-water (9:2:5:
10, upper phase). After drying, a second run was carried out with
CHCl$_3$-CH$_3$OH-CH$_3$COOH-H$_2$O (90:9:1:0.65). The spots visualized with
I$_2$ vapors, were scraped off and counted with 4 ml Picofluor (Packard
Tranylcypromine (TC) was 0.5 mg/ml; monobutyrryl-cyclic AMP was 2
mM. Data are means of 3 experiments.

For the preparation of endothelial cells see ref. 11.

Blanks (boiled homogenate), 25% of experimental values, were
subtracted from the data shown.

Similar results were observed in the perfused liver. They speculated that PGE_1 could have acted on a subpopulation of liver cells[21]. However, in a successive paper De Rubertis et al.[22] re-examined the role of PGE in the liver. Since they found that PGE_1 or PGE_2 inhibited the stimulatory effect of glucagon on cyclic AMP levels in the perfused rat liver, they concluded that the main role of PGE was to antagonise glucagon effects. These papers generated much confusion and a comment is important. Our data[19,20] are rather similar to the ones reported by De Rubertis group except that we failed to observe an inhibition of glucagon effect by PGE. Since both De Rubertis group and our data clearly show that in liver fractions PGE_1 does not inhibit glucagon effect, it is important to find an explanation to this discrepancy. The most likely explanation is that, being PGE potent vasoconstrictor agents in the rat[25], they reduce the blood flow in the hepatic circulation, thus greatly depressing not only the rate of hormone (glucagon) entry into the sinusoids but also the metabolic activity of hepatocytes.

Other discrepancies were explained where we demonstrated that PGE_1 or PGE_2 acted not on the major population of parenchymal liver cells, but on the minor population of nonparenchymal cells present in standard liver cell preparations. When nonparenchymal cells were separated from parenchymal cells by Ficoll density gradient centrifugation, we observed that PGE_1 or PGE_2 were capable of increasing cyclic AMP 20-fold. Glucagon acted mainly on parenchymal cells increasing cyclic AMP 15-fold[8]. Why in liver membranes a response to PGE_1 greater than that observed using perfused liver or standard hepatocytes can be shown? We believe that the reason is that during the preparation of liver membranes for some reason an enrichment is occurring of plasma membranes derived from nonparenchymal cells. As a matter of fact Blouin et al.[13] have shown that although nonparenchymal cells constitute only 5% of the liver mass, their plasma membranes account for at least 25% of total liver plasma membranes. It is our feeling that homogenising the liver with hypotonic media containing Ca^{2+} -as in the case of Ray's method[26] - further increases the yield of nonparenchymal cell plasma membrane.

Wincek et al.[27] reported that PGE_1 stimulated adenylate cyclase activity of nonparenchymal cell membranes although much less than we would have expected on the basis of the PGE_1 effect on cyclic AMP levels[8]. A likely explanation is that their method of liver cell preparation (employing colloidal iron) depresses the metabolic activity of cells. As a matter of fact Sweat and Yamashita[28] recently reported that glucagon increases cyclic AMP levels of hepatocytes only two fold, which compares with the 10-20-fold increase found by many authors (see ref. 20). Moreover they observed a 6-fold stimulation of adenylate cyclase of nonparenchymal cells by glucagon, which can only be explained on the basis of a very large contamination by parenchymal cells, and it is in contrast with their previous data[27].

The hypothesis was put forward that PGE_2 produced in parenchymal cells acts -as an intercellular messenger- on nonparenchymal cells.[20] The demonstration that PGE_2 is produced in parenchymal cells is in agreement with this hypothesis[9]. What is the possible meaning of this control of parenchymal cells over nonparenchymal cells? We believe, although only indirect evidence is so far available, that PGE_2 acts on endothelial rather than on Kupffer cells[27]. Since endothelial cells produce PGI_2 which acts on platelets inhibiting aggregation and on the vascular wall producing relaxation[10], there was the possibility that PGE_2 could control PGI_2 biosynthesis and therefore these two important processes. We have obtained some evidence that PGE_2 by increasing cyclic AMP levels in endothelial cells, inhibits PGI_2 biosynthesis[21] and this may influence both platelet aggregation[10] and the tone of hepatic vasculature. While in humans both these actions have been demonstrated[10] it appears that in the rat PGI_2 is important especially for the control of vascular tone. As a matter of fact we have been unable to demonstrate an inhibitory effect of PGI_2 on arachidonate-induced platelets aggregation[29]. On the other hand, PGI_2 has been shown to antagonize ADP-induced rat platelet aggregation.[10]

CONCLUSIONS

In the Figure 2 the biological role of prostaglandins in the liver is summarized.

Stimuli activating liver plasma membrane or lysosomal phospholipase A_2 of parenchymal cells[30] would result in the release of arachidonate from phospholipids, triggering PGE_2 biosynthesis. The nature of such stimuli is not clear, but hypoxia has been shown to be a potent effector[3]; on the other hand we have been unable to confirm that glucagon increases liver prostaglandins biosynthesis[2]. More work is certainly needed to identify other possible regulators of phospholipase A_2.

It is suggested[2] that once produced, PGE_2 diffuses out of parenchymal cell interacting with an adenylate cyclase coupled receptor of contiguous endothelial cells lining liver sinusoids[31]. We have shown that the receptor is on the outer side of the plasma membrane and that, as several other hormonal receptors, requires GTP[20]. One of the effects of cyclic AMP increase in endothelial cells is an inhibition of PGI_2 biosynthesis. It is not clear whether cyclic AMP acts by inhibiting phospholipase A_2 or arachidonate utilization by cyclo-oxygenase. We believe the first possibility to be more likely. We have found that MBcyclicAMP inhibits PGE biosynthesis in endothelial cell only when endogenous prostaglandin synthesis is evaluated. When arachidonate evoked biosynthesis was measured no effect of MBcyclicAMP was observed[32]. Moreover, the addition of MBcyclicAMP to endothelial cell homogenates incubated with labeled arachidonate, failed to modify the extent of conversion to 6-keto-$PGF_{1\alpha}$ (unpublished data). This is in accordance with data indica-

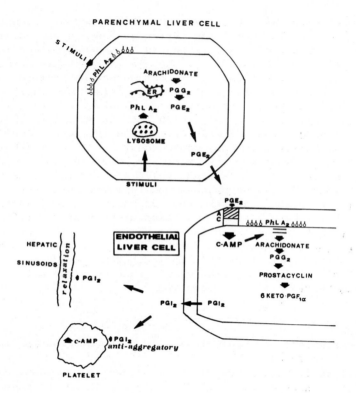

Fig. 2. Proposed role of PGE_2 and PGI_2 in the liver. Stimuli of unknown nature activate plasma membrane or lysosomal phospholipase A_2
($PhLA_2$) thus increasing the availability of arachidonate to endo-
plasmic reticulum (E.R.) cyclo-oxygenase. In the parenchymal liver
cell the major prostaglandin produced is PGE_2 (see Ref.9). Once produced, PGE_2 diffuses out and interacts with an adenylate cyclase-
coupled receptor located on endothelial cell plasma membrane. It is
suggested that cyclic AMP inhibits endothelial cell phospholipase
A_2, thus decreasing the biosynthesis of PGI_2, the major prostaglandin formed in these cells (see Figure 1).
    Since the role of PGI_2 is to relax blood vessels and to inhibit
platelet aggregation[10], the amount of PGE_2 produced by the parenchymal cell may indirectly affect PGI_2 action on hepatic vasculature
and circulating platelets. In the rat liver it is likely that the
most important action of PGI_2 is exerted on blood vessels, since it
has been observed that PGI_2 is unable to counteract platelet aggregation induced by arachidonic acid[29].

ting that cyclic AMP inhibits platelet prostaglandin biosynthesis by limiting the availability of arachidonate to cyclo-oxigenase[33,34]. These data do not agree with the observation that cyclic AMP directly inhibits cyclo-oxygenase of platelets[35].

Thus, PGE_2 by decreasing prostacyclin production in endothelial cells, would tend to diminish the vasodilator action of PGI_2, favoring instead vasoconstriction by thromboxane A_2[10]. In this way a stimulus like hypoxia[3] may increase the rate of liver circulation.

It will be of interest to ascertain whether or not prostaglandins are involved in similar mechanism in other organs. A role of PGE_2 as intercellular messenger has been suggested in the superior cervical ganglion[36,37].

AKNOWLEDGEMENTS

The original work reported here was supported by grants from the Consiglio Nazionale delle Ricerche (Rome). We thank Dr.J.Pike (Upjohn, USA) for generous gifts of prostaglandins.

REFERENCES

1. Samuelsson,B.,Granstrom,E.,Green,K.,Hamberg,M. and Hammarstrom, S. (1975) Annu.Rev.Biochem., 44,669-695.

2. Ramwell,P.W. and Shaw,J.E. (1970) Rec.Prog.Horm.Res.,26,139-173.

3. Carlson,R.P.,Flynn,J.T. and Lefer,A.M. (1977) Biochem.Pharmacol. 26,1463-1468.

4. MacManus,J.P. and Whitfield,J.F. (1974) Prostaglandins, 6,475-487.

5. Cohen, F. and Jaffe, B.M. (1973) Biochem. Biophys. Res. Commun., 55, 724-728.

6. Pace-Asciak, C.R. and Rangaraj, G. (1977) Biochim. Biophys. Acta, 486, 579-582.

7. Berry, M.M. and Friend, D.S. (1969) J. Cell. Biol., 43, 507-520.

8. Ferretti, E., Biondi, C. and Tomasi, V. (1976) FEBS Lett., 69, 70-74.

9. Bartolini, G., Meringolo, C., Orlandi, M. and Tomasi, V. Biochim. Biophys. Acta (in the press).

10. Moncada, S. and Vane, J.R. (1978) Br. Med. Bul., 34, 129-135.

11. Tomasi, V., Meringolo, C., Bartolini, G. and Orlandi, M. (1978) Nature, 273, 670-671.

12. Bunting, S., Gryglewski, R., Moncada, S. and Vane, J.R. (1976) Prostaglandins, 12, 897-913.

286

13. Blouin, A., Bolender, R.P. and Weibel, E.R. (1977) J. Cell. Biol., 72, 441-455.

14. Curnow, R.T. and Nuttall, F.Q. (1972) J. Biol. Chem., 247, 1892-1898.

15. Exton, J.H., Robinson, G.A., Sutherland, E.W. and Park, C.R. (1971) J. Biol. Chem., 246, 6166-6177.

16. Levine, R.A. (1974) Prostaglandins, 6, 509-521.

17. Kreiner, P.W., Keirns, J.J. and Bitensky, M.W. (1973) Proc. Natl. Acad. Sci. U.S., 70, 1785-1789.

18. Sweat, S.W. and Wincek, T.J. (1973) Biochem. Biophys. Res. Commun., 55, 522-529.

19. Tomasi,V. and Ferretti, E. (1975) Mol. Cell. Endocrinol., 2, 221-232.

20. Tomasi, V. (1976) Exptl. Cell Biol., 44, 260-277.

21. Zenzer, T.V., DeRubertis, S.R. and Curnow, R.T. (1974) Endocrinol., 94, 1404-1410.

22. DeRubertis, S.R., Zenzer,T.V. and Curnow, R.T. (1974) Endocrinol., 95, 93-101.

23. Tomasi, V., Poli, A., Ferretti, E. and Barnabei, O. (1975) Adv. Enzyme Regul., 13, 189-200.

24. Barnabei, O., Poli, A., Ferretti, E. and Tomasi,V. (1976) in Use of Isolated Liver Cells and Kidney Tubules in Metabolic Studies, Tager, J.M., Soling, H.B. and Williamson, J.R. eds., North-Holland, Amsterdam, pp. 422-425.

25. Malik, K.U. and McGiff, J.C. (1975) Circulation Res., 36, 599-609.

26. Ray, T.K. (1970) Biochim. Biophys. Acta, 196, 1-9.

27. Wincek, T.J., Hupka, A.L. and Sweat, F.W. (1975) J. Biol. Chem. 250, 8863-8873.

28. Sweat, F.W. and Yamashita, L. (1978) Biochem. Biophys. Res. Commun., 82, 879-886.

29. Meringolo, C. et al., submitted for publication.

30. Waite, M., Griffin, H.D. and Franson, R. (1976) in Lysosomes in Biology and Pathology, Dingle, J.T. and Dean, R.T. eds., North-Holland, Amsterdam, pp. 257-286.

31. Wisse, E. (1972) J. Ultrastruct. Res., 38, 528-562.

32. Bartolini, G. et al., in preparation.

33. Lapetina, E.G., Schmitges, C.J., Chandrabose, K. and Cuatrecasas, P. (1977) Biochem.Biophys.Res.Commun.,76, 828-835.

34. Hinkes, M., Stanford, N., Shi, M.M.Y., Roth, G.J., Raz, A., Needleman, P. and Majerus, P.N. (1977) J. Clin. Invest., 59, 449-454.

35. Malmsten, C., Granstrom, E. and Samuelsson, B. (1976) Biochem. Biophys. Res. Commun., 68, 569-576.

36. Tomasi, V., Biondi, C., Trevisani, A., Martini, M. and Perri, V. (1977) J.Neurochem., 28, 1289-1297.

37. Tomasi, V., Trevisani, A., Biondi, C., Capuzzo, A. and Perri, V. (1977) Biochem. Soc. Transact., 5, 520-523.

Lipoprotein Metabolism and Endocrine Regulation
L.W. Hessel and H.M.J. Krans editors
© ECSC, EEC, EAEC, Brussels-Luxembourg, 1979
Published by Elsevier/North-Holland Biomedical Press-Amsterdam

ON THE REGULATION OF TRIGLYCERIDE HYDROLYSIS IN HEART

W.C. HÜLSMANN AND H. STAM

Department of Biochemistry I, Medical Faculty, Erasmus University Rotterdam,
P.O.Box 1738, 3000 DR Rotterdam (The Netherlands)

ABSTRACT

The effects of insulin, glucagon and glucocorticoids on myocardial lipoprotein lipase activity are briefly discussed. The bulk of the enzyme may be
rapidly removed from the heart by heparin perfusion. It is probably mainly
localized at the endothelial surface of capillaries and is involved in the
uptake of plasma triglycerides, as described in the literature.

Another triglyceride hydrolyzing enzyme in heart is probably localized in
lysosomes or autophagosomes. After erucic acid feeding large lipid droplets
in the heart can be seen, as described earlier by a number of investigators.
Electronmicroscopy, after histochemical staining for acid phosphatase,
reveals (Fig. 1) these droplets, surrounded by reaction product. Differential
centrifugation of a heart homogenate allows the isolation of an acid
phosphatase, acid lipase and triglyceride enriched fraction, by sedimentation
between (10 min) 3000 and 30 000 x g. Electronmicroscopy reveals particles,
probably filled with lipid, and surrounded by unit membranes (Fig. 2).

Lipolysis of endogenous fat, increased by erucate feeding (Fig. 3), is
stimulated by glucagon and norepinephrine, whereas it is inhibited by
insulin (Fig. 3). Pretreatment of rats with metapyrone prior to *in vitro*
perfusion of the hearts, abolishes hormone-sensitive lipolysis. Dexamethasone
pretreatment restores hormone-stimulated lipolysis (Fig. 4), suggesting a
permissive action of glucocorticoids on the lipolysis of endogenous fat, as
was described earlier for adipose tissue by others. Therefore, a number of
arguments may be presented in favour of the similarity of triglyceride
hydrolysis in heart and adipose tissue.

INTRODUCTION

Triglyceride hydrolyzing enzymes have been described in heart. One,
involved in the uptake of plasma triglycerides from chylomicrons and very low
density lipoproteins (VLDL). It is probably mainly localized at the endothelial
lining of capillaries and is called lipoprotein lipase (LPL). A number of
investigators have reported that part of this enzyme may be rapidly removed

from the heart by vascular perfusion with heparin (compare ref. 1). Another enzyme, involved in the mobilization of stored triglycerides, is probably localized in lysosomes[1,2], autophagosomes or vacuomes[3]. It will be called tissue lipase.

The activity of the lipoprotein lipase of heart changes with the nutritional state. During fasting the activity is higher than in the carbohydrate fed state[4-9]. In agreement with its function is the observation[7] that in the fasted state, the utilization of chylomicron triglycerides by the heart is higher than after carbohydrate-feeding. This led Borensztajn et al.[8] to investigate the role of glucagon, since in starvation the serum glucagon/insulin concentration ratio has increased. They found that the administration of glucagon to fed rats increased LPL activity of heart. Also fat-feeding to rats results in a high LPL activity[10-12]. Lard-feeding results in increased plasma glucagon levels and glucagon/insulin ratios[11]. Therefore glucagon could again be responsible for the increased myocardial LPL activity. Other hormones that could be responsible for the increased activity are adrenal glucocorticoids. We have shown that a fat diet, containing erucic acid, increases plasma corticosterone levels in the rat, particularly after stress[13]. Fat-feeding in general results in the increase of adrenal weight (comp. ref. 12). De Gasquet et al.[9] have shown that two hours after the injection of glucocorticoid in fed rats the myocardial LPL activity had significantly increased. Their experiments suggest that the effects of glucagon and glucocorticoid may be additive. Since glucocorticoids increase both insulin and glucagon levels, a definite answer whether both glucagon and glucocorticoid are responsible for LPL increase during fasting, requires further experimentation. These hormone effects on LPL are relatively slow and probably involve the regulation of synthesis and transport of LPL.

Fast hormone effects can be observed on myocardial tissue lipase. In hearts, catecholamine-stimulated lipolysis has been known for many years[14-16]. We have recently shown[1] that both in the basal and in the catecholamine-stimulated states the rate of lipolysis in rat heart has strongly increased when the heart contains many large fat droplets, after feeding rapeseed oil to the animals for 3 days. Since lipolysis is inhibited by the lysosomal inhibitor chloroquine we assume that lipolysis in heart (and probably also in other organs, like liver and adipose tissue) is of lysosomal or autophagosomal origin[1]. It can be seen from Fig. 1 that electronmicroscopy of fat infiltrated rat hearts, after glutaraldehyde fixation and incubation for the demonstration of acid phosphatase activity, reveals fat filled spheres, surrounded by reaction product.

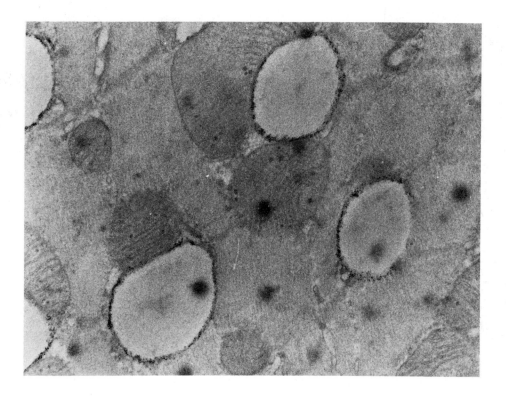

Fig. 1. Electronmicrograph of a piece of heart from a rat fed 40 cal% rapeseed oil for 3 days. Fixation in 4% glutaraldehyde in 0.067 M cacodylate buffer (pH 7.2) for 30 min at 0°C, prior to incubation for "acid" phosphatase according to Novikoff[17] with cytidine monophosphate at pH 5.0. Courtesy of Dr. J.M. van Dongen and Mr. W.J. Visser (department of Cellbiology and Histology I, Erasmus University Rotterdam).

On differential centrifugation of homogenates of the hearts of these rapeseed oil fed animals, a triglyceride and acid phosphatase and lipase enriched fraction could be isolated. Electronmicroscopy of this fraction shows unit membrane bound vesicles (Fig. 2), from which most of the fat may have had escaped during the processing. This picture strongly resembles that of the membrane bound lipid particles isolated from beef heart by Christiansen and Jensen[18]. Occasionally the apparent engulfment of a lipid droplet by a membrane-bound organelle was seen, as was seen in guinea pig lysosomal fractions isolated by Welman et al.[19]. In agreement with this pattern is the observation of Wang et al.[2] that also in normal rat hearts a lysosomal

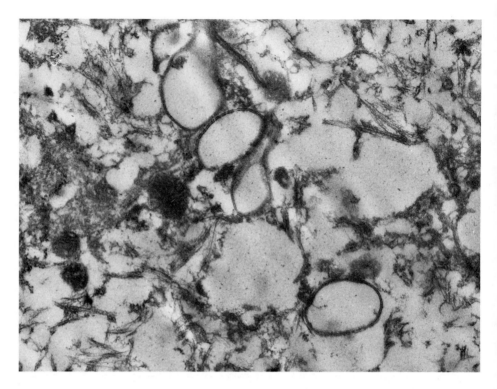

Fig. 2. Electronmicrograph of the lysosomal fraction (10 min 3000 - 30 000 x g sediment of a 10% homogenate in saline) of the heart used in Fig. 1. Fixation in 1% O_5O_4 in 0.067 M cacodylate buffer (pH 7.2).

fraction may be separated which contains triglyceride and lipase activity.

It is likely that the (secondary lysosomal) lipase activity is stimulated by Ca^{++} and/or cyclic AMP, as judged by catecholamine stimulation of the (chloroquine-sensitive) lipolytic process. That Ca^{++} may be important in stimulating lipolysis in heart comes from a number of studies. Hron *et al.*[20] observed that at low Ca^{++} concentrations glucagon or isoproterenol failed to stimulate lipolysis in perfused rat heart, although the hormones increased the protein kinase activity. Dhalla *et al.*[21] perfused rat hearts with increasing Ca^{++} concentrations and observed that at the higher Ca^{++} levels the rate of glycerol release from the heart and the level of free fatty acids in the heart increased, although cyclic 3',5'-adenosinemonophosphate levels were unaltered.

Our observation[1] that not only hormone-stimulated lipolysis in heart, but also in adipose tissue is chloroquine-sensitive, suggests that the mechanism of intracellular lipolysis might be similar in both tissues.

RESULTS

The effect of trierucate feeding on lipolysis in rat heart. We have recently reported[1] a 3-4 fold stimulation of hormone-sensitive lipolysis in *in vitro* perfused rat hearts, after feeding the animals for 3 days with 40 cal% rapeseed oil. Fig. 3A shows that compared to the hearts from control fed rats trierucate feeding (50 cal% of a 2:1 mixture of trierucate and sunflower oil; a generous gift of Unilever Research, Vlaardingen) for 3 days results in the stimulation of both basal and glucagon-stimulated lipolysis.

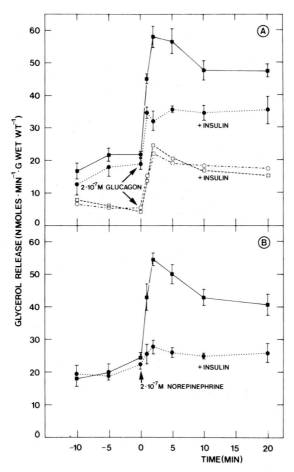

Fig. 3. The effect of insulin (0.5 mU/ml) upon glucagon (A)- and norepinephrine (B)-stimulated glycerol release from control (open symbols, n=1) and trierucate fed rats (closed symbols). The results are given in mean values ± SEM (n=4-5). For preparation and methods see ref. 16. The hormone-stimulated glycerol release in the presence of insulin was significantly different from glycerol release in the absence of insulin.

Inhibitory effect of insulin on myocardial lipolysis. Fig. 3A shows that the low rate of myocardial lipolysis in heart from control fed animals, although stimulated by glucagon, is not inhibited by the addition of insulin in the presence of 5 mM glucose. The absence of an antilipolytic effect of insulin in heart had been reported earlier by Jesmok *et al.*[22]. However, when the lipid store in the heart has increased by feeding trierucate, insulin inhibits both basal and 0.2 μM glucagon (Fig. 3A) or 0.2 μM norepinephrine-stimulated lipolysis (Fig. 3B). Hence, like in adipose tissue[23], in fat infiltrated hearts lipolysis may be inhibited by insulin.

Permissive action of glucocorticoids on hormone-stimulated lipolysis in heart. In adipose tissue hormone-stimulated tissue lipase activity requires the presence of glucocorticoid[24-26]. This also applies to heart. It can be seen from Fig. 4 that 16 h pretreatment of erucate fed rats with 20 mg metopyrone (10 mg i.p. and 10 mg s.c.), an inhibitor of corticosterone synthesis, results in the virtual absence of glucagon-stimulated lipolysis. The i.p. injection of 0.5 mg dexamethasone 4 and 2 h prior to *in vitro* perfusion of the heart fully restores hormone-stimulated lipolysis (Fig. 4), whereas 2 h *in vitro* perfusion

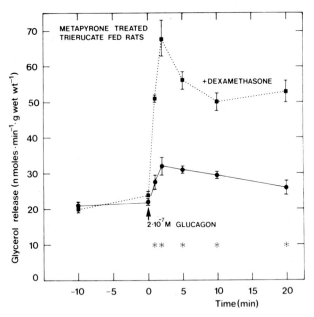

Fig. 4. The effect of dexamethasone upon glucagon-stimulated glycerol release from *in vitro* perfused hearts from trierucate fed rats, pretreated with metopyrone (see text). The results are given in mean values ± SEM (n=3-4). For preparation and results see ref. 16. * p<0.05.

with dexamethasonephosphate, prior to the addition of glucagon had no effect (not shown). Hence the effect of dexamethasone is not acute, suggesting a permissive action of the hormone.

CONCLUDING REMARKS

The finding of the similar hormone response of adipose tissue and heart, infiltrated with lipid, may be of importance in the treatment of myocardial disease. Ventricular arrhythmia has often been discussed in relation to increased long-chain fatty acid levels in plasma. For a discussion we refer to ref. 27. In that paper we demonstrated the fatty acid inhibition of (Na^++K^+)-stimulated ATPase of heart. It is likely that coenzyme A and carnitine esters of long-chain fatty acids also have a potent inhibitory effect on that enzyme[28]. Therefore, fatty acids generated in relatively high concentrations in heart cells, to which the large pool of fatty acid binding albumin is not accessible, may be strongly toxic to myocardial activity. High levels of fatty acids may be expected when there is a combination of fat infiltration and stress[13]. Hence, tools to decrease myocardial lipolysis may sometimes be of temporary help. Such a tool, used in some cases of myocardial arrhythmia, is the combined infusion of glucose, insulin and K^+. Indeed, this therapy may be expected to stimulate not only myocardial reesterification of fatty acids, but also to inhibit myocardial fat mobilization (Fig. 3).

Not only the acute antilipolytic effect of insulin may have practical consequences for the treatment of heart disease, but also the slow permissive effects of glucocorticoids (Fig. 4). Glucocorticoids promote VLDL synthesis (compare the paper presented by Brindley *et al*.; ref. 29) and probably also the uptake of plasma triglycerides by the heart, since they increase the LPL activity of heart[9]. Glucocorticoids are required for the operation of hormone-stimulated lipolysis in heart (Fig. 4), so that they might promote fatty acid turnover in heart. It will be extremely important to uncover their mode of action upon the myocardial LPL and the hormone-sensitive tissue lipase, since indications are being obtained that certain possibly atherogenic diets, such as high sucrose diets[30] and high fat diets, which may result in extreme stress sensitivity[13], both probably lead to increased circulating corticosteroid levels[29,30,11,13]. Both fructose-and fat-feeding result in increased LPL activity of heart[31,12]. Troxler *et al*.[32] observed in male outpatients significant correlations between elevated serial morning plasma cortisols and moderate to severe coronary atherosclerosis. They[32] found a significant correlation between plasma cortisol, plasma cholesterol, blood pressure and smoking -

296

the three major risk factors for coronary artery disease.

It is possible that high local levels of fatty acids play a common role in the pathogenesis of the heart diseases mentioned so far. Fatty acids have been shown to increase the vascular permeability for intravascular constituents[31], [33,34], including low density lipoproteins, resulting in atherosclerosis. Fatty acids stimulate the release of stored catecholamines in the heart[35], which may amplify their cardiotoxic effect by stimulating endogenous lipolysis. In this context it may be of interest to note the potentiating effect of glucocorticoids upon catecholamine cardiotoxicity[36]. The sudden death observed in asthmatic patients using β-adrenergic agonist containing inhalers, may often be based upon prolonged use of corticoid therapy (compare ref. 36). Finally, myocardial fibrosis may also be related to high local levels of fatty acids[12].

REFERENCES

1. Hülsmann, W.C. and Stam, H. (1978) Biochem. Biophys. Res. Commun. 82, 53-59.

2. Wang, T.-W., Menahan, L.A. and Lech, J.J. (1977) J. Mol. Cell. Cardiol. 9, 25-38.

3. De Duve, C. (1969) in Lysosomes in Biology and Pathology, Vol. 1, Dingle, J.T. and Fell, H.B. eds., John Wiley & Sons Inc., New York, pp. 1-42.

4. Hollenberg, C.H. (1959) Am. J. Physiol. 197, 667-670.

5. Cherkes, A. and Gordon, R.S. (1959) J. Lipid Res. 1, 97-101.

6. Borensztajn, J., Otway, S. and Robinson, D.S. (1970) J. Lipid Res. 11, 102-110.

7. Borensztajn, J. and Robinson, D.S. (1970) J. Lipid Res. 11, 111-117.

8. Borensztajn, J., Keig, P. and Rubinstein, A.H. (1973) Biochem. Biophys. Res. Commun. 53, 603-608.

9. De Gasquet, P., Pequignot-Planche, E., Tonnu, N.T. and Diaby, F.A. (1975) Horm. Res. Metabol. 7, 152-157.

10. Jansen, H., Van Zuylen-Van Wiggen, A., Struijk, C.B. and Houtsmuller, U.M.T. (1975) Biochem. Biophys. Res. Commun. 64, 747-751.

11. Abrumrad, N.A., Stearns, S.B., Tepperman, H.M. and Tepperman, J. (1978) J. Lipid Res. 19, 423-432.

12. Hülsmann, W.C., Geelhoed-Mieras, M.M., Jansen, H. and Houtsmuller, U.M.T. (1978) Biochim. Biophys. Acta, submitted for publication.

13. Hülsmann, W.C. (1978) Mol. Cell. Endocrinol. 12, 1-7.

14. Williamson, J.R. (1964) J. Biol. Chem. 239, 2721-2729.

15. Challoner, D.R. and Steinberg, D. (1965) Nature (Lond.) 205, 602-603.

16. Kreisberg, R.A. (1966) Am. J. Physiol. 210, 385-389.

17. Novikoff, A.B. (1965) in Intracellular Membraneous Structures, Seno, S. and Cowdry, E.V. eds., Jap. Soc. Cell. Biol., Okayama, pp. 277-291.

18. Christiansen, K. and Jensen, P.K. (1972) Biochim. Biophys. Acta 260, 449-459.

19. Welman, E., Bowes, D. and Peters, T.J. (1978) J. Mol. Cell. Cardiol. 10, 527-533.

20. Hron, W.T., Jesmok, G.J., Lombardo, Y.B., Menahan, L.A. and Lech, J.J. (1977) J. Mol. Cell. Cardiol. 9, 733-748.

21. Dhalla, N.S., Yates, J.C. and Proveda, V. (1977) Can. J. Physiol. Pharmacol. 55, 925-933.

22. Jesmok, G.J., Calvert, D.N. and Lech, J.J. (1976) J. Pharmacol. Exptl. Ther. 200, 187-194.

23. Butcher, R.W., Baird, C.E. and Sutherland, E.W. (1968) J. Biol. Chem. 243, 1705-1712.

24. Shafrir, E., Sussman, K.E. and Steinberg, D. (1960) J. Lipid Res. 1, 459-465.

25. Jeanrenaud, B. and Renold, A.E. (1960) J. Biol. Chem. 235, 2217-2223.

26. Lamberts, S.W.J., Timmermans, H.A.T., Kramer-Blankenstein, M. and Birkenhäger, J.C. (1975) Metabolism 24, 681-689.

27. Lamers, J.M.J. and Hülsmann, W.C. (1977) J. Mol. Cell. Cardiol. 9, 343-346.

28. McMillin-Wood, J., Busch, B., Pitts, B.J.R. and Schwartz, A. (1977) Biochem. Biophys. Res. Commun. 74, 677-684.

29. Brindley, D.N. et al. (1979) in Lipoprotein Metabolism and Endocrine Regulation, Hessel, L.W. and Krans, H.J.M. eds., Elsevier/North-Holland Biomedical Press, Amsterdam, pp. 241-254.

30. Yudkin, J. (1978) Lipids 13, 370-382.

31. Hülsmann, W.C. and Jansen, H. (1974) in Lipmann Symposium on Energy, Regulation and Biosynthesis in Molecular Biology, Richter, D. ed., Walter de Gruijter, Berlin, New York, pp. 322-335.

32. Troxler, R.G., Sprague, E.A., Albanese, R.A., Fuchs, R. and Thompson, A.J. (1977) Atherosclerosis 26, 151-162.

33. De Ruiter, H. (1966) in Traumatic Fat Embolism, M.D. Thesis, Amsterdam, publ. Noord-Holland N.V., Hoorn (The Netherlands).

34. Hülsmann, W.C. and Jansen, H. (1975) Biochem. Med. 13, 293-297.

35. Stam, H. and Hülsmann, W.C. (1978) Basic Res. Cardiol. 73, 208-219.

36. Guideri, G., Barletta, M.A. and Lehr, D. (1974) Cardiovasc. Res. 8, 775-786.

Lipoprotein Metabolism and Endocrine Regulation
L.W. Hessel and H.M.J. Krans editors
© ECSC, EEC, EAEC, Brussels-Luxembourg, 1979
Published by Elsevier/North-Holland Biomedical Press-Amsterdam

THE RELATIONSHIP BETWEEN GUT HORMONES, GLUCAGON, INSULIN AND LIPID METABOLISM
IN ARTERIAL WALL.

KEITH D. BUCHANAN,
Department of Medicine, Queen's University of Belfast, N. Ireland.
ROBERT W. STOUT,
Department of Geriatric Medicine, Queen's University of Belfast, N. Ireland.

Both insulin and glucagon have roles in lipid metabolism and it is
therefore possible that these hormones may have a role in the generation of
atheroma. Some gut hormones have metabolic actions including effects on lipid
metabolism although the potential importance of these hormones in this area has
been little investigated. It is the purpose of this paper to review the role
of insulin, glucagon and some gut hormones on lipid metabolism with particular
respect to the arterial wall.

ACTIONS OF GLUCAGON, INSULIN AND GUT HORMONES ON LIPID METABOLISM

Insulin has a direct effect on adipose tissue where specific membrane
receptor sites have been demonstrated. In adipose tissue insulin depresses the
liberation of fatty acids induced by the action of lipolytic hormones such as
epinephrine or glucagon. Insulin stimulates the synthesis of fatty acids in
triglycerides and enhances triglyceride synthesis in the liver.[1] It also
modifies the availability of lipoprotein lipase the major enzyme responsible
for the catabolism of circulating triglyceride[2]. The net effect of this
action is enhancement of lipogenesis and inhibition of lipolysis[3].

Glucagon in general has opposite effects on lipid metabolism than insulin[4].
Glucagon is lipolytic which results in plasma free fatty acids (FFA) levels
rising, a substrate product response which might be expected to result in
elevated hepatic production of lipoproteins. There is some experimental
evidence however that suggests that glucagon may cause a shift of FFA from
synthetic pathways of triglyceride formation to oxidative pathways of
ketone generation[5]. Glucagon has a direct lowering effect on blood lipids[6].
In the liver glucagon decreases the triglyceride lipoprotein production rate
and this cound account for the hypotriglyceridaemia noted by Amutuzio[6].

There are two further comments concerning insulin and glucagon control
of lipid metabolism which are relevant. As insulin and glucagon appear to
have in general opposite effects on lipid metabolism what may happen in any

metabolic situation is dependent on a balance between the insulin effects and the glucagon effects. In addition other hormones with importance in lipid metabolism such as growth hormone, catecholamines, cortisol and perhaps gut hormones may also modulate the effect of both insulin and glucagon. The important anti-lipolytic action of insulin could create a deficiency of FFA available to the liver for lipoprotein synthesis and therefore insulin in this capacity may be considered as a hypolipaemic hormone. However, insulin also acts directly on the hepatocyte to enhance lipoprotein production and release and could in this capacity be regarded as a hyperlipaemic hormone. Eaton (1977)[7] proposes that in any metabolic situation three factors have to be considered relevant to the net effect of insulin and glucagon on lipid metabolism i.e. changes of FFA availability, in hepatic glucagon shift or in the rate of peripheral FFA disposal. A relative abundance of glucagon over insulin promotes a glucagon shift resulting in free fatty acids being shifted away from lipid synthesis and into ketone generation whereas a relative abundance of insulin reduces FFA availability directed towards the production of lipoprotein.

Gut hormones may alter lipid metabolism in two ways. Firstly they may have a direct action on the lipocyte and secondly they mediate insulin secretion through the entero-insular axis'[8]. The potential metabolic role of gut hormones has been overshadowed by their more obvious gastro-intestinal functions. The term 'entero-insular axis' was first coined to describe the enhancement of insulin secretion provoked by an oral glucose load compared to a similar intravenous load,[9] and has now been extended to include a similar phenomenon during absorption of aminoacids[10] and also the absorption of triglycerides[11]. The mechanisms by which this phenomenon occur have not yet been completely elucidated[8] but may either be mediated through nervous factors e.g. the vagus or by the more likely mechanism through the release of gastro-intestinal hormones. There are a considerable number of gastro-intestinal hormones which will stimulate insulin secretion e.g. secretin[12], gastric inhibitory peptide[11], gastrin and cholecystokinin-pancreozymin[12]. However, it would appear at the present time that gastric inhibitory peptide satisfies all the criteria of a hormone which could mediate the physiological release of insulin during the ingestion of carbohydrate[13]. Indeed GIP may also be the mediator of the insulin response following absorption of aminoacids and triglyceride. Recently the entero-insular axis has been extended to cover the release of other pancreatic islet hormones including glucagon, somatostatin and pancreatic peptide[8].

Several gut hormones have direct effects on the adipocyte. Secretin is a lipolytic hormone[14,15]. These effects have been noted in the rat where it is considered to mediate its effect through increasing cyclic AMP levels. However, in a sensitive lipolytic assay constructed by Langslow (1973) using chicken adipocytes which are extremely sensitive to glucagon, a very poor enhancement of lipolysis by secretin was noted[16]. Vasoactive intestinal peptide also has lipolytic properties[17] but it is unlikely that gastric inhibitory peptide or purified preparations of gut glucagon-like immunoreactivity have important effects directly on the fat cell [13, 16, 18]. However, recently it has been suggested that some of these hormones e.g. gut GLI may have inhibitory effects on lipolysis[19].

STARVATION STUDIES

In our laboratory we have been intrigued that gut hormones may have important roles in metabolism and established studies to examine the circulating levels of secretin as well as insulin and glucagon during physiological events such as starvation which would encourage lipolysis. We found in nine normal subjects subjected to starvation for a 72 hour period a dramatic and significant increase in circulating levels of secretin as measured by a radioimmunoassay. (Table 1). These events were accompanied by the expected decline in plasma sugar and venous pH[20]. More extensive studies were undertaken to elaborate the relative roles of secretin and glucagon with respect to triglyceride metabolism in acute starvation[21]. During three starvation days plasma glucagon-like immunoreactivity measured with an antibody which was specific for the C-terminal region of glucagon showed significant elevation but GLI measured with an antibody specific for the N-terminal region of glucagon showed no change during the starvation period. This would suggest that the C-terminal region of glucagon has more biological significance during the starvation period than the N-terminal region. Another gastro-intestinal hormone, gastrin, which is not generally recognized to have a potential metabolic role showed no changes during starvation. Insulin surprisingly did not show the expected fall during starvation although the mean level of insulin, approximately 3 microunits/ml, prior to starvation was extremely low in our subjects. (Table 2)

TABLE 1

STARVATION IN NINE NORMAL SUBJECTS

	Control days				Starvation days			Re-feed end of day 1	Analysis of variance (P)
	1	2	3	4	1	2	3		
Plasma secretin ng/1	56 $\pm$ 6	42 $\pm$7	69 $\pm$14	51 $\pm$7	144 $\pm$53	137 $\pm$29	175 $\pm$51	52 $\pm$6	<0.01
Plasma sugar (mg/100 ml)		94 $\pm$3	92 $\pm$2	90 $\pm$3	89 $\pm$3	77 $\pm$3	71 $\pm$3	109 $\pm$3	<0.001
Venous pH		7.32 $\pm$0.01	7.34 $\pm$0.02	7.34 $\pm$0.01	7.34 $\pm$0.01	7.27 $\pm$0.01	7.26 $\pm$0.02	7.34 $\pm$0.01	<0.001

The significant values for analysis of variance compare the 8 test days; 4 of these were control days, 3 of which were during the starvation period and 1 after re-feeding.

Figures are mean $\pm$ S.E.M.

TABLE 2

PLASMA HORMONES (MEAN $\pm$ S.E.M.) DURING FASTING
FOR 72 HOURS (N=9)

	Control. Hours before fasting				Fasting hours			After 24 hrs re-feeding	Analysis of variance (P)
	-72	-48	-24	0	24	48	72		
C-GLI* (ng/1)	62 $\pm$10	50 $\pm$8	74 $\pm$14	60 $\pm$10	92 $\pm$23	94 $\pm$12	103 $\pm$19	69 $\pm$9	< 0.01
N-GLI* (ng/1)	64 $\pm$8	50 $\pm$7	68 $\pm$14	39 $\pm$7	67 $\pm$23	66 $\pm$11	71 $\pm$18	50 $\pm$7	N.S.
Gastrin (ng/1)	29 $\pm$5	32 $\pm$5	36 $\pm$6	43 $\pm$7	43 $\pm$5	39 $\pm$5	39 $\pm$6	40 $\pm$4	N.S.
Insulin (mU/1)	3.4 $\pm$0.5	3.2 $\pm$0.3	3.2 $\pm$0.5	3.7 $\pm$0.5	2.8 $\pm$0.4	3.0 $\pm$0.5	3.7 $\pm$0.5	4.2 $\pm$0.3	N.S.
Secretin (ng/1)	56 $\pm$6	42 $\pm$7	69 $\pm$14	51 $\pm$27	144 $\pm$53	137 $\pm$29	175 $\pm$51	52 $\pm$6	<0.01

* C-GLI = C terminal reactive glucagon-like immunoreactivity

* N-GLI = N terminal reactive glucagon-like immunoreactivity

Plasma triglyceride levels did not change after 24 hours starvation but began
to rise at 48 hours and were significantly higher than pre-fasting levels at
72 hours. Plasma glycerol and FFA concentrations rose steadily in parallel
during the 3 days of starvation(Fig. 1) but plasma cholesterol levels did not
change. It is suggested from these experiments that both secretin and glucagon
levels may enhance the lipolysis which is noted during the starvation.

FIGURE 1

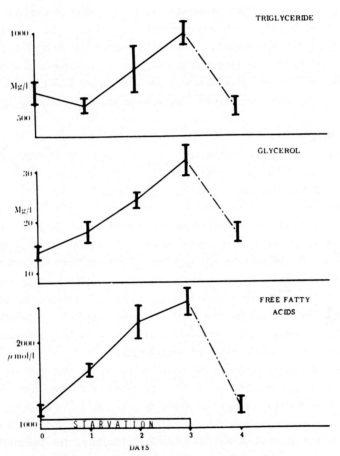

Fig. 1. Triglyceride glycerol and free fatty
acid responses to starvation. Day 4 is after
24 hours refeeding

We have extended these studies by attempting to show a direct effect of secretin on lipolysis in man by infusing secretin in doses designed to mimick the peripheral levels of secretin noted during the starvation period. Results so far are conflicting in that insulin secretion is easily stimulated by secretin and blurs any effects that secretin may have on lipolysis.

Studies reported from this laboratory concerning secretin levels in starvation have not been confirmed by other workers[22]. The reasons for these conflicting data are as yet uncertain but are probably related to the specificity of secretin radioimmunoassay. Extensive studies by us concerning the nature of the immunoreactive secretin measured during starvation have revealed that it has the same molecular weight as immunoreactive secretin which we measure under other situations but our assay does detect multiple species of secretin in tissue and plasma[23] which have not been reported by other workers.

ARTERIAL WALL

Arteries consist of metabolic active tissue which is capable of synthesizing all the major lipids. In general the lipid metabolism of the arterial wall is similar to the lipid metabolism of the adipose tissues.

There are two distinct lipases in the arterial wall[24]. One if the lipoprotein lipase actived by heparin and has its major activity in hydrolysing circulating triglyceride from chylomicrons and very low density lipoproteins, the resulting FFA being taken up into the adipose cell to be re-esterified and stored as triglyceride. The other lipase resembles the hormone sensitive lipase of adipose tissue[24]. The lipolytic activity in the arteries can be stimulated by adenyl cyclase, glucagon, cortisol and growth hormone. Although insulin has no effect on the basal rate of lipolysis it completely suppresses the stimulating effect on lipolysis of adenyl cyclase[24].

This laboratory proposed in 1969 the hypothesis that insulin could be a causative factor in atherogenesis[25]. Prompted by the knowledge that insulin could have controlling effects on lipid metabolism in the arterial wall this resulted in a series of experiments to try to establish the hypothesis. Studies in rats in vivo showed that insulin stimulated the incorporation of sodium (1-c[14]) acetate into total lipids, cholesterol and phospholipids[26]. We also showed that when rats were rendered diabetic with streptozotocin the aortas from the insulin deficient animals incorporated less glucose into the lipids of the aortas than those from control animals[27]. Following intravenous injection of insulin, there was an increased incorporation of D-glucose-U-C14 into triglyceride and free fatty acids. No effect on radioactive cholesterol was found.[28]

The above data was obtained from 'in vivo' experiments. Because of multiple variable factors in such experiments attempts were made to reassess the results on a more controlled 'in vitro' situation. The smooth muscle cell of the artery plays an important role in the process of atherogenesis[29]. Rat arterial smooth muscle cells were cultured and the effect of insulin and glucose on sterol synthesis was studied[30]. Insulin in concentrations of 10 microunits to 100 milliunits per ml stimulated the incorporation of sodium (2-C[14]) acetate into non-saponifiable lipids and digitonin precipitable sterols. However, insulin had no effect on the incorporation of labelled mevalonate into cell sterols. These experiments would suggest that the arterial smooth muscle cell is an insulin sensitive cell.

Not only does insulin have an effect on lipid metabolism in arterial wall but it can be shown that insulin has an effect on the proliferation of arterial smooth muscle cells. Insulin in concentrations well within the physiological range stimulates proliferation of cultured mammalian smooth muscle cells of the monkey.[31]

Very much less has been done relating to other hormones and arterial lipid metabolism. In experiments designed to examine the role of hyperinsulinism in the pathogenesis of atheroma, chickens were injected with long acting insulin for 19 weeks and developed lipid containing lesions in their aorta[32]. Another group of animals received only the vehicle solution of the insulin preparation. It was found that plasma cholesterol, triglyceride, and immunoreactive glucagon were all elevated in the insulin treated groups. Plasma glucagon showed a negative correlation with both cholesterol and triglyceride in the control birds. This correlation was lost in the insulin treated birds which did however show a negative correlation between blood sugar and plasma glucagon. It was concluded that hyperinsulinism in chickens is associated with excessive lipid deposition in the aorta and elevation of blood lipids. However, it is well known that glucagon occupies a more important and different role in chicken metabolism than in other animals. In the chicken glucagon is essential for life and the hormone circulates in much higher concentration.

Recent studies from this laboratory[33] examined the effects of glucagon and dibutyryl cyclic AMP, on sterol synthesis and cultured rat arterial smooth muscle. Glucagon inhibited incorporation of sodium (2-C[14]) acetate into non-saponifiable lipids and digitonin precipitable sterols. The results suggested that sterol metabolism in arterial smooth muscle cells may be influenced by hormones other than insulin but do suggest that glucagon is

306

relatively less important than insulin in this respect. We know of no studies of gut hormones such as VIP, GIP, secretin and gut GLI which may be important in lipid metabolism and their effect on lipid metabolism in arterial wall.

CONCLUSIONS

We would conclude.

1. Insulin and glucagon have important and frequently opposite effects on lipid metabolism.

2. Gut hormones may effect lipid metabolism either directly by their action on the adipocyte or indirectly through their effect on the entero-insular axis.

3. Studies in starvation would suggest a role of both secretin and glucagon in triglyceride metabolism in man.

4. 'In vivo' experiments in rats would suggest that insulin can increase lipid synthesis in the arterial wall.

5. Insulin can cause proliferation of arterial smooth muscle cells cultured from the primate and will also stimulate the synthesis of sterols within the cultured arterial smooth muscle cell.

6. Preliminary studies of the effect of glucagon on synthesis of sterols in cultured arterial smooth muscle cells would suggest that it may inhibit the synthesis of sterols but its effect is generally of less importance than insulin.

7. Very little data is available on the effect of gut hormones which may have a metabolic function such as GIP, VIP, secretin, gut GLI etc. and further studies of these interesting hormones would appear to be indicated in lipid metabolism.

REFERENCES

1.   Topping, D.L. and Mayes, P.A. (1972)
        Biochem. J. 126, pp 295-311.

2.   Bagdade, J.D., Porter, D., Jr., Bierman, E.L. (1968)
        Diabetes 17, pp 127-132.

3.   Renold, A.E., Crofford, O.B., Staufacher, W., and Jeanrenaud, B. (1965)
        Diabetologia 1, pp 4-12.

4.   Lefebvre, P. (1975)
        Biochem. Pharmacol. 24 pp 1261-1266.

5.   Schade, D.S. and Eaton, R.P. (1975)
        Diabetes 24, pp 502-509.

6.   Amutuzio, D.S., Grande, F., Wada, S. (1962)
        Metabolism 11, pp 1240-1249.

7.   Eaton, R.P. (1977)
        In Glucagon: Its Role in Physiology and Clinical Medicine.
        Edited by Foa, P.J., Bajaj, J.S., Foa, N.L. pp 533-550. Springer-
        Verlag.

8.   Dupre, J. (1978)
      In: Gut Hormones, Edited by S.R. Bloom, pp 303-309, Churchill Livingstone.

9.   McIntyre, N., Holdsworth, C.D. and Turner, D.S. (1964)
      Lancet 2, pp 20-22.

10.   Dupre, J., Curtis, J.D., Unger, R.H., Waddell, R.W. and Beck, J.C. (1969)
      J. Clin. Invest. 48, pp 745-747.

11.   Dupre, J., Ross, S.A., Watson, D. and Brown, J.J. (1973)
      J. Clin. Endo. & Metab. 37, pp 826-829.

12.   Unger, R.H., Ketterer, H., Dupre, J. and Eisentraut, A.M. (1967)
      J. Clin. Invest. 46, pp 630-645.

13.   Brown, J.C., Dryburgh, J.R., Ross, S.A. and Dupre, J. (1975)
      Recent Progress in Horm. Res. 31, pp 487-532.

14.   Rodbell, M., Birnbaumer, L., Pohl, S.L. (1970)
      J. Biol. Chem. 245, pp 718-722.

15.   Butcher, R.W., Carlson, L.A. (1970)
      Acta Physiol. Scand. 79, pp 559-563.

16.   Langslow, D.R. (1963)
      Horm. Met. Res. 5, pp 428-432.

17.   Frandsen, E.K. and Moody, A.J. (1973)
      Horm. Met. Res. 5, pp 196-199.

18.   Murphy, R.F., Buchanan, K.D. and Elmore, D.T. (1973)
      Biochim. et Biophys. Acta 303, pp 118-127.

19.   Krug, E., and Mialhe, P. (1977)
      Horm. Met. Res. 9 (6) pp 465.

20.   Henry, R.W., Flanagan, R.W.J. and Buchanan, K. D. (1975)
      Lancet 2, pp 202-3.

21.   Stout, R.W., Henry, R.W. and Buchanan, K.D. (1976)
      Europ. J. Clin. Invest. 6, pp 179-185.

22.   Greenberg, G.R. and Bloom, S.R. (1978)
      Letter to Lancet 1, pp 273.

23.   Mason, J.C., Henry, R.W., Buchanan, K.D. and Murphy, R.F. (In press)
      Biochim. Biophys. Acta.

24.   Mahler, R. (1971)
      Acta Diabet. Lat. 8, pp 68-83.

25.   Stout, R.W. and Vallance-Owen, J. (1969)
      Lancet 1, pp 1078-1080.

26.   Stout, R.W. (1971)
      Diabetologia 7, pp 367-372.

27.   Stout, R.W., Buchanan, K.D. and Vallance-Owen, J. (1972)
      Diabetologia 8, pp 398-401.

28.   Stout, R.W. (1975)
      Horm. & Met. Res. 7, pp 31-34.

29.   Ross, R. and Glomset, J.A. (1973)
      Science 180, pp 1332-1339.

30.   Stout, R.W. (1977)
      Atherosclerosis 27, pp 271-278.

31.   Stout, R.W., Bierman, E.L. and Ross, R. (1975)
      Cir. Res. 36 pp 319-327.

32.   Stout, R.W., Buchanan, K.D. and Vallance-Owen, J. (1973)
      Atherosclerosis 18, pp 153-162.

33.   Stout, R.W. (In Press)
      Diabetologia.

Lipoprotein Metabolism and Endocrine Regulation
L.W. Hessel and H.M.J. Krans editors
© ECSC, EEC, EAEC, Brussels-Luxembourg, 1979
Published by Elsevier/North-Holland Biomedical Press-Amsterdam

DISCUSSION ON PATHWAYS OF LIPID METABOLISM IN CELLS AND ORGANS

Paraphrased and annotated by H.J.M. Kempen, Gaubius Institute, Health Research
Organization TNO, Herenstraat 5d, 2313 AD Leiden (The Netherlands)

<u>Mannaerts</u>: Dr. Jeanrenaud, are the lipid droplets which you see in the liver
cells after treatment with phalloidin not surrounded by membranes?
<u>Jeanrenaud</u>: No, we see a mixture of VLDL particles and free droplets. We
noticed the same when we tested colchicine in vivo. There is first an
accumulation of VLDL in vesicles, then a coalescence of VLDL within the
membrane; after 3-4 hrs all VLDL has coalesced and then for some reason the
membrane disappears, and only droplets are left.
<u>Assmann</u>: Treatment with orotic acid or with N-acetyl galactosamine also result
in fat accumulation and impairment of VLDL secretion. In both cases this is due
to defective glycosylation of the apoprotein moieties. Could this be an
explanation also of your observations?
<u>Jeanrenaud</u>: At present we cannot exclude this with absolute certainty but the
relation with changes in cell shape point to the microfilamentous system.
<u>Galton</u>: Do these microtule inhibitors affect lipoprotein uptake, e.g. LDL
uptake in fibroblasts?
<u>Jeanrenaud</u>: We do not know about lipoprotein uptake, but they do not change FFA
uptake. Phalloidin works only in liver; its effects can be seen in fibroblasts
only after injecting it through the membrane because it does not pass by itself
through the fibroblast membrane.
<u>Galton</u>: Is there any evidence that this microtubular system can be regulated?
<u>Jeanrenaud</u>: No, we have never found effects of insulin, glucagon or cAMP either
on the polymerization-depolymerization cycle or on the actual output of
triglycerides. Only glucagon at very high concentrations was inhibitory in
vitro but this was related to a decrease in lipogenesis rather than to the
microtubular system.
<u>Kempen</u>: Did you also follow changes in secretion by chemical determinations?
<u>Jeanrenaud</u>: Yes, this gave exactly the same picture.
<u>Michell</u>: Do the animals get a severely fatty liver when they are given
phalloidin?
<u>Jeanrenaud</u>: Yes, over a period of 48 hrs their circulating triglycerides are

first reduced to almost zero, with a parallel accumulation of TG in the liver and this is followed by complete reversal of all abnormalities.

Johnston: Dr. Brindley, in fasting or diabetes the flux of FFA into beta--oxidation is strongly increased, so is there not at least a relative inhibition of fatty acid esterification?

Brindley: In these conditions the rate of fatty acid esterification can be as high as in conditions with a low glucagon/insulin ratio, provided that the supply of FFA is not limited. Under all circumstances the liver needs protection against the toxic effects of high plasma levels of FFA, and esterification is an effective protection mechanism.

Hülsmann: In addition to the regulatory role of cortisol, the rate of esterification is also determined by the intracellular level of alpha-glycero--phosphate. This is illustrated in cases of glycogenosis Type I, where one sees often more triglyceride than glycogen in the liver. In these livers the level of alpha-glycerophosphate is high, due to the lack of glucose-6-phosphatase.

Mannaerts: Some authors find high levels of alpha-glycerophosphate during fasting, when there is only little FFA esterification. So, the alpha-glycerophosphate level is not important in the acute or chronic regulation of this process.

Michell: Why are elevated rates of triglyceride synthesis associated with increased intracellular triglyceride levels? Is the secretory machinery saturated?

Brindley: The apoprotein or cholesterol synthesis may be the limiting factor in triglyceride export, and may not be geared adequately to the increase in triglyceride synthesis. Also, the energy needed for lipoprotein assembly and secretion may not be optimally available.

The liver plays an important role in the distribution of "fat-energy" among the various tissues, since it takes up FFA from the blood, and secretes VLDL. In this manner the fat-energy is made available in the form of VLDL-triglyceride rather than in the form of FFA, with the effect that the peripheral tissues can get the fat-energy optimally only by way of lipoprotein lipase. Therefore, the effect of cortisol on the fatty acid esterification in the liver has consequences for the supply of fat-energy to tissues containing lipoprotein lipase.

Kempen: Why does increased phosphatidate phosphohydrolase lead to increased production of triglyceride and not of phosphatidylcholine or phosphatidylethanolamine?

Brindley: The rate of synthesis of these phospholipids is considered to be determined by the availability of CDP-choline and CDP-ethanolamine, respectively, and the rate of production of these cofactors is relatively low and rapidly saturated. At low velocities of the phosphohydrolase, the produced diglyceride is used entirely for phospholipid synthesis; at higher enzyme activities, the excess diglyceride is channelled into triglyceride synthesis.

Michell: Could the inhibition of the phosphatidate phosphohydrolase reaction by cationic drugs like Benfluorex be caused by the direct electrostatic interaction of the drug with the anionic substrate (phosphatidate)?

Brindley: This seems unlikely, since none of the acyltransferases studied by us (using anionic acyl-CoA as substrate) was inhibited by Benfluorex.

Mannaerts: Dr. Brindley, have you tested the effect of Benfluorex on fatty acid oxidation?

Brindley: Only in rats in vivo, injected with ^{14}C-palmitate, in which the ^{14}C-CO$_2$ production by the whole animal was measured. The effect of the drug, after ethanol treatment, was insignificant.

Brunzell: Have you tested the effect of lowering the plasma cortisol level on the phosphatidate phosphohydrolase activity?

Brindley: No.

Johnston: Are you aware of any other hormones acting on this enzyme activity?

Brindley: Only in the fat cell, where adrenaline decreased phosphatidate phosphohydrolase activity. There are no other studies known to me on the liver enzyme.

Mancini: Dr. Mannaerts, can clofibrate possibly be used, not only as a hypolipidemic agent but also in the treatment of liver steatosis?

Kempen: Phyllis Novikoff has shown that clofibrate is able to reverse the orotic-acid-induced fatty liver in the rat (Lab. Invest. 36, 215-231, 1977).

Mancini: Perhaps, this drug may then be of clinical importance in the therapy of the fatty liver, occurring frequently after ileal bypass operations carried out on patients suffering from massive obesity.

Mannaerts: The rate-limiting step in the removal of triglyceride from the liver is lipolysis, not beta-oxidation. The increased capacity for beta-oxidation after clofibrate treatment would then be of limited use for the treatment of a fatty liver.

Michell: Dr. Mannaerts, you saw that fatty acid oxidation is stimulated in

liver cells of clofibrate treated rats, but urate oxidation not. Could this
mean that peroxisomes do not proliferate as a whole, but that some peroxisomal
enzymes rise in activity, while others remain unchanged?

Mannaerts: Indeed, peroxisomal protein is elevated about ten-fold, catalase
activity only for 23%, and urate oxidation not at all, suggesting selective
induction of some peroxisomal components.

Tomasi: Dr. Kempen, did you observe greater inhibition of fatty acid synthesis
by higher concentrations of glucagon?

Kempen: Yes, but a glucagon concentration of $10^{-10}M$ is already in the upper
physiological range; effects at higher concentrations are perhaps not relevant.

Mannaerts: Did you say that oleate addition blocked triglyceride secretion?

Kempen: No, but the intracellular triglyceride level was elevated, while the
triglyceride output into the medium was not. This resulted in a lower percentage secretion of this lipid.

Mannaerts: You find an inhibition of the secretion of tritiated triglyceride
after incubation with oleate. Could this be due to the inhibition of de novo
fatty acid synthesis?

Kempen: We have seen this inhibition, but during oleate incubation the tritium
incorporation into triglycerides is even increased, as a result of enhanced
esterification of tritiated glycerol in glycerolipids. So, effects on de novo
fatty acid synthesis are not necessarily related to effects on secretion of
tritiated triglycerides.

Galton: Dr. Tomasi, is there a phospholipase A_2, activated by protein kinase,
and inhibited by prostaglandins?

Tomasi: Liver plasma membranes possess a protein kinase, which is inhibited by
cyclic AMP. We are now reinvestigating the role of this kinase to see whether
it is perhaps involved in phospholipase activation.

Hessel: Why do you resist calling prostacyclin a hormone. Only because of its
short half-life?

Tomasi: This is a matter of semantics. Prostacyclin does not need to be brought
into the circulation, it works close to the site where it is produced.

Kather: Still, prostacyclin can be called a hormone, because it is released
into the blood all the time, and blood levels are maintained.

Tomasi: The prostacyclin-like immunoreactivity in the blood is partly metabolized prostacyclin. Till now, no data have been reported on an elevated level of prostacyclin itself. (cf however, Moncada et al. Nature 273, 767, 1978. Ed.).

Gliemann: Is anything known on prostacyclin production by endothelial cells in other parts of the organism; adipose tissue for instance?

Tomasi: No, unfortunately there are only data on endothelial cells, cultured from "vessel walls" (origin not specified).

Kather: I think this is the first demonstration that a prostaglandin of one cell influences the prostaglandin production of another cell.

Michell: Which of the cell's lipids is the key precursor of prostaglandin synthesis?

Tomasi: Phosphatidylinositol is the most likely precursor lipid, in view of its high content of arachidonic acid.

Kempen: Dr. Hülsmann, did you do the control experiment with metapyrone, using rats on a regular diet instead of on rapeseed oil?

Hülsmann: No.

Mannaerts and Hülsmann: The intracellular level of FFA and the lipolysis are regulated by the FFA/albumin ratio in the blood. There seems to be a vectorial stream of FFA from the artery to the lymph through the cell, with the highest FFA concentration on the lymphatic side.

Krans: You have turned on a big machinery of fat metabolism in an organ which is not designed for it. Why does fibrosis after rapeseed oil occur in the heart, and not in the adipose tissue, where also high FFA levels prevail after stimulation of lipolysis?

Hülsmann: I have no idea why; anyhow, a high level of FFA is found in the lymph coming from the heart, and this correlates with the occurrence of fibrosis at the lymphatic side of cells.

Galton: What is known about the origin of lipoprotein lipase in the heart? Does it come from the heart muscle cells, or from adipocytes in the myocard?

Jansen: The heart muscle cells contain the lipoprotein lipase; there are no adipocytes in the myocardium.

Brunzell: Chajek and the Steins find two cell types in myocardial dispergates: heart muscle cells and another cell type; the latter seems to produce the lipoprotein lipase, which can be inhibited by cycloheximide. (Biochim. Biophys. Acta 488, 140, 1977. Ed.).

Mancini: How can the toxic effects of FFA in the heart been avoided in a non-
-pharmacological manner?

Hülsmann: Acylcarnitines are strong inhibitors of the Na-K-ATPase, of the Ca-
-pumping ATPase, and of the adenine-nucleotide translocator; these effects
possibly explain the FFA-induced arrhythmia in the heart. There is an old
therapy consisting of the infusion of glucose, insulin and potassium. This
treatment is effective, since it provides alpha-glycerophosphate for re-
-esterification of the FFA and in addition, as shown in my paper, insulin
directly inhibits lipolysis.

Galton: Dr. Buchanan, most people think that lipids in arteriosclerotic plaques
are derived primarily from circulating lipids rather than de novo synthesized
in cells of the arterial wall. Do you agree?

Buchanan: Quantitatively this may be true but I am not sure that de novo
synthesis has no role to play. All the enzymes are there and at some time
during plaque formation they may start to work.

Kather: The simultaneous increase in secretin and FFA levels during fasting
does not at all point to a causal relationship between the two. Is the
situation with secretin not similar to that with glucagon in that no one has
shown a lipolytic effect in man?

Ebert: Some years ago we found a distinct lipolytic effect of secretin on human
adipocytes; under the same conditions glucagon showed no effect. (Similar
observations were reported by S. Raptis et al., Horm. Metab. Res. 1, 249, 1969,
Ed.)

-/-/-/-/-/-

EPILOGUE

H.M.J. Krans, Dept. Endocrinology and Metabolic Diseases, University Hospital, Rijnsburgerweg 10, 2333 AA Leiden, The Netherlands.

The choice of the subjects chosen in this epilogue does not have a connection with the objective value of the papers presented but is a mere direct personal reflection of the data presented in this meeting. The workshop has been named 'Endocrine Regulation of Lipoprotein metabolism'. As a member of the organizing committee and an endocrinologist I cannot resist to translate this in the question: 'where does endocrinology enter into the lipoproteins?'. The conference has confirmed that the connections between endocrine regulation and lipoprotein metabolism are complex. The insight in the modulating factors of the connections is far from complete.

Let me start with the lipoproteins. HDL is probably generated in the splanchnic area. It may be degraded in the reticulo endothelial system. Regarding the discussion over the regulation of HDL we are sorry that two participants, who intended to attend the meeting had to cancell in the last moment because they were ill. Therefore we missed Nikkilä's presentation of the endocrine regulation of HDL and the overview of the gut hormones by Rehfeld. Both papers will be included in the reports of this workshop. Some gut hormones interact with the hormones secreted by the islet of Langerhans. They may also effect specifically the splanchnical formation of HDL. The study of the specific effects of hormones on the synthesis and production of HDL is difficult until more is known about the HDL-metabolism. At this time the endocrinologists have to return HDL to the lipidologists to provide more data.

The story of the defective LDL-receptor is well known. The membrane has a hereditary defect to bind LDL and lacks endocytotic activity.

Two remarks:

1. The mechanism of the translation of a hereditary chromosomal defect into a defective (fluid) membrane is still a mystery.

2. The process of the binding and internalization of LDL is not

identical to the binding and fate of a hormone. Recognition of LDL by the receptor does not trigger primarily transfer of information through the membrane, but starts a process of endocytosis and intracellular degradation. For (peptide) hormones the importance or even the reality of entering into the cell is, however, a subject of discussion and is certainly not the most striking feature of hormone action on membrane level.

Very little is known about the way hormones interfere with the formation, regulation and intracellular handling of the LDL-receptor complex. The fibroblast studies indicate that insulin and thyroxine are involved.

The same lack of knowledge of hormonal action is apparent in the VLDL → IDL → LDL transformation process. Insulin (and glucagon) influence the formation of VLDL and insulin stimulates the disappearance of VLDL too. It has been reported in this conference that the secretion of VLDL is a process which may be regulated at the membrane level. The studies are complicated by the fact that intracellular lipid storage pools can only be visualized after phalloidin has "rigorized" the membrane. We do not know how metabolic products regulate the secretion. We do know that insulin and glucagon influence the synthesis of triglycerides and glycogen.

Lipoprotein lipases are necessary for the breakdown of VLDL. The different behaviour of fat cell LPL and LPL from other sources is clear. Endocrinology is present in the activation of adipose tissue LPL by insulin. The variation in source of LPL is not identical with long known rapidly and slowly regulated LPL-activity. The composition of the food intake may affect the LPL-activity. From studies with liposomes it is known that fatty acids damage the phospholipid bilayer. To prevent this damage the transport process of fatty acids through the membrane must be rapid. So there are still plenty holes left which have to be filled and the endocrinologist may contribute to this with his knowledge.

The subject of triglyceride formation and lipid metabolism can not be excluded when endocrine regulation and lipoprotein metabolism are discussed. The intracellular changes seen in arteriosclerosis and during hyperlipaedemia are a reflection of changed metabolism. Some factors affecting these intracellular changes are dealt with in the third part of our meeting. But no complete picture emerges yet. Some speakers concentrated themselves upon one or more steps in lipid metabolism, which they consider to be essential in the regulation of lipid metabolism (malonyl-CoA, phosphatidate phosphohydrolase and intracellular acid lipase). Others looked to specific cellular systems in the blood vessels (prostaglandins and aggregation of thrombocytes or culture of endothelial cells). Hormones modulate some steps in lipid metabolism. How they modulate is less clear.

For the study of hormonal effects on metabolic changes it is necessary to discriminate between the hormones which have an immediate effect on metabolism like most of the peptide hormones (insulin, glucagon, epinephrin etc.) and the hormones, which do often not generate immediate changes in metabolism, but can alter cellular metabolism profoundly after longstanding overproduction or deficiency (like glucocorticoids, sex hormones, thyroid hormones etc.). The effect of the first group of hormones can be studied in short time incubations. For the second group of hormones and for insight in more sustained effects of the first group of hormones, incubations of cultivated cells or in vivo experiments are necessary. But regression of metabolic properties may occur during in vitro incubations and in in vivo studies (unnoticed) parallelling changes may generate serious problems in the evaluation of the model used. The same type of problems arise when epidemiology, diseased persons or animals with genetic abnormalities are studied. The studies of hormonal effects on lipoprotein metabolism are also complicated by the fact that the turnover of the apoproteins is often a matter of days.

However, even in the group of direct acting hormones the correlation between the metabolic changes induced by the hormone and the first contact of the hormone with the cell membrane is more complicated than was thought when the first binding data were reported. The problems in binding, inactivation, internalization of hormones and the relation with membrane structure, adenylate cyclase and calcium-movements are extensively discussed in the second section.

Compilating what is known about the effect of hormones on lipoproteins, we may conclude that the role of insulin in the regulation of lipoprotein metabolism is still prominent. Catecholamines
are also important but the measurement of the (short living)
catacholamines is difficult. The role of glucagon seems reduced
compared to the ideas of five years ago. This conference has
confirmed that thyroid hormones, sex hormones and corticosteroids
are involved in the long term regulation of lipoprotein levels.
The role of growth hormone in intermediary fat metabolism, however,
remains obscure. The direct role of (some) gut hormones in lipoprotein metabolism remains dubious. They have positively an indirect effect through the interaction with the control station for
the availability of energy : the islet of Langerhans.

Besides the regulation of lipoprotein metabolism by hormones,
the opposite question may be asked: Do lipoproteins, free fatty
acids or changes in fat metabolism regulate hormonal activities?

Many questions remain unresolved but if this conference has at
least stimulated studies to integrate hormonal effects and lipoprotein metabolism one of the intentions of this conference has
been fullfilled.

SUBJECT INDEX